Understanding American COVID-19 Pandemic Beliefs, Behaviors, Politics, and Society

Understanding American COVID-19 Pandemic Beliefs, Behaviors, Politics, and Society

Herbert C. Covey

LEXINGTON BOOKS
Lanham • Boulder • New York • London

Published by Lexington Books
An imprint of The Rowman & Littlefield Publishing Group, Inc.
4501 Forbes Boulevard, Suite 200, Lanham, Maryland 20706
www.rowman.com

86-90 Paul Street, London EC2A 4NE

British Library Cataloguing in Publication Information Available

Library of Congress Cataloging-in-Publication Data on File

ISBN 978-1-66695-429-6 (cloth)
ISBN 978-1-66695-430-2 (electronic)

Contents

Preface

Virtually everyone who reads this book will have lives touched by COVID-19. Some will have lost co-workers, friends, or family members, or know someone impacted. My case is that I lost an aunt who helped raise me. Living in a COVID-19 world, she had secluded herself, had been fully vaccinated, received booster shots, and had taken all precautions. She lived with respect of the virus and lived accordingly. Unfortunately, late in the pandemic, she unknowingly became infected. That infection would trigger a massive immune response that took her life in a few days. She was literally choked to death from an overabundance of white blood cells. It was not a comfortable or peaceful passing. Her passing is just one of over a million American stories that could be told. On May 16, 2022, the United States' COVID-19 fatalities surpassed 1 million cases and continue to grow. Medical experts are now predicting even more deaths as new variants and subvariants of COVID-19 emerge. For example, the Omicron variant has proven more transmittable than the once-feared Delta variant. There is no end in sight, and a total return to "normal" will never occur for those who lost loved ones.

As the COVID-19 pandemic unfolded, it impacted almost every aspect of our lives. Our social relationships, whether within families, workplaces, schools, governments, businesses, or communities, forever changed. Social relationships, such as those with co-workers, now involve masks, social distancing, telecommunications, working from home, fewer in-person meetings, vaccinations, more extensive cleaning, handwashing, videoconferencing, and physical barriers (plastic shields) within the work environment. Within families, parents spent more time with their children, for good or bad. For some, this extended time being relatively confined resulted in stress, mental health issues, substance abuse, and strained relationships. Some of these would have occurred naturally, but not at the levels seen during and following the pandemic. As a result, businesses closed, items became scarce, people were isolated, violence increased, mental health issues gained prevalence, and our social world changed. These and new changes will continue in the future.

During the pandemic, the number of changes in social relations has been extensive. The pandemic changed many norms (rules) that guide society and social behavior. The COVID-19 pandemic had medical, societal, and political dimensions from the beginning. The pandemic's political and social dimensions are this book's focus. No single book can capture all of the dimensions of the COVID-19 pandemic, nor should it. It must be understood from multiple viewpoints. Understanding the pandemic will take years and considerable effort.

Pandemics are social phenomena that are shared and public. As Matthewman and Huppatz (2020) observed, collective adversity, such as that afforded by a pandemic, can create social solidarity. People bond together to face a common foe, in this case, the coronavirus. They have a sense of "We are all in this together," a popular slogan at the beginning of the pandemic. But with COVID-19, not every American believed they were "in this together" and charted independent responses to the virus. Some took a "me first" stance and resisted collective efforts to address COVID-19 for the larger societal good.

Much research and thought are developing in response to the pandemic. Medical research, public opinion polls, news stories, and reports are being produced at high rates. However, central questions about the pandemic remain relatively unexplored. One is why most Americans embrace medical efforts to curb the spread of the pandemic, and others consistently resist and oppose such proven measures. How did these opposing positions come about? What socioeconomic and political factors contributed to these opposing views? This book attempts to answer some of these questions about COVID-19 and the pandemic.

The approach of this book has been to pull information and data from reputable sources whose only agenda is to capture and report on the facts accurately. These sources do not have political agendas but seek the truth (contrary to individuals and groups with agendas and profit motives). Those opposed to facts will question these sources, a topic addressed in the book. Several national surveys of Americans conducted by the Annenberg Public Policy Center, Pew Research Center, Brookings Institution, Kaiser Family Foundation, and U.S. Census Bureau were relied on for this book. These are all independent non-profit policy and research organizations that adhere to standard research protocols and openly share their methods and data. None have political affiliations, which is critical to obtaining an accurate picture of the pandemic. It was thought that capturing Americans' views would shed light on where they stand on the pandemic. The Centers for Disease Control and Prevention (CDC) was also used for background information on COVID-19, fatalities, and medical interventions. In addition, information was gathered from popular sources that challenge the government's approach to the pandemic. Finally, reputable national newspapers and news services, such as the *New York Times, Washington Post,* and Associated Press, were used.

The book is multidisciplinary, drawing information from various medical, psychological, political, historical, economic, and sociological materials. It is only possible to cover the pandemic by touching bases from several fields. The focus was on the social aspects of the pandemic and less on the medical. The social sciences and humanities have mostly been "backgrounded" in favor of economic and medical approaches (Paul and Haddad 2023:227). Nevertheless, social scientists have developed and studied concepts appropriate to what is witnessed during the pandemic. A field of study labeled collective behavior (or collective action) is of particular value. Collective behavior concepts, such as rumor, crises, panic, conspiracy theories, protests, and others, are valuable tools for understanding some of the social responses to the pandemic. To this end, the organization of the book is as follows.

Chapter 1 sets the stage for COVID-19 by clarifying basic definitions of pandemics, epidemics, outbreaks, and COVID-19. Second, the biological characteristics of COVID-19 are described. Third, a timeline of COVID-19 milestones is presented. Finally, some fundamental public health strategies for limiting the spread of COVID-19 are identified.

Chapter 2 covers some of the significant consequences of the pandemic on individuals and society, including individuals' fear, health, mortality rates, and mental health. Also included are some of the social impacts of the pandemic on families, education, mental health, the workplace, and communities. Special coverage of how the pandemic has impacted people differently because of their ethnicity, racial group, and age closes the chapter.

Chapter 3 outlines major pandemics in world history, focusing on the United States. The chapter aims to identify ways prior pandemics have differed from the current COVID-19 pandemic. The chapter also covers similarities between previous pandemics and the COVID-19 pandemic. There are common behavioral patterns in resisting or embracing public health interventions that can inform the current understanding of COVID-19.

Chapter 4 outlines how focusing on collective behavior can be a helpful perspective on understanding the social aspects of the pandemic. This chapter builds on collective behavior ideas such as social unrest, rumors, panics, protests, and social movements, and basic concepts such as self-fulling prophecies, crises, and disaster responses. How these and other concepts, such as homophily and true believers, might apply to the pandemic are illustrated. Next, the chapter elaborates on the critical debate on whether the threat of COVID-19 has been over- or understated. Some groups have argued that an unjustified mass panic over COVID-19 has extensively damaged society. Others hold that COVID-19 has been understated, resulting in more avoidable infections, deaths, and a prolonged pandemic. The chapter ends with an overview of social movements that emerged during the pandemic.

Chapter 5 identifies some major social patterns and trends during the COVID-19 pandemic. These have profoundly influenced how American society has interpreted and responded to the pandemic. These include the social construction of the pandemic, individualism versus the common good, the importance of culture, and the erosion of trust in American society. The latter is elaborated on in detail with social media platforms' role in fueling myths, rumors, conspiracy theories, and misinformation about COVID-19. In addition, the degradation of the news, COVID-19 misinformation, and the general reduction in critical thinking are covered. The chapter includes a debate over trusting science to guide public health policies. The chapter concludes with a focus on how racism and inequality have played out during the pandemic. Racism and inequality, especially when it comes to health care, have surfaced in dramatic ways during the pandemic. Finally, the chapter incorporates national survey data to document American views on the pandemic.

Chapter 6 addresses how COVID-19 and the pandemic have been politicized. Although pandemics always have had a political dimension, the COVID-19 pandemic has raised the bar regarding political positioning. A section is devoted to President Trump's public comments about the nature of the pandemic and how to best respond. Strong political allegiances have, during the pandemic, polarized groups into opposing camps (tribes). Some favor public health interventions and push for more efforts in this regard. Yet others are opposed to such actions and rely heavily on their political leaders for guidance. Data throughout the chapter support the consequences of steadfastly adhering to political rather than medical advice. The roles of government and public health during the pandemic are brought to light with the findings of national surveys of adult Americans reflecting public perspectives and how these views are influenced by political affiliation.

Chapter 7 provides an overview of some rumors, myths, misinformation, and conspiracy theories about COVID-19 and the pandemic. The chapter does not cover all of these but highlights some famous examples. The examples are grouped into categories such as the origin of COVID-19, how the virus is spread, inflated morbidity rates, alternative treatments, and plots to take over the world. Myths about vaccines, one of the most important topics, is detailed. In addition, the ineffectiveness of Ivermectin and Hydroxychloroquine as treatments illustrates how inaccurate information misguides behaviors. A section is also devoted to understanding why conspiracy theories flourished during the pandemic. National survey results show how much adults believe in misinformation, rumors, and conspiracies. The surveys also demonstrate how beliefs in misinformation, rumors, and conspiracies influence responses to the pandemic.

Chapter 8 provides an overview of government efforts to minimize the spread of COVID-19. In this chapter, resistance to these efforts in the form of protests and social movements are described with examples. Examples, such as the trucker border protest and convoy to Washington, DC, are included. The history of vaccine resistance and hesitancy are reviewed. Reasons for opposition to vaccinations are identified. The chapter provides an overview of mandates and the power or lack thereof to impose them. Two major court cases are summarized on the issue of governmental authority in imposing mandates. Finally, national survey data are included in the chapter to show public opinion on the role of government and mandates.

Regardless of how thorough the approach has been, more will be known about COVID-19 as the pandemic unfolds. COVID-19 and our understanding of how it touches our lives and affects our health is ever-evolving. Of what is presented here, some of it will change. The author does not suggest that the following materials answer every question or include all the information about the pandemic. Instead, this book serves as a valuable overview of COVID-19 and gives the reader ideas on how the pandemic might be viewed.

No book is written in a vacuum; others usually support, challenge, inspire, encourage, and otherwise contribute to its creation. Among those who helped me include Dr. Donald Bross, a sounding board and source of academic inspiration while working on this book and other published research. He demonstrates unparalleled encouragement and fresh ideas regarding my work. Phil Noble introduced me to new ideas on how to approach the topic. I bounced good and bad ideas off him; he always had great angles. Dr. Scott Menard and Dr. Robert Franzese have allowed me to brainstorm ideas. The editors at Lexington Press, Emma Ebert, Dominique McIndoe, and the reviewers were exceptional. Finally, and most importantly, my wife, Marty Covey, provided uncompromising support for my research. She is the first to read and challenge my writing. With her, I've accomplished much in my career.

Chapter 1

Welcome to the COVID-19 Pandemic

"Covid is not just a cold."

Unknown Source

INTRODUCING COVID-19

In the months following December 2019, the world would know COVID-19, also called COVID, coronavirus, and SARS-CoV-2. COVID-19 is a severe acute respiratory virus. Unlike a bacterium which is comprised of a single cell that can reproduce on its own, a virus is not a whole cell but a sack of genetic material encased in a protein covering. Although a cell can reproduce on its own, a virus cannot. Instead, a virus must infect a host cell and use that cell's genetic resources to reproduce. The corona in coronavirus refers to its crown-like appearance, a circular core with spike-like projections resembling a crown. The "19" in COVID-19 refers to 2019 when the virus was detected. COVID-19 is not the first and only coronavirus, as there have been and continue to be other types of coronaviruses.

The first identification of the disease that developed into a worldwide pandemic occurred in Wuhan, China. Most authorities agree that COVID-19 originated in this region. Initially, very little was scientifically known about the COVID-19 virus. An early exception was the Chinese scientist Zhang Yongzhen, who shared the COVID-19 RNA sequence with his research team on the Internet. This posting would help the scientific world begin to develop vaccines. Unfortunately, in doing so, he violated a Chinese government directive on releasing information and placed himself at risk of government sanction.

Nevertheless, Yongzhen and his associates mapped the first complete genome of the virus that sickened and killed millions worldwide, the SARS-CoV-2 (COVID-19). How COVID-19 was introduced into the human population has been subject to speculation ranging from its source being a local wet food market in Wuhan, an accidental release from a microbiological laboratory in Wuhan, or a simple product of nature. These sources and others have fueled public perceptions and conspiracies regarding the virus's origin. However, the most recent research suggests that the coronavirus originated from an animal sold in a Chinese food market and was not purposely or accidentally a laboratory product (Maxmen 2022).

Once crossing into the human population, COVID-19 rapidly spread across the globe in months and became labeled a world pandemic. The World Health Organization identified COVID-19 as a concern on January 30, 2020, and a pandemic on March 11, 2020. By then, a large-scale worldwide pandemic was well underway. By September 2022, the pandemic had resulted in over 603 million cases and almost 6.4 million deaths, making it one of the deadliest pandemics in world history. The United States has lost over 1 million lives to the COVID-19 virus, which among the G7 wealthiest countries was the worst death tally (Barr and Shiro 2022). This should be surprising to many, as the United States is touted as having one of the best medical systems in the world.

Although declining since 2021, COVID-19 remained a leading cause of American deaths in 2022. According to Ahmad et al. (2023:489), "COVID-19, listed as the underlying cause for 186,702 deaths during 2022, ranked as the fourth leading underlying cause of death. COVID-19 was the underlying cause of 5.7% of all deaths in 2022, decreasing from 12.0% (416,893 deaths) in 2021."

COVID-19 is just one of many viruses that have impacted the world and are a forerunner of future pandemics. The world is becoming increasingly interconnected through globalization patterns such as agricultural interdependency, expanding global travel, and growing human intrusions into tropical regions where threatening viruses thrive. In addition, population growth, the overuse of antibiotics to treat illness, global warming, and the migrations of populations have all increased the risk of global pandemics. These and other patterns will expedite the spread of new and deadly viruses and corresponding pandemics (for a discussion, see Hanafi 2020). These trends make understanding viruses and bacteria scientifically important and socially significant because these trends have social, cultural, and political components. For example, group resistance to preventive measures, such as vaccinations, has ensured that some viruses have not been eliminated and continue to threaten humanity.

COVID-19 symptoms range from being almost undetectable (asymptomatic) to death. Common symptoms include high fever, headache, dry cough, and fatigue. Some individuals, such as those aged over 70 years, are more likely than others to have severe cases with serious medical issues. Serious illness is also more likely for those with underlying medical problems. COVID-19 is transmitted when people breathe in air containing the virus's droplets. It was once believed that COVID-19 could be transmitted from contaminated surfaces, but it is now known that this is not the case. Being airborne means that when people are physically close to each other, the risk of one infecting the other is increased. The risk is higher indoors than outdoors. Fluids containing the virus can also result in infection if the liquid reaches the eyes, nose, or mouth. Infected individuals are usually contagious for ten days and can spread the virus without developing symptoms. This latter fact makes it difficult to know when an untested infected person is spreading COVID-19 to others.

Coronaviruses are not new. Scientists have known about them for years, but the COVID-19 version is new. The CDC states that seven coronaviruses are known to infect humans. Of these, four of them cause the common cold (upper-respiratory-tract illness), and three cause more serious illnesses, including severe acute respiratory syndrome (SARS), Middle East Respiratory Syndrome (MERS), and COVID-19. The coronavirus has a pattern of mutating into different strains; thus, COVID-19 was and is a new variation of the basic coronavirus. The coronavirus is an RNA (ribonucleic acid) virus with a high mutation rate (Oldstone 2020). Numerous COVID-19 variants and subvariants have been introduced since the original version was identified. The major variants are Alpha, Beta, Gamma, Delta, Omicron, and subvariants (BA.1, BA.2, BA.12.1, BA.4, BA.5, and BA.2.75) and new variants are emerging, such as XBB.1.16 (Arcturus) and XBB.1.9.1. By mid-2022, the BA.5 subvariant became the most concerning to medical experts because it accounted for most COVID-19 cases. Experts are concerned about its variation from the original version of COVID-19, implying that our responses, such as vaccines, may be less effective. In addition, the virus is easier to transmit and is more resistant to antibodies.

According to medical experts, reinfections result from this evolution of variants. The general public knows the Alpha, Delta, and Omicron strains. The different strains vary in transmissibility and severity. For example, the Omicron strain was more contagious but less severe than prior strains. The Delta strain was more severe but less contagious than Omicron. As the virus mutates, new variants will emerge that, in some cases, will pose new challenges to the medical community.

EPIDEMICS, OUTBREAKS, PANDEMICS, ENDEMICS, AND PLAGUES

The terms "epidemic," "outbreak," "pandemic," and "endemic" can be confusing. An epidemic is an infectious disease outbreak that spreads quickly through a community. An epidemic is a disease that persists in a region or population with a steady occurrence rate. Epidemics are considered widespread events in populations or areas where they are not permanently present. Epidemics are new infections for populations or regions. Delanty (2021b:8) noted that epidemics are "pathological realities" and "social constructions" because "they are mediated by social and political conditions." Closely related to the word "epidemic" is the term "outbreak." An outbreak is the rapid occurrence of an infectious disease that initially impacts a relatively localized area. People sometimes use epidemic and outbreak interchangeably because they are similar. A pandemic affects people across a large region or national border. Pandemic is derived from the Greek word Patmos, meaning all people, and indicates an outbreak of a disease over a large geographical area. In contrast, epidemic refers to the involvement of a large regional segment but not global. A pandemic is simply a widespread epidemic. Because pandemics infect large populations, they are more concerning, as they can spread worldwide.

An endemic disease spreads and endures in a region or population. When a disease is endemic, people must co-exist with it. Endemic viruses stabilize and reach an equilibrium, with some people having limited immunity. Endemic diseases never really go away but persist in some form. For example, the flu is considered endemic because it is always in the world and continues to mutate. This is why there is a flu season, and a new flu vaccination is administered each year to address the latest variant. Many medical authorities believe COVID-19 is now endemic, will mutate, and will be a virus we must learn to live with. Finally, there is the term "plague." Plagues are epidemic diseases caused by bacteria, resulting in high death rates and severe illness. For example, the Black Plague was caused by a bacterium named *Yersinia pestis*, transmitted to humans by rats and the bites of infected fleas residing on those rats (see chapter 3). There are three types of plagues caused by bacteria—bubonic, pneumonic, and septicemic. The most famous was the bubonic plague which has surfaced multiple times in world history. Other calamities and evils are called plagues, such as the biblical plague of locusts that impacted Egypt as a punishment by God.

COVID-19 started as an epidemic and quickly developed into a worldwide pandemic. However, some groups and individuals believe that COVID-19 is not a "real pandemic" and suggest it is an overreaction or moral panic to a minor illness. Unfortunately, this perspective and response have led to severe and unjustified consequences for the world and ensured that COVID-19 will continue to exist and evolve.

TIMELINE OF IMPORTANT COVID-19 DATES

There have always been predictions of the next pandemic, but few, if any, people predicted or even imagined COVID-19 and its impact on the world, let alone how events would emerge. The COVID-19 pandemic continues to unfold and may take years to become settled and understood. However, there are a few noteworthy milestones in the evolution of COVID-19. The Centers for Disease Control and Prevention (2022) published a COVID-19 timeline of significant milestones. The following are a few of the key events and dates:

- December 12, 2019 - A cluster of patients in Wuhan, China, experience shortness of breath and fever.
- January 7, 2020 - Chinese authorities identify and isolate a novel coronavirus as the causative agent of the outbreak.
- January 20, 2020 - The CDC confirms the first laboratory-confirmed case of COVID-19 in the United States from samples taken on January 18 in the state of Washington.
- January 31, 2020 - U.S. Secretary of Health and Human Services Alex Azar declares the SARS-CoV-2 virus a public health emergency. The White House 2019 Coronavirus Task Force announced the implementation of new travel policies effective February 2, 2020.
- March 11, 2020 - The World Health Organization declares COVID-19 a pandemic.
- March 13, 2020 - President Donald Trump declares a nationwide emergency.
- March 15, 2020 - U.S. states begin to shut down to prevent the spread of COVID-19. New York City's public school system (the most extensive school system in the United States, with 1.1 million students) shuts down, while Ohio calls for restaurants and bars to close.
- March 17, 2020 - First human trial of a vaccine to protect against pandemic COVID-19 begins in the United States at a Kaiser Permanente research facility in Seattle, Washington. Moderna Therapeutics is the biotech company behind the vaccine.
- April 3, 2020 - At a White House press briefing, the CDC announces new mask-wearing guidelines and recommends everyone wear a mask outside the home.

- April 14, 2020 - President Trump announces his plans to withdraw U.S. support for the World Health Organization (WHO). This plan never is implemented, and some view it as scapegoating the WHO for the United States' handling of the pandemic (see Chomsky and Waterstone 2021).
- April 30, 2020 - President Donald Trump launches Operation Warp Speed, an initiative to produce a vaccine for the coronavirus as quickly as possible with the CDC as an integral member.
- December 11, 2020 - The Food and Drug Administration issues an Emergency Use Authorization (EUA) for the first COVID-19 vaccine—the Pfizer-BioNTech COVID-19 vaccine.
- December 12, 2020 - The Advisory Committee on Immunization Practices (ACIP) issues interim recommendations for using the Pfizer-BioNTech COVID-19 vaccine in persons aged 16 or older to prevent COVID-19.
- December 14, 2020 - New York nurse Sandra Lindsay becomes the first American outside a clinical trial to receive the COVID-19 vaccine.
- December 18, 2020 - The U.S. Food and Drug Administration issues an Emergency Use Authorization for the second COVID-19 vaccine—the Moderna COVID-19 vaccine.
- February 27, 2021 - FDA approves emergency use authorization for the Johnson & Johnson COVID-19 vaccine.
- June 1, 2021 - The Delta variant, first identified in India in late 2020, becomes the dominant variant in the United States. The Delta variant kicks off a third wave of infections during the summer of 2021.
- November 26, 2021 - The World Health Organization classifies a new variant, Omicron, as a variant of concern after scientists in South Africa first reported it. The variant has several mutations in the spike protein that concerned scientists worldwide.
- May 15, 2022 - The number of U.S. deaths due to COVID-19 surpasses 1 million, ranking the country as having the highest number of fatalities globally.
- August 11, 2022 - The CDC loosens mask and social distancing guidelines. These changes occur at a time when children are returning to school.
- August 17, 2022 - The CDC director, Dr. Rochelle Walensky, recommends a major reorganization of the agency based on its mishandling of COVID-19. A reorganization was necessary to streamline agency operations and speed up its ability to address pandemics. In addition, the proposed changes target the timeliness of releasing information, removing bureaucratic layers, and improving working relationships with other agencies.

- May 4, 2023 - The World Health Organization declares COVID-19 is no longer a global health emergency. It declares COVID-19 is an ongoing health issue (World Health Organization, 2023:n.p.).
- May 11, 2023 - The CDC ends the public health emergency for COVID-19 in the United States (Centers for Disease Control and Prevention 2023:n.p.).

MEDICAL PREVENTION AND TREATMENT OF COVID-19

Public health and medical responses to COVID-19 include social distancing, face masking, closures of public spaces, and physical barriers, such as plastic dividers. Other measures include air filtration and improved ventilation systems, lockdowns, contact tracing of individuals exposed to the virus, and travel and business restrictions. In addition, public health officials practiced quarantining those exposed or infected, emphasized handwashing, and implemented COVID-19 tests, temperature taking, and using disinfectant wipes, sprays, and cleaners. Public health officials labeled equipment such as plastic shields, face masks, barriers, and suits PPE, short for Personal Protective Equipment. Personal protective equipment would become standard- issue for direct care providers, first responders, and other professionals. Drug treatments include monoclonal antibodies, anti-viral drugs, and controlling the symptoms through existing drugs and interventions. Intensive care units and ventilators have assisted breathing in severe cases.

Some medications for COVID-19 have been approved for patients. The following are a few currently used, and other developing drugs show promising outcomes. Paxlovid is an anti-viral pill that targets an enzyme the coronavirus needs to reproduce. It must be taken within five days after symptoms start. It is effective in most cases by reducing the odds of hospitalization and death. Molnupiravir lowers the risk of severe symptoms of COVID-19 and death. This drug induces mutations in the coronavirus that make it non-functional. Monoclonal antibodies are medications that work differently than Paxlovid and Molnupiravir by preventing the coronavirus from replicating and, thus, reducing escalation of the disease. Given intravenously, they reduce the severity of the infection and risk of hospitalization if delivered within ten days of the first symptoms. Finally, Remdesivir is an anti-viral drug taken intravenously over three days within the first seven days of the first symptoms. Again, it reduces the risk of hospitalization and death. To date, none of these drugs prevent infection but reduce its severity.

SOCIAL DISTANCING

Public health agencies, governments, and the CDC recommended and sometimes required social distancing to control the spread of COVID-19. Because COVID-19 is transmitted by an infected person's breath being inhaled by another, creating distance between individuals had scientific support. In public settings, individuals were encouraged to space themselves at least six feet apart from others outside of their immediate family members. This social distancing changed the way face-to-face interactions occurred. Social spaces between people became larger. Social gatherings of large numbers of people were discouraged or prohibited. See-through barriers were installed to ensure social distancing. The size of gatherings was also limited to ensure social distancing. This was done by limiting the number of people permitted in indoor spaces, such as 50 event attendees. This preventive strategy would have major impacts on businesses dependent on larger groups of customers. Some people embraced such restrictions and spacing, but others openly defied social distancing measures and gathered in large groups for concerts and events. These larger gatherings became known as "super spreader events."

FACE MASK WEARING

The preventive strategy of wearing face masks has generated much social controversy, both in favor of and opposed. One of the earliest strategies to address the pandemic was wearing masks. Public officials and businesses have mandated wearing masks in indoor settings. It is safe to say that whether an individual is pro or con mask-wearing, wearing them is inconvenient and uncomfortable. Individuals have found exercise, working, movement in general, communications, caregiving, traveling, and breathing hampered by mask-wearing. The effectiveness of wearing masks depends on the materials used to make the mask and how well the mask fits the wearer's face. Surgical quality disposable masks, marked by an N-95, would be the standard for high-risk individuals. However, no mask is 100 percent effective, ranging from a high of 80 to 95 percent to a low of 38 to 39 percent. Mask-wearing has been one of the most controversial restrictions during the pandemic. The collective behavioral responses have been significant (see chapter 7).

Researchers have studied the effectiveness of masks in preventing the spread of COVID-19. One study developed an estimate of the impacts of preventive strategies on COVID-19 infection and fatality rates. A team from the Brookings Institution, Washington University in Saint Louis, and the University of Vermont developed a TRACE simulation model (Hammond and Kasman 2022). The team looked at various strategies, including mask-wearing, testing capacity, faster rollout of vaccines, social distancing policies, and others. The model showed that multiple strategies would have substantially lowered infection and death rates. In addition, implementing various strategies would have reduced the burden on the health care system and the impacts of long-term symptoms. It is important to note that some may question the model's findings, but, at this writing, no data-driven model has provided evidence that these findings are off base. Critics may not like the predictions but have yet to contradict them with any better data-driven model. Regarding mask-wearing, the TRACE model predicted:

> A significant increase in consistent usage of high-quality masks could have reduced cases by as much as two-thirds. Although masking in the United States has been politicized and efforts to increase mask usage have been controversial, our simulations demonstrate that masking remains an efficient approach to containing the spread of SARS-CoV-2 [COVID-19]. In our simulations, consistent masking by 70% of Americans during the surge would have been almost as effective as widespread closures of businesses and schools. (Hammond and Kasman 2022:n.p.)

TESTING

When COVID-19 tests became available, social implications would develop. Two basic types of COVID-19 tests have been implemented. Testing has proven to be an essential tool in addressing the COVID-19 pandemic. COVID-19 tests can detect the virus or biomarkers of COVID-19 or the presence of antibodies the body makes after getting COVID-19 or being vaccinated. Tests for COVID-19 can indicate if an individual is infected when they took the test. These tests are labeled viral because they look for an active viral infection. They involve taking samples from the nose or mouth. Two types of viral tests are rapid and laboratory (PCR). Rapid tests can be self-administered by an individual. PCR laboratory tests may take days to analyze. Hence they are less convenient than rapid self-administered tests. PCR tests are more accurate than rapid tests. A second type of test determines if an individual has ever had a COVID-19 infection. Infected or vaccinated humans create antibodies that can be detected through antibody tests. These are called antibody or serology tests that detect the blood's antibodies to COVID-19 (SARS-CoV-2). Antibodies are proteins the immune system produces to fight current and future infections. Antibody tests are not used to determine present infections but past ones.

Testing is important in reducing the spread of COVID-19 from infected to uninfected people. Testing is also of value in allowing people to rule out infections due to COVID-19 from other illnesses, which allows for more appropriate treatments. Testing is a hazard reduction measure that reduces the risk of infecting other people. This is one of the reasons why tests became required for travelers. Proof of negative COVID-19 tests became required of international travelers. Testing has generated much public debate, with some people wanting more and others arguing that testing is too intrusive and represents an overreaction. The latter group views testing as an impingement on their privacy and rights and as inconvenient. However, there is evidence that testing can be beneficial in reducing infection rates. According to one simulation model (TRACE), having better testing capacity for COVID-19 would have reduced infection rates. A significant increase in testing capacity alone could have reduced cumulative and surge infection rates by nearly one-third (Hammond and Kasman 2022:n.p.).

When COVID-19 tests became available, some people rushed to get tested whether they needed to or not. Critics would suggest that the availability of tests and the shortage of tests represented a moral panic. That is, people were unnecessarily tested out of fear. Others pointed out that test availability differed according to socioeconomic status, or racial or ethnic backgrounds. Not all individuals had access to rapid or PCR COVID-19 tests, which complicated setting base infection rates among populations. Lower-income groups needed more access to trials. The government and public health providers eventually took major steps to address inequity. Regardless of whether people wanted more or less, testing proved to be a social issue in several dimensions.

VACCINES

Developing and rolling out vaccines was one of the most effective tools to combat COVID-19. The most important public health responses would be developing and distributing effective vaccines to reduce the risk of severe infection, hospitalization, and death. Vaccines proved to be one of the most socially controversial developments during the pandemic. In the United States and much of the world, there are five basic COVID-19 vaccines. The four most prominent and approved COVID-19 vaccines in America are Moderna, Pfizer-BioNTech, Novavax, and Johnson & Johnson's Janssen. Other countries, such as China and Russia, developed alternative vaccines. The BioNTech and Moderna vaccines use a messenger RNA (ribonucleic acid) platform, which is a strand of encoded genetic material that tells human cells to produce the same spike protein that the COVID-19 virus has on its surface that allows it to invade human cells.

The human immune system responds to this protein by neutralizing antibodies and by the robust immune system hunters known as T cells. Both messenger RNA vaccines demonstrated strong immune responses during clinical trials and were well tolerated. The Novavax vaccine includes harmless pieces (proteins) of the virus that causes COVID-19. After a Novavax vaccination, the body creates an immune response to these protein pieces. The Johnson & Johnson Janssen vaccine contains a piece of a modified virus that is not the same virus that causes COVID-19. This modified virus is called the vector virus. The vector virus cannot reproduce, so it cannot cause COVID-19. Instead, this vector virus instructs cells in the body to create an immune response. All major vaccines have been proven to be safe and effective.

While the vaccines help people resist the virus, it was soon realized that "breakthrough" infections could occur in some cases. According to the CDC, until the Omicron variant surfaced, breakthrough infections of fully vaccinated people were rare and mostly happened to people with compromised immune systems. Omicron, more so than other variants, can bypass the effectiveness of vaccines. However, fully vaccinated people are less likely, as would be expected, to catch COVID-19 than the unvaccinated. Unvaccinated adults are roughly six times more likely to catch COVID-19 and 14 times more likely to die from it than vaccinated individuals (see summary by Wilson 2022).

According to the TRACE simulation model, more infections could have been prevented if the United States had had a higher uptake rate for COVID-19 booster shots. Hammond and Kasman (2022: n.p.) summarized:

> A higher take-up rate of booster shots and earlier availability for those eligible would have reduced cumulative infection rates by up to 15% of the U.S. population during the Omicron wave. Rapid increases in vaccination for children under 18 would also have led to large decreases in disease spread. Much higher investment in uptake of boosters and vaccines, including in the youngest age groups, would likely be needed before a wave to provide a substantial dampening effect.

Similar findings on the effectiveness of vaccines have been reported. Wilson (2022) summarized the Kaiser Family Foundation study results, which estimated that a quarter of a million COVID-19 deaths in the United States since June 2021 could have been prevented through vaccinations. Put differently, vaccine-preventable deaths represented 60 percent of all COVID-19-related deaths since June 2021 and 24 percent of the nearly one million deaths since the beginning of the pandemic. The Kaiser study did not include booster shots; thus, estimates are likely lower.

Other preventative steps were taken to curb the spread of COVID-19, including lockdowns and closures. These measures changed the nature of the economy, as some businesses were closed due to lockdowns. For example, restaurants closed, had limited seating, or turned to home deliveries during the pandemic. Many restaurants and physical fitness gyms did not survive, as was the case for the entertainment industry. Nevertheless, other businesses grew, such as outdoor camping and home entertainment. National and state parks became overwhelmed with visitors. Schools changed, too, as education moved from the in-person classroom to households. Some students survived, and others fell behind. Regardless, the social aspects of schooling dramatically changed with the loss of the social interactions and events typical of schools.

These public health practices would generate controversy and forms of collective behavior. During the pandemic, most people readily complied and embraced public health measures, while others ignored or dismissed them, and yet others actively opposed them. There would be panics, protests, rumors, conspiracy theories, mass movements, and other collective actions for and against public health COVID-19 control efforts. It is these collective behavioral responses that are the focus of this book. COVID-19 is a disease that harms and kills people but is also a social phenomenon. It has a social aspect that reflects groups along social, political, economic, psychological, racial, and other social structural lines. There was a lull in COVID-19 cases at the time of this writing. Some Americans have tired of restrictions and mandates. They have what might be labeled COVID-19 fatigue and have abandoned taking health precautions. The public is now tired of being unable to live "normal" lives.

COVID-19 MORTALITY RATES

Measuring mortality rates due to COVID-19 has proven to be challenging. Many factors influence how the cause of death is identified and reported. Some skeptics argue that the number of COVID-19-related deaths is overstated and exaggerated. However, others believe the number of fatalities is significantly undercounted. Issues include that methods of classifying causes of death vary, when the cause is determined, and how and if the data are reported. One of the confounding issues is whether the death was solely due to COVID-19 or did an infection trigger another cause of death, such as pneumonia. Is the COVID-19 infection the direct or indirect cause of death (see chapter 6 for elaboration)?

During the pandemic, COVID-19 caused the death rate to rise as new variants arose and people refused to get vaccinated or comply with restrictions.

There are several ways to measure deaths caused by COVID-19. None of the methods are 100 percent accurate, and all undercount the actual number of deaths due to the disease. Many factors affect the death counts, such as region, timeframe, people dying from COVID-19 without being tested, some dying from multiple underlying conditions aggravated by COVID-19, and so forth. Depending on the methods used to identify and count the cause of death, COVID-19-related deaths range from an estimated 5.93 million to 18.6 million worldwide and growing. In addition, there are COVID-19-caused deaths that are not included in the estimates due to limited testing, lack of diagnosis, and patient hesitancy or limited access to medical care. Regardless of the method, COVID-19 is responsible for many deaths in the United States and worldwide.

The World Health Organization (WHO) reported that the global death toll from COVID-19 is much higher than figures would indicate (Mueller and Nolen 2022). The WHO report calculated that the number of deaths exceeded the normally expected deaths. Excess deaths were 18 percent higher, or 10 million people, worldwide. Most of these deaths were in developing countries and within those countries' lower-income groups. In addition, several countries, such as Peru, Mexico, Russia, Egypt, and Pakistan, appeared to be undercounting COVID-19 deaths.

The United States' fatality rate is higher than other developed nations. For example, the *New York Times* compared the United States' deaths from COVID-19 to Australia's (Cave 2022). Australia enforced stricter pandemic measures than the United States. Cave concluded that many nations did better than the United States and that if the United States had responded similarly to Australia, 900,000 American lives could have been saved. Australia's death rate was one-tenth that of the United States, although a higher percentage of Australians lived in cities (known for higher fatality rates). Australia implemented stricter travel restrictions and maximized vaccine uptake before the pandemic waned. What mattered was that when polled, Australians expressed greater trust in science and government. Australians also voiced higher levels of trust in each other and said, "It is not just about me." In May 2022, 95 percent of Australians were fully vaccinated compared to 66 percent of Americans. Another study compared life expectancy in the United States with 19 other countries during the pandemic in 2020. The study found that the United States had a much larger decline in life expectancy due to COVID-19 than other higher-income countries (Masters et al. 2022). It also found that minority groups experienced disproportionately more significant reductions in life expectancy. Most COVID-19-related deaths in the United States have been for people over 70 years. COVID-19 was the third leading cause of death in the United States in 2020, and life expectancy declined by 3 years for Latinx, 2.9 years for Black, and 1.2 years for White Americans.

It was law enforcement officers' leading cause of death for two years (2020–2021). Even with that fact, some police unions sued against vaccine mandates.

Another subject that has been studied has been COVID-19's impact on the fatality rates of pregnant women. The Government Accountability Office (GAO), a non-partisan independent accounting agency, found that maternal (pregnancy-related) deaths have increased during the pandemic due to COVID-19 by 80 percent since 2018. COVID-19 contributed to 25 percent of maternal deaths from 2020 to 2021 (Government Accountability Office 2022). In addition, the report found that Black women had higher mortality rates than White and Latina women. Black women died during childbirth more disproportionately than their White and Latina counterparts. Pregnancy-related deaths for Black women increased from 44 per 100,000 in 2019 to 68.9 in 2021. In comparison, the White women's jumped from 17.9 per 100,000 to 26.1 over the same period. The latter finding is indicative of racial and ethnic disparities.

Some people have challenged what they believe is an overinflated risk of dying from COVID-19. Mercola and Cummins (2021:68) cite a CDC planning table (see CDC 2021b: Table 1), updated since 2019, that estimates the number of deaths due to COVID-19 by age grouping. They observed (p. 68), "According to the CDC—even considering the inaccuracy of testing and exigencies of fatality classification—the survivability rate is 99.997% for 0–19 years, 99.98% for 20–49 years, 99.5% for 50–69 years, and 94.6% for 70-plus years." Most COVID-19-related deaths in the United States have been for people over 70 years. Since they reported these percentages, the estimates have changed along with the age groupings. For 0–17 years of age, 20 out of a million are estimated to have died from COVID-19, with a survivability rate of 99.098 percent. For those aged between 18 and 49 years, 500 were estimated to have died from COVID-19, for a survivability rate of 99.095 percent. For those aged between 50 and 64 years, the survivability rate was 99.094 percent, and for those over 65 years, 90,000 are estimated to have died from COVID-19 with a survivability rate of 91 percent (see CDC 2021a, Table 1). Regardless of how it is calculated, according to CDC data, the chances of dying from COVID-19 have always been slim for most people except older Americans.

Other interesting calculations regarding COVID-19-related death rates include looking at the total population of the United States and simply counting the number of COVID-19 deaths. According to the U.S. Census Bureau, as of July 1, 2021, the U.S. population was 331,893,745. On May 5, 2022, the CDC reported that 993,341 people had died from COVID-19. Using the U.S. population as a base, about one person in 332 has died from COVID-19. However, missing is the idea that every American has yet to catch COVID-19 or may have had COVID-19 and been asymptomatic.

That is, they did not know they had the virus. Furthermore, some have had COVID-19 more than once. It gets messy unraveling what is occurring.

During the pandemic, the United States' COVID-19-related deaths came in waves. May 2020 was the initial wave, followed by a second wave in August 2020, then January and February 2021, October 2021 (Delta variant surge), and February 2022. There will likely be additional surges. The decrease in weekly fatalities in the summer of 2021 led some to conclude that the pandemic had ended, and then the Delta variant emerged. The later Omicron variant may ultimately be the deadliest of all variants. In the fall of 2022, deaths linked to the Omicron variant continued to occur.

The exact number of COVID-19 infections and fatalities due to underreporting is unknown (Ferreira et al. 2020). What is known is that specific populations, including older people, individuals with respiratory complications and pre-existing diseases, and those having less access to health care, were more likely to have serious cases and die from COVID-19. In addition, economically disadvantaged populations are more likely to have pre-existing conditions that increase the probability of COVID-19 infections and death.

CONCLUDING OBSERVATIONS

In December 2019, COVID-19 would surface in Wuhan, China. At the time, few understood the significance of this new coronavirus to the world. Soon COVID-19 would find its way to the United States. Although the medical community had previously dealt with coronaviruses, none compared with COVID-19. The medical and research communities quickly responded by taking COVID-19 seriously. Initially, the focus was on spread of the disease and how to contain the virus. These early efforts were futile and, at times, misdirected. COVID-19, as a virus, deserves much credit for its rapid spread as it proved highly contagious and adaptive. Complicating matters is that individual responses to COVID-19 infections can range from no symptoms to death. Individuals can spread the disease to others without indicating they are infected. The virus steadily evolved into more contagious or deadly forms (mutations) faster than medical understanding. The well-known cliches of "trying to hit a moving target" or "designing an airplane in flight" seem applicable to COVID-19.

With limited information, the medical community and governments relied on established disease prevention practices. These included face masks, personal protective equipment, testing, environmental cleaning, quarantines, social distancing, lockdowns, and closures. Some of these strategies slowed the spread of COVID-19, but others could have been more effective. Regardless, all of these would stir controversy. For some Americans, these efforts would feed preexisting political divisiveness and spark some individuals at the political extremes to embrace rumors and conspiracy theories. Some Americans' political views increasingly shaped their openness to public health pandemic control efforts. On one end were Americans who feared COVID-19 and likened the pandemic to living in a petri dish. COVID-19 dramatically shaped their daily lives in ways that they could not have foreseen. To other Americans, COVID-19, the pandemic, and its responses have been overblown at great costs to society. These individuals view the pandemic as a nuisance and an unnecessary disruption to their everyday lives.

Chapter 2

Consequences of COVID-19

> Description of the African American response to the 1793 Yellow Fever in Philadelphia: "A solicitation appeared in the public papers, to the people of color to come forward and assist the distressed, perishing, and neglected sick; with a kind of assurance, that people of our color were not liable to take the infection. . . . The first we visited was a man in Emsley's alley, who was dying, and his wife lay dead at the time in the house, there were none to assist but two poor helpless children. We administered what relief we could, and applied to the overseers of the poor to have the woman buried."
>
> Absalom Jones and Richard Allen (1794:A2)

> "Living with long COVID can be hard,
> especially when there are no immediate answers or solutions."
>
> Centers for Disease Control and Prevention (2023a)

COVID-19 AND THE WORLD

Very few aspects of society have not been touched in some way by COVID-19. From basic interpersonal to worldwide, relationships are different. At the interpersonal level, daily interactions have changed because of masks, physical barriers, social distancing, and other restrictions. For decades, social psychologists have recognized that non-verbal communications are essential to understanding and interpreting information. COVID-19 adaptations changed the rules and context in which people interact by restricting non-verbal information (cues). Examples are numerous, such as how remote learning dramatically changed student-teacher interactions.

Going to the grocery store or bank became a different experience with social distancing, barriers, and masks. It became more challenging to identify people wearing masks. The following are a few ways COVID-19 impacted societies and the world.

On the world scale, the pandemic was a major disruption worldwide. A notable recession and widespread shortages of food and other supplies occurred. Shipments of goods waited offshore, resulting in supply chain disruptions and panic hoarding. Educational systems at all levels were modified and locked down. Travel, especially international, was curtailed or prohibited. China, New Zealand, Australia, Italy, Spain, and to a lesser degree, the United States imposed travel bans to hamper the spread of COVID-19. Travel bans in some countries, such as Australia and New Zealand, were easier to enforce than in the United States. Complicating matters was the observation that travelers were not always honest about their symptoms and more vested in getting to their destination. Events, especially in the entertainment industry, were canceled or postponed. The size of gatherings was limited or prohibited. Businesses in some sectors cut back or were permanently closed, resulting in financial crises for owners and employees. All these and others led to social, economic, and political disruption. One of the major challenges for decision-makers during the pandemic was balancing "economic with medical considerations" (Zielonka 2021:71). Regardless of where the lines were drawn, people were unhappy.

FEAR

One of the consequences of the pandemic has been fear. It has been perhaps the most important emotion during the pandemic (Offe 2021:33). There is no doubt that COVID-19 has generated fear, which is common when the social order is disrupted. People feared getting sick, dying, or spreading the virus to others who might become seriously ill or die. Individuals feared making family members and friends deathly ill, especially children and older adults. During the pandemic, anxiety and fear were co-partners in social life, as individuals constantly weighed the risks of actively participating in society and face-to-face social relationships. Some of this fear and anxiety exceeded the risks from the coronavirus, and some were justified, as COVID-19 isolated individuals from loved ones and friends. However, some question whether this fear was warranted, such as Mercola and Cummins (2021:67), who wrote, "Fear is ultimately what strips us of our human rights and drives a society into totalitarianism, and the only way to circumvent such a fate is to bravely resist fear." They added, "Today, one of the biggest sources of fears is a global pandemic—one that allegedly came about naturally, and to which we have no known defenses—or so the official story goes."

Following the World Trade Center attack on September 11, 2001, New York's emergency rooms were quickly overwhelmed with patients. In 2020, the same pattern occurred with the rapid spread of COVID-19. National newscasts flooded the media with vivid images of New York's hospital hallways packed with patients. Reporters interviewed medical staff who felt overwhelmed and helpless in controlling the disease that was making many patients seriously ill. Reporters also filmed temporary morgues set up throughout the city. The media shared horrific images of the sick and dead, and it should be no surprise that many Americans would view these as terrifying.

However, some believed this fear of COVID-19 was unjustified and was a moral panic. A moral panic because it was, in their view, an intense fearful overreaction to COVID-19. For example, using cause-of-death data tables, Bagus, Peña-Ramos, and Sánchez-Bayón (2021) concluded that the fear of death from COVID-19 was unwarranted (see chapter 5). In the same vein, Siegel (2020:xiii) observed that "despite the real, ever-present danger from Covid, the overall climate of fear was inflated well out of proportion to the risk and the reality and was its own core danger to society." He later added:

> With over 8 million cases of tuberculosis every year worldwide, 5 million new cases of AIDS, over 300 million cases of malaria, and over 1 million deaths due to each, Americans rarely worry about these diseases. In the United States, approximately 40,000 people die of influenza every year, a statistic that went unnoticed until it was the flu turned on the wheel of hype. (Siegel 2020:7)

On the flip side of fear is optimism bias, which is the belief that bad things are more likely to happen to others than ourselves. For example, people can have an optimism bias when they believe automobile accidents, cancer, heart failure, disease, house fires, violence, and other adverse events only happen to others. Optimism bias may help people overcome negative emotions; it can also lead people to underestimate the chances that COVID-19 will infect them. Van Bavel, Baicker, Boggio, et al. (2021) noted that optimism bias could lead people to dismiss or ignore public health warnings about the risks of COVID-19. Balancing between being overwhelmed by fear and anxiety and optimism bias can be difficult. With COVID-19, that balance is challenging, as the range of individual responses to COVID-19 infections varies.

Whether the fear of COVID-19 is justified or not, fear shaped everyone somehow. Besides the direct fear of COVID-19 infection, some Americans feared what impact pandemic mandates and restrictions would have on their lives. Offe (2021) labeled this secondary fear. This secondary fear was that such measures would negatively impact education, jobs, interpersonal relationships, businesses, and daily life. For the fearful, their lifestyles changed as they took precautions to protect themselves and others. The psychological toll of fear weighed heavily for some. For the fearless, living with restrictions and mandates they thought unnecessary also weighed heavily on some. In addition, the fearful interacted with those who failed to appreciate or comply with COVID-19 precautions, resulting in strained social relationships and discomfort for both.

COVID-19-RELATED HEALTH ISSUES

Some people get terribly ill from COVID-19 and require hospitalization, while others are asymptomatic and barely become ill. Symptoms may appear 2–14 days after exposure to the virus. People with COVID-19 may experience any number of the following symptoms in any combination: high fevers or chills, cough, fatigue, shortness of breath, difficulty breathing, muscle or body aches, sore throat, congestion or runny nose, loss of taste or smell, headaches, diarrhea, nausea, and vomiting. These symptoms are similar to allergies, colds, influenza, and other common infections. This makes it difficult to determine if it is a case of COVID-19 or some other infection unless a test is conducted. In more severe COVID-19 cases, trouble breathing, confusion, inability to stay awake or wake up, persistent pain in the chest, pale gray or blue skin and lips, high fevers, and poor skin tone. Respiratory problems requiring assisted breathing support characterize the more severe cases. The news media has shared multiple accounts of patients and their families with serious health issues. Images of people in crowded intensive care units, hallways of overcrowded hospitals, temporary care structures, storage units for the deceased, and patients on ventilators flooded the news during peaks of COVID-19 infections.

Besides the immediate consequences of COVID-19, a growing body of research finds that the coronavirus causes brain damage, such as "brain fog," and negative neurological symptoms. The virus's attack on the brain could be long-term and result in memory loss, reduced blood flow, and confusion, among other symptoms. In addition, an increasing number of studies are linking COVID-19 to diabetes. Diabetic individuals are more vulnerable to severe illness and have higher death rates from COVID-19. There seems to be agreement that uncontrolled diabetes impairs the immune system and decreases the individual's ability to withstand a COVID-19 infection. Likewise, some medical researchers are linking COVID-19 infections with later development of type 2 diabetes.

Studies have linked COVID-19 to various health issues, some involving the heart. For example, in April 2020, in the United Kingdom, physicians witnessed increased reports of previously healthy children presenting severe inflammatory syndrome with Kawasaki disease–like features (i.e., rash, fever, swelling of feet and hands, swollen lymph glands, irritation and redness of whites of eyes, and inflammation of mouth, lips, and throat). The cases occurred in children testing positive for COVID-19 infection. This condition is called Multisystem Inflammatory Syndrome (MIS-C), which is rare. COVID-19 has also been associated with myocarditis, which is heart muscle (myocardium) inflammation. According to the Mayo Clinic (2023:n.p.), this "inflammation can reduce the heart's ability to pump blood and cause chest pain, shortness of breath, and rapid or irregular heart rhythms (arrhythmias)."

The long-term effects of COVID-19 are currently unknown. However, long-term health issues have been reported for individuals who have had COVID-19 infections (for an overview, see Proal and VanElzakker 2021). These long-term health consequences include fatigue, loss of smell and taste, headaches, pain, paralysis, and other medical issues (see Moyer 2022). Whether these are directly due to COVID-19 or immune systems is being investigated by medical researchers. For example, in a study of over 273,000 COVID-19 survivors, 37 percent reported medical symptoms three to six months after infection (Taquet et al., 2021). One estimate concluded that as many as 31 million working-age Americans might have long-COVID-19 symptoms (see Bach 2022a; Sanchez et al. 2022). A Brookings Institution report estimated that as many as 1.6 million full-time workers could be out of work because of long-term COVID-19. This accounted for 15 percent of the labor shortage in January 2022. As of August of the same year, it is estimated that 16 million working-age Americans likely have long-term COVID-19. Of these, 2 to 4 million are out of work (Bach 2022b). A later Brookings Institution study found that reduced immigration and COVID-19 deaths resulted in a post-COVID workforce reduction of approximately 1.4 million workers (Bauer et al. 2023:n.p.). A recent study of over 31,000 previously COVID-19-infected adults was conducted in Scotland (Hastie et al. 2022). The researchers found that some respondents reported long-COVID-19 symptoms lasting up to 18 months. Of the previously COVID-19-infected (symptomatic) respondents, 6 percent had not entirely recovered and 42 percent had only partially recovered. Those reporting long-COVID-19 symptoms said they had persisting impairments of daily activities, breathlessness, palpitations, chest pains, and confusion. So little is understood about long-term COVID-19 that more research is needed.

One of the most dramatic impacts of the pandemic on individual healthcare has been the postponement of routine and needed medical care. People and medical providers have delayed or canceled medical interventions and examinations for various reasons. Medical issues such as heart disease, diabetes, liver disease, and cancer have been put aside because of strained medical resources or COVID-19 restrictions. Additionally, some have questioned the emphasis on treating COVID-19 cases over other serious health concerns. The treatment of COVID-19 cases has limited access to routine and acute health care. Siegel (2020:216) held that COVID-19 became the primary medical concern to the detriment of other major health issues. He wrote:

> Only COVID illness mattered; Covid hospitalizations and deaths were on our radar screen. Deaths from suicide because of how Covid disrupted a person's life were not sexy; it was not a Covid death. Teeth that fell out or became infected because no dental care was available were somehow detached from Covid. Heart attacks due to blood pressure, cholesterol, or diabetes went untreated or blurred together with Covid deaths where the heart was involved in both cases.

The emphasis on COVID-19 and stress on the healthcare system created a medical backlog that will continue for years. Drug overdoses also rose partly because of the use of deadly fentanyl. In addition, some have speculated that drug use has increased due to isolation and depression and a reluctance to contact emergency responders in overdose cases.

A significant consequence of the pandemic was exposing the health systems and inadequacy and inherent inequalities. Delanty (2021a:viii) observed that the pandemic "has exacerbated inequalities, xenophobia, and racism." These and other dimensions of any quality played out in the healthcare system. Some groups have had a history of reasonable access to healthcare, while others have yet to. People of color do not have the same access to healthcare as White people. The wealthy had better access than the lower-income populations. The preventative benefits of good diets, access to care, better education, and other factors collectively labeled as the social determinants of health are favorable to some populations and unfavorable to others. Thus, when infected, those populations with less favorable healthcare fared worse than others, as indicated by different infection, vaccination, and mortality rates.

The COVID-19 pandemic has had a disproportionately negative impact on the health of Black and Latinx communities. Evidence shows that people in diverse communities and minorities will experience more significant adverse health consequences from COVID-19 (Sanchez et al. 2022). In 2020, Black and Latinx individuals, on average, experienced 2.9- and 3-year decreases in life expectancy, respectively, primarily due to COVID-19 deaths (Arias et al. 2021). In 2020, Black and Latinx individuals, on average, experienced 2.9– and 3–year decreases in life expectancy, respectively, primarily due to Covid-19 deaths (Arias et al. 2021). This was approximately 2.5 times more than the decrease for White individuals. Similar findings have been reported by Masters, Aron, and Woolf (2022), whose comparative study of the United States and 19 other countries found that life expectancies were shortened during the pandemic and varied by racial group. Native Americans and Latinx groups were hit the hardest at the pandemic's beginning but were later surpassed by White populations. For Asian Americans, life expectancy decreased by 1.8–1.9 years, Latinx populations by 3.7 years, and non-Latinx Black populations by 3.2 years. The sharpest decline was for indigenous (Native American) populations of 4.3 percent (4 years for women and 4.75 years for men). In addition to these two groups, research has found that other groups have a higher risk for long COVID. Tsampasian, Elghaazaly, Chattopadhyay, et al. (2023) reviewed COVID-19 studies and found that people over age 40, those with previous health issues, who had experienced severe COVID-19 infections, were unvaccinated, were female, were obese, had immunosuppressive conditions, and/or had mental health issues, had a higher risk of long COVID-19.

One of the implications of COVID-19 is the financial cost of serious infections. Some patients have needed Intensive Care Unit care followed by extended hospital stays and then rehabilitation. The costs per stay depend on factors such as the seriousness of the infection, prior medical conditions, length of stay, hospital rates and fees, state cost controls, and other factors. One study estimated the costs for an average COVID-19 hospitalization by state (Hardy 2021). An independent non-profit developed a tool that compared costs for severe COVID-19 and less severe cases by state. According to the study, Nevada was the most expensive at a $472,213 average for severe hospitalization cases, and California was at $111,213 for less severe COVID-19 hospitalizations. Maryland had the lowest average costs of $131,965 and $31,339 for serious and less severe hospitalizations, respectively. Others, such as the *Detroit Free Press*, question these amounts and believe the average cost is closer to $17,000 per case (see Valverde 2021). Regardless, the benefits of investing in prevention are notable. When the vaccination price is compared to hospitalization, the benefit rests with getting the vaccine. Oldstone (2020:xvi) wrote of the use of disease research and COVID-19:

> A safe estimate is that for each dollar invested by the government and basic research to study these diseases, a return of at least 1,000- to 10,000-fold has been realized for those now financially productive instead of requiring long-term care. We need to find out the real long-term costs of Covid-19 (long covid). We do know that some survivors of Covid-19 have lasting physical and mental challenges.

PSYCHOLOGICAL CONSEQUENCES OF COVID-19

A significant consequence of the pandemic has been social isolation. Virtually everyone has been affected by social isolation during the pandemic. Some initial strategies for limiting the spread of COVID-19, such as quarantines, social distancing, confinement, reliance on meetings via the Internet, separating nursing home residents, and lockdowns, all contributed to isolating individuals. Considering that humans need social connections (relationships), the psychological consequences of isolation have been significant. Some people experienced a loss in their daily routines and activities.

Unsurprisingly, COVID-19 has had negative psychological consequences for many people, whether infected or not. The isolation, stress, social disruption, and altered personal relationships have resulted in a decline in mental health for some Americans. Some individuals report being traumatized during the pandemic and depressed, as their lives had been disrupted at many levels. Arora, Grey, Östlundh, Lam, Omar, and Arnone (2020) systematically reviewed academic journals to find studies of mental health outcomes during COVID-19. Studies identified Post-Traumatic Stress Disorder (PTSD) at 33% as the most prevalent psychological disorder. PTSD was followed by anxiety (28%), stress (27%), and depression (22%). Healthcare workers had psychological outcomes similar to those of the general population. In a similar vein, a Brookings Institution national survey of 1,015 adults found that many Americans lost a sense of control over their lives. This was especially true for women and young people between the ages of 18 and 34 years (Busette 2022).

Long periods of social isolation for individuals from lower socio-economic backgrounds placed them at higher risk of having mental health issues (Ferreira et al. 2020:13). Older adults who are at the highest risk of severe symptoms of COVID-19 were some of those most impacted by social isolation (Van Bavel, Baicker, Boggio, et al. 2021). For example, scenes of isolated older adults residing in nursing homes limited to interacting with their families through windows and barriers were commonplace. However, others believe older Americans' mental health fared better than younger people. For example, an American Association of Retired People story noted that some experts found that older people rated coming out of the pandemic with better physical and mental health than those aged 16 to 24 years (Hochman 2023:9).

An additional concern during the pandemic has been the mental health of adolescents isolated from peers and external social activities. Centers for Disease Control and Prevention 2021 data show that 37 percent of surveyed high school students experienced poor mental health during the COVID-19 pandemic (CDC 2022b). Forty-four percent of students felt persistently hopeless over the year. Fifty-five percent indicated they had experienced emotional abuse by a parent or other in the home. Eleven percent reported physical abuse, such as hitting, beating, or kicking in the house. These percentages were higher than pre-pandemic figures. Those adolescents with more robust connectivity to their schools fared better. However, with closed schools, connectivity was harder to establish for many youths.

Further evidence of mental health issues can be found in survey data. During June 24–30, 2020, 5,412 U.S. adults completed a web-based survey. Of the respondents, 40.9 percent reported at least one adverse mental health condition, and 10.7 percent said they had considered suicide seriously within the last 30 days (Czeisler et al. 2020). These and others are indicators of social strain. However, some studies on mental health during the pandemic have found mixed results. In a Brookings Institution study, Dobson, Graham, Hua, and Pinto (2022) found varied results after reviewing mental health data from multiple national data sets before and during the pandemic. They observed that some studies indicated increased depression and anxiety during the pandemic, but other studies found little change since the pandemic. The authors suggest caution when interpreting mental health indicators and the importance of not relying on a single data source.

Often co-occurring with mental health issues are those of substance abuse. There is little doubt that substance abuse increased during the pandemic. Early in the pandemic, it was found that the frequency of alcohol consumption during lockdowns increased by 14 percent (Pollard et al. 2020). Alcohol-related deaths also rose during the pandemic. According to a National Institute on Alcohol Abuse and Alcoholism survey, alcohol consumption increased shortly after the pandemic started, especially among women, people with minor children at home, and Black Americans (Barbosa et al. 2021). Among respondents drinking alcohol between February and November 2020, the researchers found increased consumption and excessive consumption were maintained from April through November 2020. Significant findings included (Executive Summary:1):

- Using the estimated 166,052,940 people aged 21 or older nationally who drank in 2019, this translates to an increase from February to November 2020 of 1 billion more drinks per month, with 14.6 million more people exceeding drinking guidelines and 9 million more people binge drinking in November 2020 compared with February 2020.
- The proportion exceeding drinking guidelines between February and November 2020 increased by 54% for women and 32% for men. More women than men surpassed recommended drinking guidelines between April and November 2020.

- Between February and November 2020, binge drinking increased by 42% for women and 32% for men.
- The most significant increases in consumption from February to November were for Black and Hispanic women (173% and 148%, respectively), Black men (173%), men of other non-white races (209%), and women with children younger than age 5 (323%).

COVID-19'S IMPACT ON FAMILIES

The pandemic has had significant social impacts on the family. Cherlin (2021) summarized a few of the changes families experienced. He observed that families became more isolated and women's roles as caregivers became more intense, as children remained home for longer time spans. He noted that homeschooling became more common, and women had higher job losses than men. Birthrates declined, and families either canceled or postponed plans to have children. The same pattern occurred during the 1918 influenza pandemic. Increased death rates led to decreased births nine months later (Aassve et al. 2020). A similar slowdown seems to have occurred during the COVID-19 pandemic. Lindberg, VandeVusse, Mueller, and Kirstein (2020), using a 2020 national survey, found that more than 40 percent of women indicated that since the pandemic, they had changed their plans about when and how many children they planned to have. In contrast, 17 percent of women reported they wanted to have children sooner or more of them because of the pandemic. A third of the women reported having to delay or cancel sexual reproductive health services or had trouble getting birth control because of the pandemic. These patterns were not equally distributed for women and were experienced differently depending on their racial and ethnic group membership.

Within households, family relationships changed. Parents and children involuntarily had more time together in confined spaces. Increasing numbers of parents worked from home, and their children stayed home rather than physically attending school—the proximity of living together as families affected behavior. The likelihood of tension and stress among family members increased over prolonged periods. Stress indicators include domestic violence and child maltreatment (Van Bavel et al. 2021).

The loss of a parent to COVID-19 impacted some families. For example, the CDC published a study on October 7, 2021, in the journal *Pediatrics* that reported more than 140,000 U.S. children under the age of 18 years had lost a parent, custodial grandparent, or grandparent caregiver who provided the child's home and met basic needs (Hillis et al. 2021). Worldwide the same pattern occurred, as an estimated 5.2 million children lost a parent or caregiver to COVID-19 during the first 19 months of the pandemic (Unwin et al. 2022). Any loss of a parent results in altered relationships within the family.

Other important functions performed by families became issues during the pandemic. For example, the family serves as the primary provider of food. For some families, food insecurity increased from pre-pandemic levels. Another function of families is to provide shelter. Parker, Horowitz, and Minkin (2021) conducted a Pew Research Center national survey of American adults and found that a rising share of them say the availability of affordable housing is a major problem in their area (for a first-year overview of Pew Research Center opinion surveys, see Deane, Parker, and Gramlich 2021). Specifically, those indicating that affordable housing was a major problem in their communities rose from 39 percent in 2018 to 49 percent in 2021 during the pandemic, a 10 percent gain.

COVID-19'S IMPACT ON EDUCATION

School closures, mask-wearing, social distancing in schools, severe staff shortages, remote instruction, absenteeism, and other policies dramatically impacted education success and attainment. School closures resulted in a deeper involvement of families in their children's education. This was not always convenient or easy, especially for single parents. Single parents had to balance work, childcare, and now education. The inability to attend school has impacts beyond class curriculums and learning. School closures affected the ability of children in low-income households to secure food and access health services. Public schools provide food and health services that became unavailable during the pandemic. This resulted in some children missing meals and medical care. School closures widened educational inequalities between children from different socioeconomic backgrounds (Blundell et al. 2020; Fisher and Bubola 2020; Maestripieri 2020).

School policies regarding COVID-19 proved controversial. Critics of school closures point out that there is no relationship between closures and COVID-19 case counts. In addition, medical evidence has consistently found that younger children have a lower risk of severe COVID-19 infections than adults. The issue is less about young children becoming seriously ill and more about them transmitting COVID-19 to school staff, other adults, and family members. Rather than being based on public health factors, decisions by local school boards to close or remain open were based on political orientation. Democrats tended to support school closures, and Republicans wanted schools to stay open.

School closures underscored racial gaps in education. White students were likelier to have in-person educational opportunities than children of color.

Public schools with high percentages of Black and Hispanic students had a greater tendency to close, which in practice furthered racial disparities (Russell and Patterson 2021). According to one study, in the fall of 2021, most private schools (95%), compared to fewer (40%) public schools, stayed open for in-person learning (Russell and Patterson 2021). A higher percentage of White children attend private schools than children of color. For some children, in-person schooling is a better option than remote, and falling test scores suggest remote learning has set many children back in their education.

A Brookings Institution summary report on the impact of the coronavirus pandemic on education found that schools have experienced severe staff shortages, closures, high absenteeism, and quarantines (Kuhfeld et al. 2022). In addition, the report noted that educators and students struggled with mental health issues, stress, higher rates of violence and misconduct, and lost instructional time. Kuhfeld, Soland, and Lewis (2022) used data from 5.4 million students in grades 3–8. They tracked the pandemic's impact on student math and reading test scores before (fall 2019), following the initial onset (fall 2020), and over a year (fall 2021) into the pandemic. They found that average test scores had a sizable drop. The gap between low-poverty and high-poverty elementary schools increased by 20 percent in math and 15 percent in reading. Elementary school students from lower-income households fell further behind those from higher-income households. The drop in test scores is consistent with other research.

A Pew Research Center study of 1,316 teenagers and their parents conducted from April to May 2022 found that most teens (65%) preferred in-person over virtual or hybrid learning (Anderson et al. 2022). The authors reported that racial differences were found regarding preference. White (70%) and Hispanic (64%), more so than Black teens (51%), preferred school to be entirely in person. Teens living in higher-income households also had a greater tendency to prefer in-person learning. The study's authors also reported that a few (16%) teens feared that they had fallen behind in their schoolwork during the pandemic, but most did not.

However, some data suggest that COVID-19 did not always result in adverse educational outcomes. Using data from 25 states, Harris and Chen (2022) found that high school graduation rates slightly increased during the pandemic in 2020 and returned to a prior level in 2021. However, they discovered a 16 percent decline in high school students transitioning into post-secondary education. Factoring in subgroup membership, graduation rates increased for students with disabilities, English learners, and Black students. However, college entry for students of color declined. They noted that reduced high school standards might account for some high school graduation patterns.

Nevertheless, research has found that the national achievement scores of grade school children have declined during the pandemic. According to the National Assessment of Educational Progress, 9-year-olds lost ground in math, and reading scores were the lowest in 30 years. Moreover, these declines spanned across all income levels and races, especially for lower-performing students (Mervosh 2022).

Finally, many students missed traditional school activities and special occasions such as proms, homecomings, sporting events, and graduation ceremonies. Losing these and other extra-curricular activities was difficult for some students and led to depression.

COVID-19 EMPLOYMENT AND ECONOMIC FALLOUT

According to the U.S. Bureau of Labor Statistics (2022), millions of Americans lost their jobs due to the pandemic. However, job losses were uneven across the economy. Maestripieri (2021:2) observed, "The variance and job losses in terms of demographic characteristics depend on sorting between different sectors: the affected sector showed a predominance of youth, minorities, women and low-skilled workers, usually employed with temporary contracts or in precarious working conditions, including solo self-employment." Those individuals in high-paying jobs were less likely to lose their jobs and could telework.

The pandemic has shown the world what jobs are essential: those that produce food, provide healthcare, educate children, and transport goods, supermarket workers, refuse collectors, and cleaners. As a result, people working in these sectors were less likely to lose their jobs. According to a Pew Research Center study, in 2020, about three in ten lower-income adults (28.2%) experienced unemployment at least some of the year (Kochhar and Sechopoulos 2022). Likewise, 13.8 percent of middle-income adults and 7.8 percent of upper-income adults had at least a spell of unemployment in 2020.

Financially, the COVID-19 pandemic job losses affected households. Parker, Horowitz, and Brown (2020) surveyed 4,917 American adults in April 2020. Overall, 43 percent of the respondents indicated that the pandemic negatively impacted their household finances. The pandemic hit lower-income harder than middle- or upper-income households. They also discovered that 32 percent of upper-income, 42 percent of middle-income, and 52 percent of lower-income respondents reported that someone in their household had lost a job or taken a pay cut during the pandemic. Over half (53%) of the lower-income respondents indicated they could not fully pay their monthly bills compared to 19 percent of middle-income and 7 percent of upper-income respondents. Overall, 47 percent said they had rainy-day funds to cover their expenses for up to three months. Only 23 percent of lower-income respondents said they had emergency funds covering costs for three months. Differences were noted between ethnic and income groups on rainy-day funds, with people of color having fewer emergency funds.

According to their survey data, some ethnic groups experienced higher job losses than others. Hispanic adults (61%) said they or someone in their household had lost a job or taken a cut in pay due to the coronavirus outbreak. About half of the Black and White adults said their household had experienced job losses or pay cuts. Parker, Horowitz, and Brown (2020) identified other negative financial impacts on households, such as the ability to save for retirement. These impacts were not experienced equally by all groups, as lower-income, minority, younger, and less educated adults, and women had rougher financial conditions during the pandemic.

Later in the pandemic (January 24, 2021), the Pew Research Center surveyed a national random sample of 10,334 U.S. adults to learn more about American financial outlooks and how personal finances have changed since the beginning of the pandemic (Horowitz et al. 2021). The survey found lower-income adults reported saving less, older adults were delaying retirement, and 4 in 10 said someone in the immediate family had lost a job or wages. Half of the adults that lost jobs had taken on debt to pay bills. Horowitz et al. (2021) found that personal finance ratings varied "widely" across racial, ethnic, and socioeconomic groups. They found differences among groups in savings, spending, ability to pay bills, concern over debt, food insecurity, retirement savings, delayed retirement dates, and financial goal attainment. Hispanics, Asian and Black Americans, lower-income adults, and those under 30 were more likely to report that someone in the household had lost a job or taken a pay cut due to the pandemic. About four in ten (39%) said their family's financial situation had improved compared with a year ago; 32 percent of those with middle incomes and just 22 percent of lower-income adults indicated the same. Lower-income adults (74%), most Black and Hispanic adults, and those with a high school diploma or less education said their finances were in fair or poor shape. The researchers said about four in ten Americans indicated they were spending less money than usual since the pandemic began, especially among upper-income adults. Some 53 percent of Americans with upper incomes said they had been spending less money, compared with 43 percent of those with middle incomes and 34 percent with lower incomes (Horowitz et al. 2021).

Finally, another Pew Research Center report, using U.S. Census and Pew Research Center survey data, by Kochhar and Sechopoulos (2022:4), found that from 2019 to 2020, the median income of lower-income households decreased by 3 percent, and the median income of middle-income households fell by 2.1 percent. The authors (p. 4) noted that "the median income of upper-income households in 2020 was about the same as in 2019." However, again, the researchers concluded that the degree of impact depended on labor market turmoil during the pandemic.

COVID-19 AND WORKPLACE CHANGES

For some Americans, the pandemic shifted the workplace from the office to the home. Business and building closures resulted in some white-collar jobs moving to the workers' residences. A 2021 International Labour Organization (ILO) estimate reported that 93 percent of the world's workers had experienced some form of temporary or permanent workplace closure during the pandemic (International Labour Organization 2020). Two years into the pandemic, Parker, Horowitz, and Minkin (2022) surveyed 5,889 American adults working part- or full-time and having only one job or a job they consider their primary job. They found six out of ten workers reported working mainly from their homes. This percentage declined from earlier in the pandemic when 71 percent said they worked mainly from home. Even with workplaces reopening, the percentage of adults preferring to work at home increased from earlier in the pandemic. In addition, 64 percent indicated that balancing work with personal life by working at home was easier. However, 60 percent indicated they felt less connected to co-workers. Socioeconomic status seems to play a key role in working from home. Adults with upper incomes and/or higher levels of education were more likely to work from home. As the pandemic continued, health concerns over COVID-19 decreased while the preference for working from home increased.

During the pandemic, women were likelier to lose their employment in what some have labeled a "pink recession" (see Matthewman and Huppatz 2020). The pandemic has impacted working women in other ways. According to Harvard economist Claudia Goldin, the pandemic significantly impacted working women. The pandemic has stressed working women because they kept their jobs but needed to provide additional care to children and older adults (Goldin 2022). More than men, women have taken the brunt of increased child caregiving responsibilities. This is due to increased childcare and the closure of schools and daycare centers. With homeschooling, women caregivers have taken on more supervision of children. Increased workplace flexibility due to the pandemic will benefit women and men but decrease face-to-face interactions among co-workers. Goldin speculated that decreased face-to-face co-worker interactions might harm the careers of women and men working from home.

COVID-19 IMPACTS ON LOCAL COMMUNITIES

Parker, Horowitz, and Minkin (2021) surveyed 9,676 American adults in October 2021 to better understand their views on where they prefer to live and the impact of COVID-19 on local communities. During the pandemic, adults' preference for urban living declined from 23 percent in 2018 to 19 percent in 2021. Their preference for suburban living increased from 42 to 46 percent over the same span, and their preference for rural living stayed almost unchanged. They concluded that the coronavirus had something to do with the decline in the appeal of city living. More importantly, the Parker et al. (2021) study respondents indicated that the pandemic had driven people in the community apart. Overall, 47 percent said the pandemic had divided their community apart, 39 percent reported there was not much difference, and 13 percent thought it had brought people closer together. In addition, about a quarter of the adults indicated the pandemic had health and economic impacts on their communities, and those living in urban areas felt the pandemic impacts more acutely than those from suburban and rural areas. These views on the pandemic's impact on local community health and economics were influenced by racial and ethnic group membership. For example, more Black respondents saw COVID-19 as a significant economic and health problem than other racial and ethnic groups. Parker et al. also found that more than a third of U.S. adults (36%) believe it will take over two years for their local community to return to how it was before the COVID-19 outbreak or that their community will never return to normal.

One of the community impacts of the pandemic affected individuals that were homeless. The pandemic impacted homeless individuals on multiple fronts. They have poorer health and a greater risk of illness. During the pandemic, people experiencing homelessness had limited availability to prevention measures, such as face masks, sanitary supplies, and vaccinations. When they became ill with COVID-19, they often lacked access to medical care. They were impacted in another important way. Vandenberghe and Verán (2021:179) noted, "For the homeless, the street disappeared as a space of survival." With lockdowns of businesses, especially restaurants, rubbish and trash bins, which are food sources, became empty. Panhandling and other sources of financial support disappeared as people abandoned the streets. Undocumented immigrants disappeared from public spaces to avoid being more easily identified and harassed by law enforcement.

Some communities, specifically cities, experienced outward migration. Migration from major cities to suburban and rural settings occurred on a grand scale. According to U.S. Census data, 56 American cities of over a million experienced a decline in population during the pandemic (Frey 2022a;

2022b). This pattern can be attributed to jobs that can be performed from rural locations because more workers can telecommute and work from home.

Parker, Horowitz, and Minkin (2021) conducted a Pew Research Center national survey of American adults in 2021. The study found that perceptions of problems during the pandemic differed by race and ethnicity. For example, 42 percent of Black adults said crime was a major problem in their community, compared with 30 percent of Hispanic adults, 24 percent of Asian adults, and 17 percent of White adults. Black (42%) and Hispanic (41%) adults saw drug addiction as a major problem in their area; White adults (34%) and an even smaller share of Asian American adults (20%) said the same. Black adults are more likely than their White and Hispanic counterparts to see drug addiction, crime, and racism as major community problems. In urban areas, the issues included in the survey tend to be seen as more of a problem than in other community types.

There is evidence that community violence increased during the pandemic. A Centers for Disease Control and Prevention report issued May 10, 2022, indicated that gun-related homicides surged by 35 percent during the first year of the pandemic. In a *New York Times* article, Rabin and Arango (2022) reported that gun-related deaths surged during the pandemic. They noted that national statistics and experts have concluded that gun-related death rates have been the highest ever recorded and had the most significant percentage increase over the first year of the pandemic. Low-income communities and Black Americans experienced the most significant increases in gun-related death rates. Most of the rise occurred for Black males. Experts attribute the trend to increased firearm purchases following the election, lockdowns, and social isolation due to the pandemic.

COVID-19 AND RACE

Evidence indicates that people of color, minorities, and migrants have higher rates of COVID-19 infection than White upper- and middle-class Americans. Some vulnerable minority communities have experienced a more rapid spread of COVID-19 and corresponding death rates (Best 2021; Maestripieri 2021). Best (2021:10–11) summarized, "According to the most recent CDC estimates, Black communities experience higher infection, hospitalization, and death rates than their White counterparts." There are a variety of reasons why this would be the case. Joseph (2021:8) wrote:

> Typically, administrative burdens are the most burdensome for those who are elderly, lower income, people of color, immigrants, lack access to computers and computer literacy, and have limited English proficiency. For individuals

> who fit in intersecting categories, inability to navigate the system puts them at even more of a structural disadvantage. When you add these burdens to systemic racism, a distrust of the medical system, and concerns about detention/deportation, communities of color—citizens and immigrants—continue to be left behind despite being the hardest hit by the pandemic.

Several studies have reported that the pandemic has devastatingly impacted Black and Latinx Americans (Masters et al. 2022). According to a Brookings Institution report, since the pandemic, Black and Latinx Americans have seen 2.9- and 3-year declines, respectively, in their life expectancies due mostly to COVID-19 deaths (Barr and Shiro 2022). The disproportionate impact on these two groups can be attributed to limited access to health care and insurance, environmental exposure to unhealthy conditions, such as poor water quality, food insecurity, and lack of nutritional food. Latinx populations are 3 times and Blacks are 1.7 times less likely than White Americans to have health insurance. According to Barr and Shiro (2022), among 25 socioeconomic groups, the lowest vaccination rates were for uninsured individuals.

In addition, Black and Latinx Americans were more likely to live in zones where air quality was poor. COVID-19 is a respiratory virus. Barr and Shiro cite research reporting a correlation between air pollution and COVID-19. Finally, one in ten American families had food insecurity before the pandemic. Food insecurity increased during the pandemic. This is exacerbated by the observation that factors affect the health information accessible to minorities. This point was made by Ferreira, José Sá, Martins, and Serpa (2020:3) with their observation, "The manipulation of information, poor content quality and difficulties in accessing communication and information technologies affect individuals with fewer resources and enhance illiteracy, making them more likely to ignore the health warnings developed by the governments."

There has always been a class system regarding health care in the United States. Medical research on COVID-19 has shown that minorities, compared to Whites, have worse outcomes resulting from COVID-19 infections. Considerable research has found that certain groups, such as those with pre-existing conditions, ethnic and racial minorities, and older adults, have a higher risk of infections and fatalities. The shortage of medical treatments, such as intensive care unit beds, vaccines, ventilators, and drugs (such as sotrovimab), has forced medical personnel to prioritize (triage) treatments by developing guidelines (risk calculators). Some of these calculators include minority status and age. This practice has led to legal challenges and politicization of access to health care (see Richmond 2022).

Research has found that socioeconomic status and race are associated with levels of trust in social institutions, such as the healthcare system (see chapter 5). Racial and ethnic minorities have historical and contemporary experiences of discrimination in healthcare, leading to distrust. Commentators often point to the Tuskegee syphilis experiments that exploited Black men as a prime example of why the healthcare system is seen as untrustworthy. Van Bavel, Baicker, Boggio, et al. (2021:463) summarized, "Members of these communities may be more likely to be wary about the public health information they receive, less willing to adopt recommended safety measures and potentially more susceptible to 'fake news.'"

Another racial and ethnic dimension to the pandemic is how fear of COVID-19 has generated racist and ethnocentric behaviors and attitudes toward minority groups. Race and ethnic group membership in the United States have always mattered regarding health care, and COVID-19 is no exception. Van Bavel, Baicker, Boggio, et al. (2021:462) believed that how people experienced fear and threat, in the case of COVID-19, has ramifications on how people felt and reacted to others, especially out-groups. They noted that being threatened with disease (COVID-19) is frequently associated with higher levels of ethnocentrism, intolerance, and negative attitudes towards out-groups, such as immigrants, ethnic and racial minorities, and foreigners. During the pandemic, prejudice and discrimination became increasingly visible and common. Exploring this subject, the Pew Research Center conducted a study to better understand American experiences with racial and ethnic discrimination since the beginning of the COVID-19 pandemic. The center surveyed 9,654 randomly selected American adults from June 4 to 10, 2020. Almost all American adults had a chance of being included in the study.

The study found that most Asian Americans (58 percent) and 45 percent of Black Americans reported that people were more likely to express racist views toward their group since the coronavirus outbreak. In addition, Asian and Black Americans were more likely than other groups to report negative experiences since the pandemic's beginning (Ruiz et al. 2020). These experiences included discomfort, being subjected to jokes or slurs, and/or being threatened. Almost 40 percent indicated it was more common for people to express racist views about people who were Asian Americans than before the pandemic. This pattern was also found for Hispanic and Black Americans. Concern among Black adults varies considerably by age. About half of Black Americans younger than 50 (51%) worry about people being suspicious of them because of their race or ethnicity if they wear a mask or face covering; 30 percent of Black adults ages 50 and older said the same. This reflects an enduring American negative stereotype that young Black Americans tend to be criminals; hence, if they wear a mask in public, they may be contemplating criminal behavior. In contrast, some Black, Asian, and Latinx American adults reported getting support since the beginning of the pandemic.

Race and ethnicity surface regarding hospitalization rates among different American groups. Horowitz (2020) reviewed the Centers for Disease Control and Prevention data that shows Black Americans had higher hospitalization and death rates than other ethnic and racial groups. Although Black Americans represent about 13 percent of the population, according to the COVID Tracking Project, they were 24 percent of the COVID-19 deaths for which racial or ethnic information was available as of June 2, 2020 (Gramlich and Funk 2020). The reasons for this pattern are subject to debate and, according to Horowitz (2020), are divided along political party lines. Reasons include living in densely populated areas (cities), pre-existing health conditions, lack of access to adequate medical care, and public-facing (exposed) jobs. This list could add a lack of trust in government and healthcare providers due to a history of mistreatment of Blacks by White American–dominated healthcare and medicine. However, according to Kramer (2021), there is survey data that shows Protestant Black Americans who attend church regularly do have confidence in the guidance they receive from public health officials, such as those from the Centers for Disease Control and Prevention (CDC), or their primary care doctors (77 percent and 80 percent, respectively).

Political orientation matters in how people view higher Black American hospitalization rates for COVID-19 (Horowitz 2020). For example, most Democrats (73%) compared to Republicans (34%) are more likely to say higher hospitalization rates are due to circumstances beyond the control of Black Americans. Most Republicans (64%) say the higher rates are due to people's choices and lifestyles. It is important to note that some members of Black and Hispanic communities resist vaccinations for practical reasons such as it will cost them money (52%), they cannot get time off from work, or they will lose work time because of vaccine side effects (Attwell 2021). In the realm of conspiracy theories, a small group (6%) of people believe the COVID-19 vaccines were designed to control the size of the Black and Hispanic communities. At the same time, 13 percent are unsure, and 81 percent say this is false (Annenberg Public Policy Center 2021a).

Finally, the global pandemic may also create opportunities to reduce religious and ethnic prejudice and discrimination. Crises and disasters sometimes bring out the better sides of people. In many communities, volunteers, medical staff, neighbors, and individuals helped others, regardless of ethnicity, race, age, or gender, to address COVID-19 and general issues. As Van Bavel, Baicker, Boggio, et al. (2021:462) noted, "Coordinated efforts across individuals, communities, and governments to fight the spread of disease can send strong signals of cooperation and shared values, which could facilitate the reorganization of previously considered out-groups and in-groups into a single community with a common destiny."

COVID-19 AND OLD AGE

The pandemic has played out differently for people depending on their age. The adverse medical and health consequences of COVID-19 infections for older people are well established. Older people had the highest vulnerability to infection and death rates from COVID-19. In addition, one of the earliest outbreaks with increased fatalities was in a nursing home in Washington. In comparison, the young have experienced COVID-19 differently than older people in terms of having fewer serious infections and lower fatality rates.

The COVID-19 pandemic shaped the way society characterizes older people. A study by Ng and Indran (2021) reviewed a 12-billion-word news media database of 30 million news articles referencing older people. They found that during the pandemic, older adults' negative age-based stereotyping (framing) increased seven times compared to the familial frame. Before the pandemic, positive topics represented about 61 percent of the subjects but only 35 percent during the pandemic. Ng and Indran concluded that the negative stereotyping of older people during the pandemic was linked to their being portrayed as more susceptible to COVID-19 and the virus being mostly an old person problem. Ng and Indran (2021:64) wrote, "Since the outbreak, older adults have been framed continually in public discourse as a monolithic group of frail, helpless, and vulnerable individuals." In addition, older people were portrayed as a burden to society because they were the most likely to get seriously ill or die from COVID-19.

CONCLUDING OBSERVATIONS

The COVID-19 pandemic has altered almost every aspect of social life, and some contend that it will never return to "normal." Loved ones have been lost, people have experienced serious bouts with the virus requiring intensive medical care, economies have been hampered and damaged, relationships strained, and so on. Americans rediscovered that socioeconomic status and race matter in how the COVID-19 pandemic has been experienced. Socioeconomic status matters when accessing health care, the workplace, unemployment, and resources needed to cope with COVID-19 and daily living. Some experts have concluded that less obvious collateral damage occurred to health and education during the pandemic (for a discussion, see Masroor 2020; Neal 2020). The overall cost of the pandemic has been enormous and continues. Cutler and Summers (2020) estimated that by the summer of 2021, the pandemic had cost an estimated 16 trillion dollars. They estimated the lost gross domestic product, health losses from premature deaths, and long-term health and mental impairments. They likened the COVID-19 pandemic's adverse economic impact to the Great Depression. This estimate undoubtedly has grown as the pandemic continues and evolves.

Despite numerous negative consequences previously highlighted that have resulted from the pandemic, there have been a few positive developments. One has been a reduction in fossil fuel use and consequently slowing down the rate of global warming. With reduced travel, air pollution has been reduced. Families have spent more time together. COVID-19 is now not at the forefront of society, and most people do not obsess over it in daily life, as they did when the pandemic was at its height. Our bodies can generally fend off the disease better due to effective vaccines and enhanced immunity. Communities have come together to take care of the vulnerable. Rapid advances in medicine and research have occurred that will help in future pandemics. Awareness and responses to mental health issues have increased (see Pescosolido and Lee 2021).

The COVID-19 pandemic is an example of what can be expected. A pattern of disease pandemics has occurred in recent decades and is likely to continue with globalization and population growth. For example, the world experienced Influenza H5N1 in 1997 and 2005, SARS in 2003, H1N1 in 2009, MERS in 2012, the Ebola epidemic since 2014, and COVID-19. With COVID-19, only some existing norms apply. The virus, what we know about it, people's understanding, and their responses all change over time. COVID-19 is a moving target with more changes predicted in the future.

Chapter 3

A Brief History of Pandemics and Vaccines

"It was about the beginning of September 1664, that I,
among the Rest of my Neighbours,
heard in ordinary Discourse that the Plague was but again in Holland;
for it had been very violent there,
and particularly at Amsterdam and Roterdam, in the Year 1663,
whither they say, it was brought, some said from Italy,
others from the Levant among some Goods,
which were brought home by their Turkey fleet;
others said it was brought from Canada;
others from Cyprus. It mattered not, from whence it come;
However, all agreed, it was come into Holland again."

Daniel Defoe, *A Journal of the Plague Year* (1722:1)

OVERVIEW OF SELECTED PANDEMICS

Viruses like COVID-19 have shaped and continue to shape human societies (Delanty 2021b:2; Kolbert 2020). Viruses have decimated military forces, killed millions, changed the class structure of medieval Europe, and shaped the outcomes of wars. Viral pandemics have disrupted trade, facilitated the European conquest of the New World, suppressed world exploration, and played havoc on societies and cultures. Viral pandemics continue to destabilize and reduce populations in contemporary times. While some viruses only lead to small outbreaks and epidemics, others become major pandemics and spread over large regions. Some of the major pandemics and plagues in history include the multiple waves of the Black Plague, smallpox, the 1918 influenza virus, seasonal influenza, poliomyelitis, measles, and yellow fever. In addition, West Nile, Human Immunodeficiency Virus (HIV) or AIDS, Ebola, Severe Acute Respiratory Syndrome (SARS), and Middle East Respiratory Syndrome (MERS) have occurred. Now COVID-19 can be added to this list.

To help frame the social aspects of the COVID-19 pandemic, it is helpful to briefly review how societies have dealt with pandemics. While the circumstances of these pandemics and plagues differ, it is possible to identify similar patterns of social responses. As expected, collective responses to pandemics are determined by time and place. Collective beliefs, values, norms, institutions, direct experiences, and medical knowledge influenced how societies interpreted, understood, and responded to pandemics. For example, Perlstadt (2016) used a collective behavior approach to analyze the 430–426 BCE plague of Athens and the Cult of Asclepius. This plague, likely typhoid fever, was a little understood and unusual event in the lives of the ancient Athenians. Perlstadt shared the Athenian historian Thucydides's account of the plague. Thucydides identified escalating phases of collective behavior in his description of the plague that included "rumor, panic, despair, not observing rituals, and general lawlessness" (Perlstadt 2016:1048). In response to the plague and the inability to effectively address it, a new belief system arose that Athenians referred to as the Cult of Asclepius. The Cult of Asclepius was a reformative social movement leading to new, meaningful, and lasting reforms to Athenian medical practices and religious beliefs.

Table 3.1 lists some of the most significant pandemics and the estimated number of resulting fatalities. A few selected pandemics and plagues, such as the Black Plague, smallpox, 1918 influenza, polio, measles, and Human Immunodeficiency Virus (HIV), will be reviewed in detail later, setting a historical foundation for understanding collective behavior and COVID-19.

A BRIEF NOTE ON THE HISTORY OF VACCINATIONS

The practice of immunizing people against disease dates back many centuries. Before hypodermic needles were invented, medical practitioners used variolation to immunize people. For example, evidence exists that as early as 1000 CE, the Chinese used variolation (inoculation) to prevent smallpox. Variolation is the practice of introducing live viruses to a person by smearing a sample of a virus or similar virus into an open skin cut. By doing so, the variolation was thought to give the individual a less severe infection so that their body could fight it and become immune. Variolation was practiced in China, Africa, and Turkey well before the practice spread to Europe and the Americas.

Table 3.1. Selected Worldwide Common Era Pandemics

Major Epidemics, Pandemics, and Plagues	*Estimated Fatalities*
Black Death (Second Plague) 1347–1351	200 million
Smallpox 1520	56 million
Spanish Flu 1918–1919	40–50 million
Plague of Justinian 541–542	30–50 million
HIV/AIDS 1981–Present	25–35 million
Columbian Exchange Epidemics (Smallpox and other diseases) 1492–1550	20 million or 80–90% of indigenous populations in the Americas
The Third Plague 1855	12 million
Coronavirus (COVID-19) 2019	5.78 million (USA 900 thousand)
Antonine Plague 165–190	5 million
17th-Century Great Plagues 1645	3 million
Asian Flu/H2N2 1957–1958	1.1 million
Russian Flu 1889–1890	1 million
Hong Kong Flu 1968–1970	1 million
Cholera Outbreak 1917–1923	1 million
Japanese Smallpox Epidemic 735–737	1 million
19th-Century Great Plagues 1817–1923	600 thousand
Swine Flu 2009–2010	200 thousand
Yellow Fever late 1800s	100–150 thousand
MERS 2019–Present	850 thousand
SARS 2002–2003	770 thousand
Ebola 2014–2016 (outbreaks)	11.3 thousand

Source: Cartwright, Mark. 2020. "Black Death." *World History Encyclopedia,* last modified March 28, 2020. Accessed at: https://www.worldhistory.org/Black_Death/.

In 1796, Dr. Edward Jenner was considered the founder of vaccinology when he inoculated a boy with cowpox to prevent smallpox. Two years later, a smallpox vaccine would be developed. Before his work, variolation using live smallpox virus had been used in Asia, Africa, Europe, and the American colonies to prevent more serious cases of smallpox. In 1853, the British parliament passed the Vaccination Act that made infant smallpox vaccinations mandatory. This mandate would generate controversy and opposition, although the smallpox vaccine had major benefits for humans compared to the years before it was introduced (John 2020). Isaacs (2021) noted that in 1885, over 80,000 vaccine dissenters paraded through Leicester, England, carrying banners, a child's coffin, and an effigy of Dr. Jenner. Similar opposition developed in the United States and Canada.

Other vaccines for different diseases would be developed. In France, Louis Pasteur led the development of vaccines for rabies (1885), cholera (1897), and anthrax (1904). In Germany, Robert Koch's research in infectious diseases was critical to understanding diseases. In 1923 Alexander Glenny's work led to the development of a vaccine for diphtheria. A vaccine for pertussis, a killer of infant children, would be developed in 1948. Over the years between 1950 and 1985, Dr. Albert Sabin (live attenuated oral) and Dr. Jonas Salk (inactivated) developed polio vaccines.

All vaccines, whether for shingles, pneumonia, chicken pox, tetanus, measles, influenza, whooping cough, or other diseases, vary in effectiveness. Some, like tetanus and chicken pox (shingles later in life), require periodic boosters. On the other hand, some vaccines, such as for polio and smallpox, are 100 percent effective for the life of the vaccinated. With COVID-19, periodic boosters have been necessary because antibodies generated by COVID-19 vaccines' effectiveness decline over time, and new COVID-19 variants and subvariants are evolving. This latter fact will require modifications to existing and new vaccines.

The past two decades have seen the application of molecular genetics and its increased insights into immunology, microbiology, and genomics applied to vaccinology. As a result, vaccines for hepatitis B, seasonal influenzas, and others have been created. Current successes include the development of recombinant hepatitis B vaccines, the pertussis vaccine, and new techniques for seasonal influenza vaccine manufacturing. In addition, medical researchers used molecular genetics to engineer COVID-19 vaccines.

THE BLACK PLAGUE

The Black Plague killed an estimated 200 million people from 1347 to 1352. The disease is often referred to as simply the plague. Historically, there have been multiple Black Plagues. The disease is caused by a bacillus bacterium (*Yersinia pestis*) transmitted by fleas hosted and carried by rodents. Recent research has also identified fleas and lice in human clothing and bedding as transmitting the disease. Specifically, clothing and bedding of plague victims that contained infected lice and fleas would not be discarded but recycled for use by others. Therefore, these items facilitated the spread of the disease to humans.

The plague's origin has been traced to Central Asia to infected rats that traveled to Genoa, Italy, via trading ships. From there, the disease spread throughout Europe along trade routes. There are three basic types of the plague, bubonic (lymph nodes), pneumonic (pulmonary), and septicemic (bloodstream). Each was present at roughly the same time. Although each has different symptoms, they were lumped together as the Black Death or Plague. The bubonic plague was the most common form during the 14th century. Bubonic plague causes swelling of the groin and armpits (lymph nodes). The 14th-century pandemic was labeled the Black Plague because infected individuals would develop black sores (buboes) on the skin. Called buboes, the swelling looked like black bumps and hence the name. Those individuals suffering from the disease ran high fevers, vomited, were dehydrated, and had respiratory failure, joint pains, and other debilitating physiological effects. Mortality rates ranged from 30 to 75 percent of infected cases. Death was quick and often occurred within 72 hours. The other two types of plague are usually fatal in all cases.

Medieval citizens sought explanations for what caused the plague and speculated that putrid air, decaying bodies, swamps, or excrement were the source of the disease. Many attributed the plague to supernatural forces, namely God or the gods. Some people believed that God was punishing society for sinful behaviors. Others attached the disease to the work of the devil. Earlier in history, some thought it was caused by supernatural phenomena, such as a 345 CE visible comet. Others thought astrological alignments were linked to the disease. In some regions, marginalized groups, such as Jewish people, people with disabilities, Roma, and "outsiders," were identified as the source of the disease. The bubonic plague unleashed massive violence in Europe, including the murder of Catalans in Sicily, and clerics and beggars in some regions, and the persecution of Jews (Cohn 2012). Jewish people were massacred or forced to flee some regions. It is common for pandemics to have scapegoats, who are often marginalized groups.

Medieval society and physicians had no concept of microscopic organisms like bacteria and viruses. Thus, physicians were helpless to treat plague patients. Physicians tried unsuccessful treatments, such as bloodletting, fumigation, and consuming modified vinegar, potions, and pastes. The only defense was to escape to the country and isolate themselves, which those with the resources did. However, these migrations unknowingly spread the disease to the countryside. Mark (2020b) noted that the only effective way to slow the spread of the disease was to quarantine the sick, similar to today's COVID-19 practices. Quarantine was developed in the 14th century when ships were required to isolate for 30 days to ensure they were not plague-ridden. This later was expanded to 40 days, hence the term "quarantine" (Mark 2020b). Praying for protection or relying on amulets were other responses. In addition, charitable organizations, many church based, arose to treat the sick. Eventually, the plague ran its course, as rats and human populations died off. Improved sanitation also helped slow the disease.

There would be other outbreaks over the years but none of the magnitude of the 14th-century plague. In 1894, the bacterium *Yersinia pestis* was isolated and identified as the cause of the Black Plague. During the same year, Waldemar Haffkine developed the first vaccine for bubonic plague. Before the development of this vaccine, some of the treatments for and responses to the Black Plague included:

- Animal cures
- Potions, fumigations, bloodletting, and pastes
- Flight from infected cities to rural areas
- Persecution of marginalized communities
- Religious cures, such as prayers and sacred amulets (charms)
- Quarantine and social distancing

The socioeconomic consequences of the Black Plague were significant for medieval Europe. The plague accelerated the social changes ending the medieval feudal society. High mortality rates among the peasantry resulted in a scarcity of manual labor. Some cities and rural areas were devastated, but others seemed relatively untouched. Widowed women gained some property rights depending on where they lived. A shortage of farmers, abandonment of towns, peasant rebellions, and questioning of authority fueled the demise of serfdom. People challenged governmental and church authority, as both had little impact on the spread of the disease.

Over the centuries, the plague would come in waves across Europe. Following the surge in the 1660s, the English author Daniel Defoe (1722) wrote about the 1665 London plague. Although a fictional account, the book *A Journal of the Plague Year* contains many historical facts that provide insights into how Londoners responded to the bubonic plague of 1665. People did not know what caused the plague but took precautions beyond praying. According to Defoe, Londoners kept certain animals out of city limits, killed suspected animals, lit bonfires at night, sequestered the infected, aired out things known to have been used by plague victims, painted red crosses on doors of infected households, and shut down gaming tables, public dancing rooms, puppet shows, and other businesses (Defoe 1722:31). The Lord Mayor of London also implemented numerous restrictions regarding guards, nurse-keepers, notices of sickness, and burial of the dead. Defoe also wrote of alternative treatments, which he tied to quackery, foolery, and profiteering. Some of these responses, such as shutting down businesses, quarantining, quackery, and cleaning areas, sound remarkably similar to the COVID-19 pandemic.

When thinking about the Black Plague, most people associate it with the Middle Ages and Europe and Asia. However, the Black Plague also surfaced in Hawaii and San Francisco in the late 19th and early 20th centuries. The plague had an outbreak in 1898 in Honolulu and eventually found its way to the major port of San Francisco. In Honolulu, authorities targeted Asian neighborhoods and blamed residents for what White residents viewed as an Asian problem that needed controlling through isolation and other restrictions. White Americans burned Asian communities and buildings, forcing the evacuation of residents, resulting in their becoming homeless. At the time, little was understood about the real cause of the plague, and theories about miasma (bad air) had survived from the Middle Ages. Racism was rampant in Hawaii and later San Francisco, as some referred to the plague as the "rice eaters disease." The United States had a long history of racism against Asian Americans and had, in 1882, passed the Chinese Exclusion Act that barred Chinese Americans from the benefits of US citizenship. The plague did little to improve race relations.

In 1900, San Francisco had its first known fatality due to the Black Plague (Randall 2019). To address the Black Plague, city officials walled off the Chinatown section of the city. An eight-foot-tall wall and barbed wire were used to quarantine Chinese American residents. As expected, there would be pushback from the Chinese American community. In addition, efforts were made to clean up areas of the city and eliminate rats suspected of transmitting the disease, although no one knew how. It would be later discovered that infected fleas transmitted the disease to humans.

Butler (2022) highlighted some American social reactions to the Black Plague. She noted that local newspapers and businesses were concerned that acknowledging the presence of the Black Plague would hamper and disrupt the local economy. Public health officials implemented measures, such as a quarantine of Chinatown, to control the spread of the disease. However, the press questioned the motives of public health officials and accused them of simply wanting more funding. Butler shared a *San Francisco Call* newspaper headline stating, "Plague Fake is Part of a Plot to Plunder." Evidence of political pressure surfaced when the mayor and Board of Health soon lifted the Chinatown quarantine. Other deaths due to the plague would soon surface but were either kept from the general public or considered misdiagnoses. Public opinion would not change.

Important summary observations about the Black Plague include:

- It created great social strain, fear, social and political disruption, depression, and personal loss. It "fueled" social unrest (Turner 2021:139).
- Some people isolated themselves from social contact, and others moved to the countryside. Social distancing was invented in response to the Black Plague (see Turner 2021).
- The storage and burial of corpses exceeded system capacity.
- It was transmitted through trade routes.
- It was destructive to the medieval economy and political structures.
- It created labor shortages (Delanty 2021a).
- People attempted desperate cures, such as the Vicary Method of attaching a live chicken's shaved buttocks to infected swollen lymph nodes. Then, when the chicken displayed signs of illness, it was believed it was drawing the disease from the body.

- Prejudice and discrimination surfaced as minority groups were blamed for causing the disease. For example, early Christians were blamed for causing and spreading the plague during Roman times, and during the Middle Ages, Jews were blamed throughout Europe. Scapegoating the Jews for the disease is similar to blaming Asians or Middle Eastern peoples (Mark 2020c). In the United States, Asian Americans were blamed for the disease.
- Some people prayed for cures and treatment.
- Some citizens were reluctant to comply with quarantine restrictions, which could last 40 days.
- Altruistic caregivers were present and took personal risks to help the infected.
- Some medieval cities implemented pest houses outside city walls where plague victims were housed and the infected could be cared for (similar to isolating patients in separate care units).
- Physicians used face coverings when treating patients, although they did so to reduce odors associated with the infection or to prevent inhaling miasma (bad air) and thus prevent infection. In contemporary times, masks continued to be worn but were of little value when compared to public health sanitation measures.

Mark (2020b) noted that during the Middle Ages, quarantines and what is now known during the COVID-19 pandemic as "social distancing" had little effect on stopping the spread of the disease. He added that, unfortunately, people were reluctant to stay isolated or quarantined from the cities and ports during the waves of the Black Plague.

The Black Plague has two underlying characteristics in common with the COVID-19 pandemic. Both were characterized by failures of the populations to appreciate the seriousness of the disease until it was too late—also, failures of governments to respond to it on time. Before the recognition of germ theory, it is understandable that people would interpret the plague in terms of the prevailing religious ideology. However, in the modern era, the failure of governments and populations to respond quickly with practical measures remains bewildering (Mark 2020b). Other comparisons between the Black Plague and other pandemics have been made, such as HIV (Strong 1990).

SMALLPOX

In its time, smallpox was known as the most terrible of all the ministers of death. Likewise, it has been characterized as the greatest killer of human beings (Hopkins 2002). The origin of smallpox is as an infectious disease caused by one of two virus variants, Variola major and Variola minor. Variola major kills one out of three people who become infected. Variola minor kills about 1 in 100 infected people. Its origin is unknown, but experts agree it has been infecting human populations for thousands of years (CDC 2021c). The early symptoms of the disease are usually a high fever and vomiting. As the disease progresses, severe and painful rashes and ulcers appear all over the body. The rashes swell with fluid, forming blisters that eventually open, leaving scars. Those surviving may be blinded and are left seriously scarred. The disease is spread through contact with infected individuals or from contaminated objects. Historically, trade routes, wars, and colonization have spread the disease.

Roughly 30 percent of individuals infected will die, with children having higher mortality rates. It is estimated (see Table 3.1) that approximately 56 million people died from smallpox in the 1520 pandemic. Smallpox was an epidemic disease in the American colonies. It had a devastating impact on Native American groups, essentially wiping out some tribes. In the past, some cultures, such as in South and Central America, had much higher mortality rates due to a lack of immunity to the disease when Europeans introduced it. "Smallpox alone, in the 20th century, killed an estimated 300 million individuals, about three-fold as many people as all the wars of that century" (Oldstone 2020:5).

Before variolation and inoculations, those people with smallpox were separated from others and quarantined to limit their social contacts. Similar to the Black Plague, some people fled from known areas of infection to avoid contact with the ill. The Chinese are believed to have developed the first effective treatment for the disease in the 1500s via inoculation (Needham 2000). There is also evidence that other parts of the world, such as Africa, the Middle East, and India, at least in folk medicine, had relied on this practice for centuries (McNeill 1975). Inoculation (variolation) was a method in which pus from an infected person's smallpox sores (pustules) was applied to an open scratch or skin cut, or inhaled through the nose. After variolation, people usually develop the symptoms associated with smallpox, such as a fever and a rash. The hope was that the infection would be a milder form of smallpox. Milder cases were often the rule, but a small percentage of people died from the disease following inoculation. After intentional smallpox exposure, fewer people died from smallpox than those naturally infected.

Knowledge of the benefits of inoculation found its way to Europe and the American colonies in the early 18th century. The eradication of smallpox faced resistance 200 years ago (Oldstone 2020:37). Conis (2015) observed that as news of the new procedure spread, it was met with mixed reactions of dread and enthusiasm. Some people were open and excited to prevent one of the most terrifying diseases. However, others thought exposing their healthy bodies to disease matter from infected people or animals (cowpox) was repulsive. The British were less resistant to accepting inoculations for smallpox than people on the Continent, where the practice was limited by religious views (McNeill 1976).

Some colonial Americans believed that inoculations interfered with God's will and represented a wanton spreading of the disease. However, the religious leader Cotton Mather and his associates inoculated people amid great controversy in 1721. Mather is credited as being the first to introduce inoculation for smallpox in the colonies during an outbreak of the disease in 1721. It is generally believed he learned about inoculation (variolation) from his West African enslaved servant Onesimus and wrote, "He told me that he had undergone the operation which had given something of smallpox and would forever preserve him from it, adding that was often used in West Africa" (Niederhuber 2014:1).

With an outbreak of smallpox raging through Boston, Mather approached the medical community with the idea of inoculation and immediately faced hostile resistance. Only one doctor, Doctor Boylston, openly supported Mather's efforts. Arguments against inoculation included that it ran contrary to established medical practices, such as purging and bleeding, and it was based on folklore (African and not European). In addition, people believed it harmed innocent people, violated God's will, and the practice would spread the disease even faster. However, data collected by Dr. Boylston and Mather supported the procedure's effectiveness. Nevertheless, emotions ran high. Niederhuber (2014:1) described some of the high emotions at the time:

> On a November day in 1721, a small bomb was hurled through the window of a local Boston Reverend named Cotton Mather. Attached to the explosive, which fortunately did not detonate, was the message: "Cotton Mather, you dog, dam you! I'll inoculate you with this; with a pox to you." This was not a religiously motivated act of terrorism but a violent response to Reverend Mather's active promotion of smallpox inoculation. The smallpox epidemic that struck Boston in 1721 was one of the deadliest of the century in colonial America but was also the catalyst for the first major application of preventative inoculation in the colonies. The use of inoculation laid the foundation for the modern techniques of infectious diseases prevention, and the contentious public debate that accompanied the introduction of this poorly understood medical technology has surprising similarities to contemporary misunderstandings over vaccination.

Eventually, inoculation became increasingly accepted, and Mather was proven right.

The history of the development of the smallpox vaccination is important to what would follow. In 1768, Thomas Dimsdale treated the Russian empress Catherine the Great, her son, and the court. Unfortunately, in some cases, these inoculations caused fatal infections or failed to provide protection. Some of the inoculated individuals spread the disease to others. Nevertheless, others would inoculate themselves to protect themselves from the disease.

A few years later, General George Washington recognized the value of inoculation. Acknowledging that smallpox infections could destroy an army, in 1776, he ordered (mandated) the inoculation of all of the soldiers (McNeill 1975). At the time, many medical community members resisted inoculation and relied on traditional medicine based on outdated assumptions. Humoral treatments, such as purging and bleeding, dominated medical thinking.

Real progress in smallpox inoculation would occur in England at the end of the 18th century. It was common knowledge in parts of England that milkmaids who caught cowpox never contracted smallpox. In addition, it was known that an English farmer inoculated his wife and children with pus from a cowpox pustule, and none of them caught smallpox. Word of mouth of this incident spread across the countryside and eventually reached the physician Dr. Edward Jenner. Dr. Jenner studied and experimented with cowpox inoculations and announced his findings in 1798. Jenner faced immediate opposition to his inoculation of patients with the cowpox virus. Oldstone (2020:64) wrote, "Opponents argued that vaccination was a revolting practice, that to infect a healthy person with repugnant material from an animal was an outrage, that vaccinated victims sprouted horns and looked like cows, and that one was interfering with God's way since vaccination was not mentioned in the Bible." Oldstone added, "This opposition was mounted by those in the medical and business professions and religious leaders." Nevertheless, the practice of inoculation for smallpox by using the cowpox virus grew.

In 1966, the World Health Organization embarked on a 10-year worldwide smallpox vaccination campaign that faced acceptance and resistance in parts of the world. In some regions, members of the vaccination teams were killed, held captive, or injured by vaccination-resistant groups. However, by 1979, authorities declared that the smallpox disease had been eradicated. However, when weaponized, smallpox is a weapon of choice for biological warfare because most people born after 1971 have not been vaccinated against smallpox. The threat of biological warfare using smallpox as a weapon in 2001 motivated the federal government to require select American workers in healthcare, government officials, the military, and emergency services to get vaccinated.

Oldstone (2020:75) described how some of the designated workers, especially healthcare workers, resisted smallpox vaccinations using the following arguments:

> First, about 20% of the population cannot be vaccinated because disease or medication, eczema, other skin lesions, or pregnancy compromises their immune

> systems. This group also includes young children and a large population who take medication that suppresses the immune system. Second, general apathy has accompanied the decreased urgency to vaccinate, that is, the philosophy of "it is not likely to happen to me." Third, conservative or libertarian opposition says that vaccination should be a self-choice and not one of a general public health concern, in line with suspicion of government dictums. Fourth, the unlikely possibility remains that vaccines may be contaminated or expose recipients to secondary bacterial infections. Fifth, economics do not favor vaccine production.

To this list could be added potential side effects from vaccination, which occur in one in a thousand cases and deaths in one in a million (Oldstone 2020:76). However, these are small risks compared to the horrors of smallpox.

Smallpox summary observations include:

- Public resistance (much more pronounced) to smallpox inoculations was similar to opposition to COVID-19 vaccinations.
- Smallpox devastated the economy and social structures, and it became a pandemic.
- Established medical institutions resisted and relied on traditional medical approaches that sometimes made patients worse, had no benefit, or helped spread the disease.
- Smallpox during the Roman Empire was blamed on Christians, who were subsequently persecuted.
- Some religious groups resisted vaccinations and viewed smallpox as God's will. Similarly, contemporary religious groups, such as a Jewish sect in New York City and Christian Scientists, have resisted COVID-19 vaccinations on religious grounds.

The eradication of smallpox, except for some of the virus stored in two locations (Russia and the United States), can be attributed to a sustained worldwide effort to eliminate it, a one-dose effective vaccination, and the involvement of local health officials in its eradication.

1918 INFLUENZA (SPANISH FLU) PANDEMIC

The 1918 influenza pandemic, or the Great Influenza Epidemic, also known as the Spanish Flu (so-called because it was first openly reported by Spain, not because it was the source of the pandemic), was a deadly worldwide disease (Mark 2020b). The term "influenza" stems from the Italian word for influence and refers to the influence of the stars. It is estimated that as many as 500 million people worldwide were infected with the 1918 virus (Oldstone

2020). An estimated one-fifth of the world's human population was infected, and 2 to 3 percent died. Worldwide, it is estimated that between 50 and 100 million people died, and of these, an estimated 675,000 were Americans, making it one of the deadliest pandemics in history.

More people died during the 1918 flu pandemic than the total number of military and civilian deaths due to combat occurring during World War I. "Most, nearly 80 percent of US Army war casualties, were caused not by bullets, shells, or shrapnel but by influenza" (Oldstone 2020:361). Deaths from the epidemic of influenza virus over the years 1918–1919 outpaced WWI's by fourfold. Over this one year, an estimated 40 to 50 million people died from influenza compared to 9 to 11 million military (combat) deaths over four years of war. Worldwide, the 1918 pandemic killed more people than the combined WWI, WWII, Korean, and Vietnam wars. One estimate of the 1918 influenza pandemic using modern population numbers would result in a staggering 400 million deaths today (Loomis 2018:194). Three other major influenza pandemics in 1957, 1968, and 2009 were mild, with worldwide estimates of 1 to 1.5 million deaths (Oldstone 2020:356).

The 1918 pandemic differed significantly from all previous influenza pandemics and ones that followed because for the first time young and healthy adults quickly succumbed to the disease. In the past and subsequent influenza pandemics and epidemics, the very young and the elderly died (Oldstone 2020:356). Although the 1918 influenza pandemic arrived and disappeared in under two years, it enormously impacted social, health, political, military, and economic institutions. However, the 1918 influenza pandemic was seldom referenced in the following years.

Scientists and historians have concluded that the 1918 influenza virus most likely came from an army camp in southwest Kansas. It would quickly expand to other army bases, such as Fort Riley, Kansas, and eventually make it across the country and into Europe. During 1918, the United States was engaged in WWI and needed soldiers to go overseas, whether sick with the flu or not. Thousands of U.S. soldiers were deployed to Europe to fight in WWI. The U.S. military did not want to damage troop morale, so much information about the disease and its spread was suppressed. The transportation of large numbers of infected troops to the European front expanded the flu to other regions. Large gatherings of people for domestic events also spread the disease across the United States. Siegel (2020:169), referring to COVID-19 protests, observed, "Yesteryear's draft rallies and parades, which spread the dreadful flu during WWI, were today's protest in large gatherings."

The 1918 flu pandemic came in four waves, the first in 1918 and the fourth in 1920. Most infected experienced sore throats, headaches, and fevers in the first wave. The first wave was relatively mild compared to later waves. The second, third, and fourth waves were more serious and frequently complicated by pneumonia, a significant cause of death. The CDC concluded that the 1918 pandemic was caused by an H1N1 virus of avian origin (Robinson 2021). The following is a summary timeline of the 1918 influenza pandemic.

CENTERS FOR DISEASE CONTROL AND PREVENTION 1918 INFLUENZA PANDEMIC HISTORIC TIMELINE (EXCERPTS)

- April 1917 - U.S. enters World War I with 378,000 personnel in the armed services.
- March 1918 - More than 100 soldiers at Camp Funston in Fort Riley, Kansas, become ill with flu. Within a week, the number of flu cases quintuples.
- May 1918 - Hundreds of thousands of soldiers travel across the United States and the Atlantic Ocean each month as they are deployed for World War I.
- September 1918 - The second wave of flu emerged at Camp Devens, a United States Army training camp just outside of Boston and at a naval facility in the area. A second wave of flu peaks in the United States between September and November. This second wave is highly fatal and responsible for most of the deaths attributed to the pandemic.
- October 1918 - The 1918 flu pandemic virus killed an estimated 195,000 Americans during October alone. In the fall of 1918, the United States experienced a severe shortage of professional nurses because of the deployment of large numbers of nurses to military camps in the United States and abroad and the failure to use trained African American nurses. The Centers for Disease Control and Prevention (2018b:n.p.) noted, "The Chicago chapter of the American Red Cross issues an urgent call for volunteers to help nurse the ill. Philadelphia is hit hard with the pandemic flu viruses—more than 500 corpses await burial, some for more than a week." Overwhelmed, officials use cold-storage plants as temporary morgues and a manufacturer of trolley cars donates 200 packing crates for use as coffins. Chicago and many other cities across the United States closed theaters, movie houses, and night schools and prohibited public gatherings. San Francisco's Board of Health requires any person serving in public spaces to wear masks and issues a strong recommendation to all residents to wear masks. New York City reports a 40 percent decline in shipyard productivity due to flu illnesses amid World War I.
- November 1918 - The end of World War I enabled a resurgence of influenza as people celebrated Armistice Day and soldiers began to

demobilize. Salt Lake City officials place quarantine signs on the front and rear doors of 2,000 homes where occupants have been struck with the flu.

- December 1918 - Public health officials begin education programs and publicity about the dangers of coughing and sneezing; and the careless disposal of "nasal discharges." A Committee of the American Public Health Association encourages stores and factories to stagger opening and closing hours and for people to walk to work when possible instead of using public transport to prevent overcrowding.
- January 1919 - A third wave of influenza occurs in the winter and spring of 1919, killing many more. This third wave subsides in the summer. However, many San Antonio citizens have begun complaining that new flu cases are not being reported, fueling another influenza surge. Seven hundred and six cases of influenza and 67 deaths are reported in New York City, triggering fear of a recurrence of severe flu activity.
- February 1919 - Influenza appears to be nearly eradicated in New Orleans as the number of reported cases drops. Illinois passed a bill to create a one-year course to become a "practical nurse" to address the nursing shortage the pandemic had exposed.

Source: Modified from a Centers for Disease Control and Prevention 2018 article, "1918 Pandemic Influenza Historic Timeline."

During the 1918 pandemic, Americans and public health agencies acknowledged the effectiveness of quarantines (Mark 2020b). Despite mixed messages and directives from officials, general compliance with severe restrictions was generally excellent, as most people thought it helped the WWI war effort. In addition, there was greater acceptance of governmental intervention in private lives. Furthermore, many people had the firsthand experience of losing a family member or friend to influenza, thus, were open to cooperating with public health directives. However, compliance with quarantines, mask-wearing, and other measures was only sometimes followed. For example, Oldstone (2020:366) cited the examples of the cities of Philadelphia and Saint Louis:

> Philadelphia allowed public gatherings, open schools, churches, and assemblies. Local authorities hosted a grand citywide parade in support of a WWI loan bond drive. Over 12,000 Philadelphians died from the infection within four months of that gathering. In contrast, physicians in St. Louis persuaded city officials to register influenza cases two days after the first illness was detected. The city government shut down schools, churches, theaters, and public gathering places, then initiated strict quarantines with infected persons confined to their homes. Compared to Philadelphia, St. Louis had half as many cases.

In Saint Louis, public health authorities implemented lockdowns and social distancing, which reduced the number of influenza cases and death rates compared to other cities not having similar practices. However, this all changed, and when Saint Louis lifted restrictions, influenza cases soon skyrocketed. The pattern of the timing of implementation and stoppage of restrictions would have similar ramifications for other American cities (for a discussion, see Loomis 2018:200–201).

Some precautions for the 1918 influenza pandemic were unique for the time, and others are similar to COVID-19 measures. For example, the following United States Navy guidance, titled "Precautions Against Influenza," sheds light on the public health thinking during the 1918 pandemic (see Angeny n.d.) (numbers added):

1. Influenza is spread through discharge from the eyes, nose, and mouth. Therefore, avoid persons with coughs and colds.
2. If obliged to cough or sneeze yourself, when near another person, turn the face or cover the mouth and nose with a handkerchief: such handkerchief should afterward be sterilized by boiling or destroyed.
3. Avoid standard drinking cups.
4. Do not expectorate promiscuously.
5. Do not stand close to others while conversing or talking directly to them.
6. Discharges from the mouth are disseminated while talking.
7. Avoid poorly ventilated rooms and see that living and sleeping quarters are well ventilated.
8. Avoid crowds, especially inside.
9. Spend as much time as possible in the open, especially in the sunshine.
10. Dress warmly and avoid having wet feet. Keep regular hours.

These guidelines addressed social distancing, avoiding large groups, good ventilation, avoiding ill people, and are similar to modern CDC precautions regarding COVID-19. Medical responses were minimal during the 1918 influenza pandemic, as experts knew little about the virus. In addition, during the 1918 pandemic, most Americans strongly supported wearing masks. However, masks were ineffective because of poor wearing practices and the materials used to make them. Over 90 years later, a World Health Organization Writing Group (2006) reviewed the 1918 pandemic and found that social-distancing measures did not stop or appear to reduce disease transmission dramatically.

There was resistance in some circles to prevention measures, such as mask-wearing. For example, an anti-mask organization named the Anti-Mask League of San Francisco formed to protest a city ordinance requiring people to wear masks during the pandemic (Dolan 2020). The San Francisco Board of Health repealed the ordinance in less than a month. The league would end shortly but reappeared to protest a second ordinance. Issues raised by anti-masking organizations included the uselessness of masks and impingements on personal liberties. In addition, some resisters noted that mask mandates ran against the grain of democracy. Modern commentators have highlighted the similarities between anti-mask and resistance efforts during the 1918 and COVID-19 pandemics (see chapter 8).

According to McNeill (1975), medical personnel and facilities were overburdened when the 1918 influenza hit and medical services broke down. This is precisely what happened when COVID-19 struck; however, unlike COVID-19, the 1918 influenza passed rapidly, and routine human life resumed within weeks. COVID-19, on the other hand, has endured over two years with no end in sight. The 1918 influenza virus was poorly understood, and no effective drugs or vaccines were used to treat the flu or secondary infections. Instead, non-pharmaceutical interventions were used, such as quarantine, good hygiene, disinfectants, isolation, face masks, and limits on the size of public gatherings.

Since there were no anti-viral medications to slow its spread, caregivers relied on aspirin, Vicks VapoRub, mustard plasters, clean linens, hot soup, and other relatively ineffective remedies. Newspapers printed advertisements for unproven (quack) medical treatments promoted by people to profit quickly from desperately ill people. As Robinson (2021) concluded, one consequence was that ineffective therapies resulted in high demand for trained nurses and, consequently, nursing shortages. The demand for nursing and medical care providers was similar to COVID-19 demands and shortages. Robinson identified the need for more nurses, partially due to many serving overseas in WWI, shortages of doctors, hospital beds, and equipment resulting in delays in addressing other medical needs of patients. Robinson also noted there was no available vaccine for both, at least initially for COVID-19. The strength of nurses and their commitment to duty were reported in 1918, which was a common theme in the national media during the COVID-19 pandemic.

Over 100 years ago, following the end of the pandemic, *Science* magazine published an article on the lessons from the 1918 influenza pandemic (Soper 1919). The author, George Soper, concluded that three factors affected the spread and prevention of the pandemic. One factor was that people needed to appreciate the risks of infection. Second, it ran against human nature for people to confine themselves in strict isolation to protect others. The third factor was that people sometimes acted unconsciously as a continuing danger to themselves and others. Some experts might reach similar conclusions about the COVID-19 pandemic.

POLIOMYELITIS (POLIO)

Poliomyelitis (polio) is an infectious viral disease that affects the central nervous system and can cause temporary or permanent paralysis and, in rare cases, death (Oshinsky 2006). How do individuals become infected with polio? "The portal of entry for poliomyelitis viruses is the alimentary track via the mouth" (Oldstone 2020:171). The polio virus spreads from person to person and can infect a person's spinal cord resulting in paralysis. Most at risk of polio infections are children between 5 and 10 years, but the virus can infect older people (Loomis 2018).

The most common consequence of viral poliovirus infection in humans is an asymptomatic, usually mild, and short-lived disease. Although most people who become infected show no symptoms or recover within a week, the illness progresses with severe consequences in a small fraction of cases. According to the CDC, most people (72%) who get polio will not show any visible symptoms. One in four people who get the polio virus will have flu-like symptoms, including fever, sore throat, fatigue, constipation, headache, vomiting, nausea, and stomach pain. These infected individuals recover within a few days, with symptoms disappearing between 2 and 5 days later. The brain and spinal cord can be harmed in more severe cases, affecting between one and five out of a thousand people. For serious cases, symptoms include the sensation of needles and pins in the legs, meningitis (1 in 25 people), a severe infection of the covering of the spinal cord or brain, and paralysis in parts of the body (1 in 200 people). Finally, death due to paralysis (inability to breathe) can occur in rare cases. Those children with polio may appear fully recovered yet can experience muscle pain or paralysis as adults, referred to as post-polio syndrome.

The polio virus has existed since antiquity, as evidenced by the early Egyptian and other ancient civilizations. The first documented major poliomyelitis outbreak in the United States occurred in Vermont in 1894 (see Oshinsky 2006 for an overview of polio in America.). The contagious nature of polio was not established until 1905. For most of history, people did not know how polio was transmitted and lived in fear. In 1916, New York City experienced an outbreak of polio that caused clashes between health officials and the public. Some parents were fearful that their children would catch polio by having contact with outsiders. Parents sometimes resisted public health interventions by hiding their children from authorities. Sounding remarkably similar to the current COVID-19 pandemic, Oldstone (2020:166) wrote:

> Under the sway of panic, people looked with skepticism and suspicion at government health offices. The selectmen of many villages, whose doctors were struggling with the impossible and failing to stop the epidemic or save patients

> from paralysis, resorted to homemade martial law. Movie theaters were closed to children under 16 years of age. Swimming pools were closed. Children exposed to polio infection or in an area where a case was found were to be isolated for two weeks at home. Isolation could be best controlled in middle-class and wealthy families, but poor children unable to be isolated were often forcibly taken to hospitals.

The polio virus generated great fear in the general population until vaccinations were developed. During the late 1940s and early 1950s, polio outbreaks occurred throughout the country during the hot summer months. In response to these outbreaks, terrified parents isolated their children and kept them away from swimming pools, roller rinks, lakes, beaches, movie theaters, and other public venues (Brink 2021). This fearful parenting impacted the mental health of children and their parents. Communities and neighborhoods would ostracize families or children diagnosed with polio (Loomis 2018). Parents monitored their children for any signs of the disease. Public concern for polio expanded in the 1930s through the 1950s until a vaccine was introduced in 1955. According to Carroll (2020), polio was feared most by Americans, second only to the atomic bomb.

Much of the public interest in polio grew due to President Franklin D. Roosevelt being diagnosed in 1921 with polio. He lost the use of his legs due to polio. Initially, he concealed his paralysis because he did not want to appear weak to voters. Plus, there was a stigma attached to those having the disease. As the nation's leader, President Roosevelt was instrumental in launching the National Foundation for Infantile Paralysis, later named the March of Dimes. Motivated by an extreme public fear of the disease, a sense that something needed to be done, and President Roosevelt's visible support, the March of Dimes became very successful as a social movement organization (SMO). According to Brink (2021), Americans responded to this SMO by volunteering and donating to find a cure. Volunteers went door to door asking for donations, and many businesses displayed cardboard stands where people could insert dimes into slots. Funds were raised by traveling exhibits of people using iron lungs, and posters of children using braces were standard. The March of Dimes also recruited celebrities, such as Judy Garland, Marilyn Monroe, Mickey Rooney, and Elvis Presley, to raise funds and promote the vaccines.

After years of research, Jonas Salk and associates developed the first polio vaccine in 1955. Salk's vaccine used a formalin-inactivated virus. A second vaccine using a live-attenuated virus was developed by Albert B. Sabin and administered in the former Soviet Union and Eastern Europe in the late 1950s. The parents of 600,000 children volunteered to participate in Sabin vaccine trials (Brink 2021). The Sabin oral vaccine would be licensed in the

United States in 1961. The two vaccines would compete for medical and public acceptance. Salk's inactivated polio vaccine (IPV) is the only polio vaccine in the United States since 2000. Depending on a person's age, it is given by a shot in the arm or leg. Sabin's oral polio vaccine (OPV) is used in other countries because it is cheaper and easier to administer, especially in remote areas where healthcare is limited. Almost all children (99 out of 100) who get all the recommended vaccine doses will be protected from polio.

Most Americans were united in addressing polio. When vaccines became available, most adults did not resist getting their children vaccinated because the consequences of the disease were dramatic and physically evident in many cases. In some communities, school nurses administered vaccinations, and most people were happy to get vaccinated. Unfortunately, those individuals not being vaccinated suffered from polio infections. On July 17, 1959, United States Surgeon General Leroy E. Burney reported that nine out of ten new polio cases occurred among persons who had not been vaccinated (Homola 1963).

Like all vaccine rollouts, despite the solid public fear of polio, there was some public resistance to the vaccines. Sociologists Lang and Lang (1961:270–271) wrote of this resistance:

> When the development of the Salk vaccine was first publicly announced, many persons opposed the desirability of mass inoculation against polio. Some scientists were skeptical; they argued that there was not yet conclusive proof of the vaccines providing lifelong immunity against all kinds of polio; that many people had already developed a lasting immunity; that there was always the risk of mishaps, of triggering an outbreak in a person already exposed. Having critically appraised the situation, they urged utmost caution. A second group had no firm evidence on which to base their opinion against vaccination. Still, they refused to go along because none of their friends seemed to think it worth the trouble to get a vaccination. Still other persons clambered against mass inoculations on the assumption that this was a plot—on the part of Roosevelt supporters active in the anti-polio drive or of profit-greedy laboratories or the Russians—to push Americans into accepting a risky policy. They may have expressed generalized distrust of authority and medical authority in particular.

Other pockets of polio vaccine resistance existed. For example, some chiropractors did not view polio vaccines as necessary and openly opposed vaccine campaigns. They dismissed the link of infections to contagious pathogens (the virus). Instead, they adhered to the basic chiropractic principle that all diseases originated in the spine. They concluded this even when the number of cases rapidly dropped when polio vaccines were introduced. According to Carroll (2020), the *Journal of the National Chiropractic Association* recommended that vaccines should not be taken and adjustments to the entire spine should be given during the first three days of polio infections (for discussion, see Homola 1963). These spinal adjustments would be sufficient treatment for the disease.

The rollout of the polio vaccines was successful but also chaotic. Demand for the vaccines was high from the beginning. People formed long lines to get vaccinated out of fear and undeniable faith in science and medicine. According to Arnold-Foster (2021), the polio vaccine campaign in 1950s America has mythical status as a straightforward success. However, it was confusing and chaotic, and the government underestimated the vaccine demand. She observed that the federal government failed to plan for the rollout effectively, and information about where and how to get vaccinated was absent. In addition, racial inequities regarding access to polio vaccines were present in Jim Crow America, as Black children lined up for their vaccines outside of segregated White schools while White children were vaccinated inside. Some Black Americans, weary of White-dominated medicine, hesitated to get vaccinated. The March of Dimes, aware of racial factors, recruited Black celebrities, such as Ella Fitzgerald, Louis Armstrong, and Sammy Davis Jr., to promote vaccinations among Black communities (Brink 2021).

There were medical setbacks that caused the public to be vaccine-hesitant. In April 1955, physicians began to observe cases of paralytic polio in vaccinated children. The paralysis was occurring in the vaccinated arms. All of the cases had vaccines prepared by Cutter Laboratories in California. By May 1955, polio vaccines were suspended so that the cause could be identified. Although never proven, it is likely specific production procedures were not followed that led to compromised vaccines. Some of the missteps of the polio vaccine rollout and the fierce competition between Sabin and Salk led to changes in governmental oversight of vaccines. Regulatory processes were implemented to ensure appropriate testing and monitoring of vaccines and other drugs. Such oversight measures also helped manage liability claims against vaccine and drug manufacturers.

With the effectiveness of polio vaccines being well established, the possibility of the virus being eliminated is viable. However, there are several barriers to this occurring. Oldstone (2020:152) observed, "Problems of eradication were related to poverty; remote geography with pockets of viral persistence, poor sanitation, and contamination of water supply; breakdown of healthcare due to war or government collapse; and physical attacks on healthcare workers administering the vaccine." A case in point is what happened in Nigeria when an outbreak of polio occurred and spread—according to Oldstone, religious and political leaders advised a mostly uneducated Muslim population not to get polio vaccinations developed in the West. In 2004, Nigerians traveling to Mecca for Hajj likely spread the disease to others, eventually infecting individuals as far away as Indonesia.

Oldstone (2020) outlined why polio has yet to be eliminated globally. He observed that in most cases, polio circulates invisibly as infected individuals do not show clinical signs of infection. Accessibility is another issue, as parts of the world are difficult to enter, and thus, vaccinations are not provided. Loomis (2018) noted that polio is only found naturally in four countries, Afghanistan, Nigeria, Mozambique, and Pakistan, due to poor health infrastructure and vaccine resistance by religious and political groups, such as the Taliban. To this list can be added the United States (New York), Israel (Jerusalem), and England (London), as new polio cases surfaced in 2022. These outbreaks of polio have been linked to unvaccinated individuals or, in some sporadic cases, individuals that had oral vaccinations. According to an Associated Press story (Cheng 2022), the oral vaccine may lead to polio infections in sporadic cases (2–4 cases per 2 million doses). This is why some countries have halted the use of the oral vaccine. Those countries solely using injected vaccines have eliminated polio. The oral polio vaccine has been credited with the dramatic decline in worldwide cases. A new oral vaccine has been developed in response to recent polio infections, but the supply is limited. Public health experts are concerned that opponents will further use these rare oral vaccine cases to resist vaccinations during the COVID-19 pandemic. Dr. Scott Barrett, Columbia University, reflected on this concern and was quoted as saying:

> What is different now is a reduction in trust in authorities and the political polarization in countries like the U.S. and the U.K. The presumption that we can quickly increase vaccination numbers may be more challenging now. (cited by Cheng 2022:n.p.)

Other barriers to elimination include civil wars. Civil wars and roaming soldiers prohibit healthcare workers from vaccinating people. In addition, it is unsafe for healthcare workers to enter and administer the vaccine in some areas where militias, rebels, and civil wars pose dangers. For example, in Pakistan and Afghanistan, healthcare workers have been killed for immunizing children (Cheng 2022). Finally, in some countries with poor hygiene and numerous persons who are chronically infected with other viruses that cause diarrhea and gastrointestinal problems, administrations of the vaccine may not stay in bodies long enough to be effective due to diarrhea (rapid removal of oral vaccine) or because of other infections in the gut. Finally, in the United States, anti-vaccine groups continue to resist vaccines. In addition, because polio is now rare, younger parents have been complacent in getting their children vaccinated. As a result, an out-of-sight and out-of-mind attitude has led to occasional local outbreaks of the disease, such as recent ones in New York and California.

MEASLES

Measles is a serious viral disease that is very contagious. Measles has been documented as early as the 9th century. Humans are the only natural host for the measles virus. Measles can result in significant complications and possible death. Measles begins as a fever followed by a cough, red eyes, and a runny nose. Eventually, a red rash of tiny spots starts at the head and spreads throughout the rest of the body. The measles virus spreads through the air when an infected person coughs, talks, or sneezes. The measles virus can infect individuals through the cell linings in the mouth, throat, nose, and eyes. The virus can stay in the air for as long as two hours, so anyone not vaccinated can potentially catch the disease. Up to 90 percent of people exposed to the virus are estimated to become infected unless vaccinated. Individuals infected with measles can spread it to others four days before and four days after the rash appears. Once it has begun, no treatment exists to stop or limit a measles virus infection. Before the development of measles vaccinations in 1963, people quarantined and segregated those infected. According to Oldstone (2020:123):

> Measles is one of the most contagious viruses passed among humans and can cause severe disease. Before extensive vaccinations began throughout the United States, even as late as the 1960s, over 500,000 individuals a year were infected, and more than 400 died. Included annually were over 48,000 hospitalizations, with numerous cases of brain infection (encephalitis) resulting in 7,000 patients with seizures and over 2,000 children with severe brain damage requiring hospitalization in mental institutions. However, by the end of the 1970s, when immunizing vaccination became routine, measles virus infections decreased by 90%, as did its sequela.

Before vaccinations were available in 1963, 3 to 4 million Americans became infected with measles yearly. Roughly 48,000 of these cases required hospitalization, and 400 to 500 died. With the vaccination program implemented in the United States, there has been a 99 percent reduction in measles cases. However, about 1 in 5 unvaccinated people infected with measles will be hospitalized. In addition, unvaccinated pregnant women who become infected run the risk of premature births and low birth weight babies.

Measles is severe for children younger than five years, pregnant women, individuals with compromised immune systems, and adults over age twenty due to complications such as ear infections, diarrhea, pneumonia, and encephalitis. Encephalitis can result in death, deafness, and intellectual developmental disabilities. The odds of childhood death from measles are low, ranging from 1 to 3 per 1,000 infections, but are unacceptable. "Currently, of the approximately 200 million cases per year of measles on our globe, over 500,000 persons die, a shameful figure considering the availability and low cost of effective vaccines" (Oldstone 2020:125).

Before vaccines, most American children had measles by age 15. In 1963, a vaccine was developed, and since 1968 has been the only vaccine used to prevent measles. Measles vaccines are 95 percent effective when both doses are taken. The vaccine provides long-term protection, although some humans have a genetic profile that makes them unresponsive or poorly responsive to the vaccine and, thus, not protected from the infection (Oldstone 2020:125). Today, the vaccine is usually combined with mumps and rubella and is called an MMR or combined with varicella (chicken pox), an MMRV.

The federal government aimed to eliminate measles by 1982, but that did not occur. However, the number of cases has dramatically dropped through extensive vaccination efforts. Measles in the United States was declared eliminated through the vaccination program. However, there are occasional measles outbreaks in the United States for various reasons. For example, measles outbreaks occurred in Los Angeles in 1977 and San Diego in 2008. These outbreaks highlighted the challenge of getting everyone vaccinated.

Measles and the MMR vaccine, similar to COVID-19, have always had myths, rumors, and misinformation. According to the Infectious Diseases Society of America (2022), some of the ideas about the vaccination for measles are myths and not factual. A few selected myths and facts about the MMR vaccine are:

- Myth: The measles, mumps, and rubella (MMR) vaccine causes autism. Fact: There is no evidence that MMR causes autism, but a great deal of evidence shows it does not cause autism. Nevertheless, some parents adhere to this myth, resulting in outbreaks and serious consequences, such as loss of hearing, blindness, and even death for some children.
- Myth: The measles vaccine does not prevent severe illness and death—the number of measles deaths dropped long before the vaccine was introduced, and it is no longer deadly. Fact: The measles vaccine prevents thousands of deaths each year worldwide. Globally, there was an 84 percent decrease in measles deaths between 2000 and 2016 as the vaccine became more widely available—many more than 200 million deaths were prevented.
- Myth: The measles vaccine can be deadly. Fact: There have been no deaths shown to be related to the vaccine in healthy people. There have been rare fatalities from vaccine side effects among immunocompromised children, so they are recommended not to get the vaccine.
- Myth: The MMR vaccine can cause measles. Fact: The vaccine does not cause measles. All measles vaccines are made from the virus. One

type of vaccine is made from a dead virus, and the other is from a weak virus that does not cause the disease but causes the immune system to recognize the virus and develop immunity to it.

These myths and facts about the MMR demonstrate a typical collective behavior pattern common to vaccines over history. The pattern is that false rumors influence perceptions about vaccinations. What drives these rumors and myths is often values and emotions rather than facts. In the case of the MMR and MMRV, the evidence is clear that the vaccine helps prevent measles and related severe illness or even death.

Despite the proven effectiveness of measles vaccines, there are pockets of resistance to the vaccine. Oldstone (2020) identified reasons people refuse or do not get the vaccine. For example, some people are apathetic because they have not seen or heard of anyone getting measles for years. For some groups, religious beliefs or individual concerns that the government and public health cannot be trusted influence some people. Some resisters contend that children already get too many vaccinations, and some rely on advice from alternative medical providers not to get measles vaccinations.

HUMAN IMMUNODEFICIENCY VIRUS (HIV)/AIDS

Acquired Immune Deficiency Syndrome (AIDS) is a lethal disease caused by the Human Immunodeficiency Virus (HIV). There are two types of HIV viruses, Type I (HIV-1) and Type II (HIV-2). In the 36 years since the initial case report, of the more than 75 million HIV infections, nearly half of them have died (Oldstone 2020:295). According to the CDC, roughly 80,000 to 100,000 Americans in the United States are newly infected annually. In addition, over 250,000 individuals are estimated to be infected but unaware that they are carriers that can spread HIV infections. Before anti-viral treatments, 80 percent of those infected died slowly and painfully.

HIV is spread through body fluids such as semen, blood, vaginal fluid, and breast milk. Other methods of transfer include needle sharing and unsanitary medical equipment. Once infected, the virus gives the individual flu-like symptoms for a few days and suppresses the immune system over the long term. The suppressed immune system allows other diseases to flourish, such as pneumonia, herpes, and tuberculosis. Later, lymphomas, Kaposi's sarcoma, and other diseases may emerge. Many of these will lead to death or at least debilitating lives.

Similar to COVID-19, conspiracy theories regarding the origin of HIV were soon circulated. Some conspiracies promoted the idea that HIV was a government plot that targeted specific populations, such as communists, homosexuals, or Black Americans. The Russian government capitalized on the opportunity to blame the U.S. government with a propaganda strategy titled INFECTION. The Russians planted false information and paid for advertising to place the blame on the U.S. military (see Oldstone 2020). Another conspiracy theory came from gay communities that the U.S. government introduced HIV to eliminate gay people. A comparable conspiracy theory emerged, but the target was Black Americans. Prior negative experiences of Black Americans and medical research helped this conspiracy theory sound plausible. With all these, no factual evidence ever surfaced to support these conspiracy theories. However, that did not keep some people from believing and spreading them as facts. Ultimately, after years of research, both types of HIV were traced to monkeys in Africa.

Other similarities between COVID-19 and HIV and AIDS have been present. One is fear of the infected. Haitians and Haitian Americans have been discriminated against because of an association between them and AIDS. Gay people, whether infected or not, have been discriminated against because they were viewed as carriers of the disease. HIV infections became a new negative social status with social implications. Discrimination against those with infections occurred in the workplace and classrooms. Blaming the victim for their infection became a common social reaction. People with infections not only had to deal with their declining physical health but also mental health issues. The research found that people with HIV infections had higher depression, post-traumatic stress disorder, substance abuse, emotional distress, and suicide rates. It was common for people living with AIDS to feel guilt and feel rejected.

The HIV epidemic has been significant enough in the United States that President Donald Trump, in his February 2019 State of the Union address, called for a government-run health program to eliminate the HIV epidemic in the United States within ten years. Worldwide, HIV is significant and resulted in an estimated 25 to 35 million deaths (Table 3.1), many occurring in Africa. In addition, the impact of HIV on the families and economies of numerous developing countries, especially in Africa, has been enormous. Although progress has been made in treating the disease, HIV remains a worldwide health concern.

OTHER IMPORTANT VIRUSES

COVID-19 is not the only coronavirus posing a threat to humans. There have been other coronaviruses over the decades, including H1N1 (1933), H2N2—Asian Flu—Influenza "A" (1957), H3N2—Hong Kong Flu (1968), SARS (2003), H1N1 (2009), and Middle East Respiratory Syndrome—MERS (2012).

The recent H1N1 pandemic in 2009 came in waves. H1N1 vaccines were developed and approved, and a federal campaign encouraged citizens to get vaccinated to halt the spread of the disease. In 2009, the World Health Organization announced the end of the H1N1 pandemic. In 2012 MERS found its way into the human population in Saudi Arabia. MERS is a severe respiratory illness with a high rate of death (35%). Other viruses that have reached epidemic and potentially pandemic levels include Lassa Fever, Ebola, West Nile, Zika, Monkeypox, and Hantavirus. These viruses pose essential threats to humans and are constantly monitored for outbreaks. In addition, all can disrupt social relationships in the communities, regions, and countries where they emerge.

CONCLUDING OBSERVATIONS

It is important to note that new viruses are being introduced to humans through various routes. One means of introduction is for a virus to modify its genetic material. For example, COVID-19 has mutated into new variants, such as Delta and Omicron, and subvariants, such as BA.4 and BA.5. These variants and subvariants change how the virus behaves. Another route is when humans increase their contact with vectors or other humans that carry different viruses. For example, human expansion into tropical rainforests may introduce new viruses. Countless viruses reside in remote regions that could potentially infect humans. Infected individuals may become more susceptible to viruses (pathogens' harmful effects) when their immune systems are weakened. New potentially harmful viruses are discovered, researched, or developed in laboratories. The ability to modify existing viruses has value and potential risks to humans.

General observations regarding prior societal responses to plagues, pandemics, and epidemics can be made. While the contexts in which societies experienced pandemics, plagues, and diseases were dramatically different than the modern context for COVID-19, there are historic patterns worthy of note.

- Pandemics and plagues have caused societies to change dramatically. Civilizations have risen and fallen due to plagues and pandemics (Diamond 2005; McNeill 1976; Oldstone 2020).
- People have always sought explanations for why diseases occur spiritually or naturally. In antiquity, mass-scale outbreaks of diseases were attributed to the gods and their revenge on humans. During the Middle Ages, Christianity thought diseases were God's punishment for sinful

behavior. With COVID-19, while a coronavirus causes the disease, some individuals have attributed it to political plots, elites, and conspiracies.

- Related to searching for causes is the social pattern of placing blame on groups or individuals for being the source of the pandemic. Scapegoating or blaming marginalized groups is a common thread. Racism and ethnocentricity have been common behaviors and attitudes surfacing during pandemics.
- Epidemics and contagion reinforce prejudices and enhance stigmatization processes: against the Jews (the 1347–1350 plague), against the poor in the Renaissance (the plague, typhus), against Irish immigrants in the 19th century (cholera), against the poor in the 19th and 20th centuries (tuberculosis), against the four Hs (homosexuals, Haitians, hemophiliacs, and heroin addicts) in the 1980s (HIV/AIDS), against Africans (Ebola), against Chinese and Asians (bird flu, SARS, and the coronavirus), against the "stranger," the "foreigner," or the "other" (see Ferreira et al. 2020:10). With COVID-19, some political leaders accused Muslims, Asians, and people from developing countries as transmitting it.
- Although exposed to pandemic diseases, some people do not become seriously ill. However, similar to asymptomatic COVID-19 individuals, some get infected by viruses and do not have major medical consequences but are dangerous to others as transmitters. This has promoted the unintentional spread of diseases by humans.
- Quarantining and isolating sick individuals has been practiced for centuries to control epidemics and pandemics. Quarantining and isolation were practiced by those who could isolate, such as medieval aristocracy. Escape to the countryside was an option for the well-to-do. Ships from foreign ports were required to quarantine for 30 to 40 days to ensure that they were not passing on the plague. This was a form of social distancing.
- Pandemics have led to collective behavior, such as protests, social movements, and migrations of populations. Some pandemics have also restructured societies, creating opportunities for some and losses for others. For example, the Black Plague of the Middle Ages led to major changes in medieval social structure, such as the development of skilled workers and businesses and the rise of the middle class.
- Whatever responses to pandemics have been implemented, be it quarantines, isolation, vaccines, or travel restrictions, a segment of society will circumvent or resist measures to control the disease. Public health officials have been viewed as intrusive when they have, rightly or wrongly, attempted to prevent the spread of diseases.

- Misinformation, some of it based on ignorance, beliefs, political agendas, and/or self-interest, is always present in any pandemic, plague, or epidemic. Misinformation about treatments and vaccines has led some people to avoid one of the most effective tools for ending disease, vaccinations. By some people resisting or avoiding effective vaccines, some diseases will continue to harm human beings throughout the world. According to Oldstone (2020), the spread of vaccine misinformation has resulted in the deaths of hundreds of millions of people. He likened this behavior to playing with fire.

Chapter 4

The Pandemic and Collective Behavior

"He who permits himself to tell a lie once, finds it much easier to do it a second and third time, till at length it becomes habitual; he tells lies without attending to it, and truths without the world's believing him. This falsehood of the tongue leads to that of the heart, and in time depraves all its good dispositions."

Thomas Jefferson, *Letter to Peter Carr*, August 19, 1785

"Serious misfortunes, originating in misrepresentation, frequently flow and spread before they can be dissipated by truth."

George Washington, *Letter to John Jay*, July 6, 1796

COVID-19 AND COLLECTIVE BEHAVIOR

The COVID-19 pandemic has resulted in major social, economic, and political upheavals. Social scientists have observed that the pandemic represents an ideal context for social research and important subject matter for sociologists (Dingwall et al. 2013; Matthewman and Huppatz 2020). The pandemic has been a global experiment, as entire countries have locked down, social reforms have occurred, supply chains have been disrupted, jobs lost, profits made, new markets developed, and other changes have occurred. Some of these changes go beyond the bounds of traditional society, organizations, and institutions. COVID-19 has a social dimension to it and, in the minds of some, is a social disaster (Connell 2020) or crisis (Walby 2021; 2022). Others suggest the pandemic has been overstated (Frijters et al. 2021; Mercola and Cummins 2021; Siegel 2020).

COVID-19 is both a medical and social phenomenon. Thus, the social sciences can provide insights into understanding the pandemic. Sociologists sometimes focus on spontaneous and unstructured behavior. When they do, they focus on what is labeled collective behavior (dynamics). Collective behavior, a particular field of sociology, is concerned with the formation and activities of crowds, fads, protests, panics, rumors, crises, mass hysterias, riots, crazes, and social movements. Many of these forms of collective behavior have been abundant during the pandemic. "Collective behavior includes an enormous array of behaviors, processes, structures, and the context, and it encompasses parts of many sociological subfields" (Marx and McAdam 1994:1). Collective behavior looks at actions taken by groups of people that differ from established social norms. Collective behavior focuses on a logic involving "emergent group behavior in settings where cultural guidelines are nonspecific, inadequate, or in dispute, or lacking altogether" (Marx and McAdam 1994:3).

Collective behavior refers to social processes and events outside and inside the existing social structure (Evans 1975; Miller 2014). Collective behavior is often spontaneous and includes a variety of behaviors and events. The collective behavior approach focuses on four groupings of people: the crowd, the mass, the public, and social movements. In addition, it pays attention to other phenomena, such as protests and rumors. Group dynamics always drive collective behavior, and in the modern age, it can be virtual because individuals involved may never have any physical contact with other participants. In some instances, collective behavior can result in individuals behaving in ways they never thought they would or should.

Understanding the social structure is crucial in interpreting how society has responded to the pandemic. "Social structure . . . consists of a set of statuses defined by relatively stable relationships that people in various positions have with each other" (Lang and Lang 1961:6). In a nutshell, COVID-19 and responses to it have disrupted the existing social structure in some crucial ways. The pandemic altered, added, or eliminated many social norms. The result was the creation of fertile grounds for social unrest and corresponding forms of collective behavior, such as crowds, protests, rumors, propaganda, and social movements.

SOCIAL CONDITIONS CONDUCIVE TO COLLECTIVE BEHAVIORS

Before the pandemic started, social conditions for collective behaviors were ripe. The United States was in an election year with uncertainty about the future. Several factors contributed to uncertainty and unrest. For example, mass shootings involving four or more victims were increasingly common. In 2019, 475 people were killed in mass shootings. This number increased in 2020 to 521 and in 2021 to 705 people. These shooting events were broadcast on national media resulting in public discomfort. In addition, severe multiple weather events, such as hurricanes, flooding, and droughts, impacted the nation and several regions. In 2019, a government shutdown lasted the longest in American history. The shutdown disrupted the lives of millions. Depending on the economic sector, some individuals and businesses thrived or suffered significant losses. Many workers lost their jobs or were economically impacted. Entertainment, travel, education, and the service industries were hit particularly hard.

Laid-off workers were unable to pay bills and mortgages. Protests over the mistreatment of minorities by law enforcement in some cities led to riots and a social movement for police reform. Radical right-wing groups demonstrated to promote their cause in some cities. Left-wing groups also made the headlines with their protests. The controversy stirred over constructing a border wall, with groups taking both sides of the issue. The war in Afghanistan continued after over 20 years of involvement with no end in sight. Post-truth politics now govern America, so sorting out the truth has never been more challenging. No matter what issue was at hand, all of this contributed to a sense of uncertainty, stress, and unrest among the American public.

With these trends, events, and developments, Congress, the president, and other elected officials provided little evidence of leadership in joint problem-solving and moderation in the country. Compromise, moderation, and effectiveness were supplanted by extremism, blaming, and opposition to good policies for the sake of political affiliation. All this fueled political polarization that accomplished little other than serving as a role model for some Americans. Polarization led to an abandonment of moderation, trust, and cooperation. Compromise and moderation became signs of weakness, negative characteristics, and social or political liabilities for elected officials. None of this polarization reduced social uncertainty, stress, unrest, and anxiety and set the context for the pandemic. This political polarization in the country promoted the division between those Americans who complied with COVID-19 mandates and those who resisted.

Social scientists note that social systems and routine behaviors become disrupted when significant elements of the social order break down, such as in American society before the pandemic. Traditional norms (rules) erode and are not in place in response to new situations and crises, such as when the pandemic surfaced. The spread of COVID-19 was a new situation, as most pandemics require new adapting methods. For Americans, polarization played an essential role in shaping collective responses. The dominant culture, as reflected by the government and public health directives, was either complied with or opposed. Most Americans complied with public health recommendations and directives. However, other Americans felt that these directives ran counter to their American cultural values, such as freedom of choice, and opposed them initially. As Marx and McAdam (1994:19) observed, "Subordinate persons [those feeling powerless] may be unable to obtain what they feel they are entitled to—freedom, dignity, equality, tolerance, or opportunity if they accept the dominant culture." They consequently resist as an exercise of power and control, which fuels more social unrest. This pattern has been evident throughout the pandemic.

CHARACTERISTICS AND TYPES OF SOCIAL UNREST

Writing over 50 years ago, the sociologist Herbert Blumer (1975) proposed five types of social unrest. He suggested one form of unrest was based on insecurity and a wariness of the future. During social unrest, people are more likely to move around in unpredictable and normless ways to avoid something without knowing what they are trying to find or avoid. A significant characteristic of social unrest is excited feelings, usually vague apprehension, fears, and insecurity. Such excited feelings are conducive to rumors, exaggerated views, and perceptions (see Blumer 1975:25). Finally, a characteristic of social unrest is psychologically unstable people suffering from disturbed impulses and feelings. To Blumer, this unrest was an unfocused fear of what lay ahead.

An example would be the Y2K (year 2000) speculation that the world might come to a halt when the year 2000 occurred. Another would be the fear regarding the H1N1 virus in 2009 when dire warnings about its potential to kill many people were proposed. However, neither Y2K nor H1N1 materialized as some predicted. This type of unrest might be applied to COVID-19 because some feared the long-term and unknown consequences of the coronavirus. Although coronaviruses have occurred, the COVID-19 virus behaved differently and spread faster and easier.

To Blumer, a second type of social unrest is characterized by frustration and protests about present circumstances. People and groups responding to this type of social unrest mobilize into action, such as protesting policies, people, or events. Protests against or for school closures, mask mandates, proof of vaccination, travel restrictions, and the like could be considered to address this type of social unrest. A third type of social unrest is a flight from the present when conventional lifestyles and philosophies no longer speak to or meet current needs. Embracing alternative lifestyles or joining religious or utopian communities are examples of addressing this form of unrest. With COVID-19, the closest example of addressing this type of unrest would be the reliance on alternative treatments, such as those individuals or groups that embrace unproven substances to treat COVID-19 (see chapter 7). The fourth type of social unrest has high expectations to do something for society to make major societal changes. For example, efforts to dismantle traditional public health care or eliminate all vaccines could be considered responses to this type of unrest. Likewise, promoting public health or vaccinations for all could be doing something for society to address unrest driven by the general health of society. To Blumer, the final type of unrest is characterized by despair and fatalist withdrawal from society. With COVID-19, some individuals withdrew or severely limited their outside contact with others. Others were isolated in protest to mandates and public health directives.

THRESHOLDS OF COLLECTIVE BEHAVIOR

The threshold concept helps understand social responses to the COVID-19 pandemic and corresponding collective behaviors. According to Granovetter (1978), the threshold is important for understanding collective behavior. Granovetter (1978:1420) defined threshold as "the number or proportion of others who must make one decision before a given actor does so; this is where net benefits begin to exceed net costs for that particular actor." Tang and Liu (2010:20–21) observed, "To understand collective behavior, researchers in social science and behavioral studies have used the threshold model, in which an actor adopts one action when the number of his [or her] friends taking action exceeds a certain threshold." The concept can be applied to several aspects of the pandemic and related policies. For example, an individual's responses to COVID-19 rumors, protests, vaccinations, wearing masks, and compliance or non-compliance with mandates are likely influenced by an individual's perceptions about how many other people are responding. The threshold (number) of immediate friends and family members' responses matters to the individual and how she or he responds. For example, using this concept, we would expect individuals to be more willing to wear masks if others around them are also wearing them. The individual would most likely conform to social expectations and norms. Likewise, if others are not wearing masks, there would be a tendency to conform and not wear masks.

The threshold is where the perceived benefits to an individual of doing the thing in question, such as protesting a school closure, exceed the perceived costs (Granovetter 1978). For example, some individuals may be wary of being vaccinated until a proportion (threshold) of people are vaccinated without having negative health consequences. Depending upon their ethnicity, educational level, age, friends' perspectives, medical history, and advice from media sources and other factors, different adults will have different thresholds. In the case of vaccinations, for some individuals, the threshold of hundreds of thousands of people dying from COVID-19 and even more getting seriously sick to the point of requiring hospitalization was insufficient for them to become vaccinated. Even with rigorous clinical testing prior to the release of the vaccines, they never reached the threshold, while others with lower thresholds were quick to get their vaccines.

The threshold for getting vaccinated during the COVID-19 pandemic is difficult to identify for several reasons. This is because COVID-19 impacted different populations at different times and in different ways. Urban residents were the first groups infected at high rates along the coastal states. Over time, the infection rates shifted to rural areas. For some Americans, the number of infections or deaths mattered less than being given a small financial incentive for getting vaccinated.

COLLECTIVE BEHAVIOR PERSPECTIVES APPLIED TO THE PANDEMIC

From the beginning, COVID-19 and the pandemic have created a situation of ambiguity. COVID-19 affected humans in ways that previous coronaviruses had not. Initially, no one knew its origin, how it was spread, and how to control it. Emergent Norm theory defines collective behavior as responding to new or ambiguous social situations. According to this perspective, ambiguous situations can result in adaptive responses. It focuses on behavioral responses to situations where no pre-existing rules (norms) or expectations apply. COVID-19 created enough ambiguity to result in new behaviors. At the pandemic's beginning, so little was understood about COVID-19 that social norms on responding were absent. For example, when, how, and where to wear masks or social distance norms had to be created. These norms did not naturally evolve but were imposed quickly by governments, public health agencies, and businesses. As a result, new norms (expectations for behavior), new ways of interacting, and new social relationships quickly evolved.

In the case of COVID-19, the media and government messaging were ambiguous by sending mixed messages from the beginning about the virulence and consequences of the coronavirus. Depending on the source, COVID-19 was either no big deal or a deadly infection. Falling back on traditional understandings and behaviors is common. However, in the case of COVID-19, this only occurred for various reasons—few people in society had experienced severe pandemics. Americans had never experienced lockdowns, social distancing, and wearing masks. Few credible guidelines were available, and those present changed as more was learned about COVID-19.

Another collective behavior perspective focuses on social strain. Without question, COVID-19 introduced social strain at all levels of society. Labeled value-added theory, this perspective defines collective behavior as a response to social strain (Miller 2014). When deterioration or failure of the social structure occurs, such as when natural disasters, wars, or pandemics come about, the levels of anxiety, hostility, emotions, and desire for change increase; these can result in collective behaviors. People under social strain mobilize to eliminate or address this social strain. These behaviors often occur outside of regular and routine channels of behavior. Structural strain arises when people lack the knowledge and skills to cope successfully with a problematic situation, such as COVID-19.

RUMORS AND COVID-19

One of the most important social aspects of the pandemic has been the abundance of COVID-19 rumors. Rumors have differing definitions, such as a claim, statement, or opinion shared with others needing a discernible source or authority for its truth. The origin of a rumor is often unclear and often spread by word of mouth or social media. A rumor is a statement, claim, or story circulating without confirmation or certainty about the facts. Rumors can be factual or made up from false information. A rumor may be true but often turns out to be false, an exaggeration, or a spinning of facts. Decades ago, social scientists Gordon Allport and Leo Postman (1947/1965:ix) defined rumor as "a specific or topical proposition or belief, passed along from person to person, usually by word of mouth, without secure standards of evidence being presented."

This definition remains useful but must accommodate changes in sharing rumors online and in mass communications. Commonly rumors are promoted between people and groups in face-to-face circumstances but with the development of social media and the internet, rumors are not restricted to face-to-face interactions (word of mouth). They can be readily shared with vast audiences through these new communications tools. Rumors can be spread quickly over the internet and via Facebook, e-mail, Instagram, TikTok, podcasts, Twitter, and other social media platforms. Social media platforms and biased news programs have capitalized on the pandemic by advancing rumors about COVID-19. Biased news sources are also important spreaders of COVID-19 rumors. With COVID-19, everybody has heard a rumor about the virus and how best to respond. In a sense, many adults spoke about COVID-19 as if they were knowledgeable when they were not. They heard or read something that could be true or false and passed it on to others.

CONDITIONS FOR THE SPREAD OF RUMORS

Rumors typically tend to flourish under certain conditions. Some of these conditions were present before and during the pandemic. A favorable condition for rumors is the extent to which people believe the social structure can address problems and crises. With COVID-19, some groups lacked confidence in the social structure, specifically the government, to handle the pandemic. During the pandemic, some Americans' mistrust of basic institutions increased, and they became increasingly susceptible to believing rumors. The openness of American society to a range of communications promoted the generation of COVID-19 rumors. Marx and McAdam (1994:29) noted that "open societies [such as the United States] are paradoxical in this regard." They added, "Their very openness is conducive to greater trust, but at the same time, they provide an abundance of resources for private groups to communicate rumors."

Uncertainty about the future can be stressful, and to reduce anxiety, people often seek information to determine what is likely to happen. They seek information from multiple sources. When traditional social controls over information are lacking, ineffective, or absent, rumors help fill information voids. Rumors quickly develop and spread (Lang and Lang 1961). When originators (sources) and spreaders of rumors are anonymous, there is little incentive to ensure the accuracy of information. Instead, there is a tendency for them to exaggerate. Originators and transmitters involved in spreading rumors may distort information without being concerned about being negatively sanctioned. There is little accountability, and false rumors are seldom withdrawn or corrected, and take independent lives. Rumor transmitters (sources) are seldom held responsible for adverse consequences. Thus, there can be a cavalier approach to spreading rumors and misinformation. Like gossip, rumors may be entertaining, dramatic, and further agendas.

Rumors flourish when a ready (susceptible) audience is present. With COVID-19, an eager market existed for whatever true or false rumors were made available. Americans had a strong need for information about

COVID-19. Prior experiences and beliefs made some Americans more receptive to rumors if those rumors supported their preexisting beliefs. Rumors are subject to social expectations, and people tend to rely on sources of information that they are familiar with that reinforce their perspectives. In addition, the relevance of the rumor to the individual's and group's concerns is important. Rumors that do not affect people or groups are less likely to develop and spread. COVID-19 rumors did touch virtually all aspects of many people's lives and livelihoods and consequently were important and intense. Rumors about COVID-19 seem to conform to Allport and Postman's (1947/1965) fundamental law of rumors which proposed that the intensity of a rumor is due to the subject's importance to people and the availability of information. Miller (2014:109; see also Allport and Postman 1947/1967:33–34) wrote:

> The intensity of rumor is the product of the importance of the subject to the individual and the ambiguity of the evidence about the topic at issue. In other words, rumor is most likely to occur when people are intensely interested in a topic and little definite news or official information is available. Conversely, rumor is unlikely when people have little interest in a topic and/or official information is plentiful.

With COVID-19, the public need for information increased as the virus spread worldwide. Early in the pandemic, COVID-19 was an insignificant virus for many Americans until it hit a nursing home in Kirkland, Washington, in April 2020. Multiple deaths among the residents and staff at the long-term care facility sparked alarm over the potential harm of the virus. The national media covered the story, but little could be communicated other than images of body bags being removed by emergency staff and reports of rising death counts. For some Americans, these images would leave a lasting impression.

PURPOSES OF RUMORS

Rumors serve many purposes. A rumor is a process in which people develop shared definitions of unstructured and ambiguous situations. Rumors create simplistic views of complex or uncertain situations. Rumors help people make sense of unclear or unusual events (Allport and Postman 1947/1967). COVID-19 provided an excellent opportunity for rumors to flourish, as the pandemic was unusual. Rumors provide a sense of certainty and agreement. Rumors reduce tension at the psychological and sociological levels by providing explanations for events and processes. Rumors meet the personal needs of individuals, such as their careers, ego needs, being valued as a source of information, feeling important, and facilitating personal gain. Rumors serve to "bring the orientations of others sufficiently in line with one's own to make the collective activity possible" (Lang and Lang 1961:81). Rumors fill the need for information and provide certainty about the situation—rumors close information gaps when society, culture, or authorities offer inadequate event explanations. For example, during the initial appearance of COVID-19, so little information was available that some people turned to alternative sources, much of which was based on rumor.

Rumors aim to mobilize individuals and groups to act or form desired opinions. In the case of the pandemic, rumors were used by some to support and others to circumvent public health and government policies. People often turn to sources they previously relied on for information, such as social media platforms, cable news, and social networks. Technological advances, such as the internet and social media, expedite the flow of rumors and information at unprecedented speed and range. Rumors are often generated and advanced through the internet by nominally identified individuals, sometimes through avatars (artificial beings). Prior to the internet, rumors were highly localized and slow to expand. Rumors were typically limited to communities, neighborhoods, families, and small friendship groups and only survived briefly. COVID-19 became just another story from the same, sometimes biased, sources.

CHARACTERISTICS OF RUMOR PROCESSES

Rumors have commonly shared characteristics, such as that motives and conditions for transmitting rumors are not purely individual but operate within cultural and social contexts. Rumors originate, are transmitted, and are influenced by cultural and social contexts in which they arise (Lang and Lang 1961:66). Allport and Postman (1947/1965) noted that people who spread rumors seldom ask for clarification or verification of the source or facts about a rumor. Rumor spreaders tend not to be critical thinkers but are unquestioning and prone to take rumors as truth. Rumors can help crystallize differences due to the cleavages in social and cultural structures. Just as the emergence of a rumor signifies a certain distrust and dissatisfaction with traditional sources of information, so also the specific path a rumor takes reveals the existence of divisions within a social setting (Lang and Lang 1961:76). With COVID-19, rumors about the strength of the disease, the risks it posed, and ways to treat it were subject to many rumors. While many rumors start with a kernel of truth, they change as they spread. What might start as a fact changes from person to person, and the message is altered with each transfer. This process is called distortion.

Allport and Postman (1947/1965) observed that as information became distorted, three changes might occur: details might be lost, called "leveling"; there might be a greater organization of materials (content) around a dominant theme, or "sharpening"; and messages were presented in ways that were consistent with pre-existing individual and cultural views, or "assimilation." With leveling, as rumors are spread, they become shorter, and much of the original information is lost in translation and transmission. With sharpening, some details are retained, and others are lost. This is selective perception based on the individual's (transmitter's) interests and prejudices. For example, in the case of COVID-19, individuals with strong political views incorporated those views in what information they retained and shared during the pandemic. Assimilation means people tend to be selective hearers and transmitters of information. In the rumor process, individuals and groups choose between competing definitions of the situation and alternative explanations and select some definitions over others. In some cases, Americans believed what they wanted to believe rather than what the facts indicated, which is consistent with the process of assimilation. Either individuals became fearful and paranoid about the COVID-19 virus and altered their lifestyles or believed in rumors that much of the pandemic was fabricated and overblown and resisted changes. Klapp (1972:251) observed:

> Because people are excited, they spread rumors rapidly and indiscriminately, and because they are suggestible, they pass along the most outlandish stories as fact. Because people are critical and irrational, they spread rumors that usually contradict established authorities' views and statements. Rumors are seldom accurate, but they are intentionally consistent—a consistency that is based not on critical consideration but on paranoid logic.

People generally have little interest in researching and verifying whether rumors are true or false. If the rumor fits their predispositions and worldview, they are more likely to accept it as truth. There are many examples of this pattern in the United States. For years, a rumor was spread that Barack Obama was not qualified to be president because he was not a natural-born citizen. Individuals who disapproved of his candidacy and eventually being elected as president, referred to as "birthers," promoted this rumor. This rumor persisted even despite verified facts to the contrary. The birthers were willing to dismiss the facts to promote their motive of removing President Obama from office. Failing this, rumors, such as the president being a Muslim, would emerge. Even when the rumors were discredited by the facts (evidence), some who opposed President Obama held on to their inaccurate beliefs. This pattern was repeated during the pandemic. For example, that COVID-19 is a "hoax" illustrates this pattern.

COVID-19 AND PANDEMIC RUMORS

Beginning with rumors (see chapter 7 for examples of COVID-19 rumors), the pandemic has fueled several rumors. These rumors have minimized or overestimated COVID-19 and its symptoms. For example, there have been pipe-dream rumors such as, "A cure has been found," "It is a minor infection and no big deal," "We will have a cure in weeks," and others. Rumors about the risk of COVID-19, such as how deadly the virus is or how it is no worse than the common cold, have been shared. There have been wedge-driving rumors, such as some groups of people being responsible for causing the disease, such as Asians or Jewish people. Several rumors have been spread from friendship networks. Everyone knows someone miraculously cured by a home remedy or alternative medicine. Rumors about where they thought they caught COVID-19 are commonplace.

Rumors about products used to promote or discourage the use or consumption of specific products are called product rumors. Product rumors often sound plausible (Miller 2014). American history is replete with examples of product rumors that take on a life of their own and have done significant damage to the reputations of products and businesses. For example, product rumors include a claim that a man fell into a vat at a Coca-Cola plant and dissolved in the soda. Another was that someone with Hansen's disease (leprosy) worked at a Chesterfield cigarette factory, potentially passing the disease to smokers. Another product rumor was AIDS being spread through fast-food restaurants (for a good discussion, see Miller 2014:95).

Regarding COVID-19, product rumors regarding vaccines have been numerous. For example, the rumor that vaccines were insufficiently tested or contained microchips that can be used to track people's locations was spread. To this could be added the product rumor that human fetuses are used in the manufacture of vaccines or live viruses are present in the vaccines that has been advanced. There are other rumors with no clinical evidence, such as the effectiveness of unproven drugs such as ivermectin and aspirin being effective treatments for COVID-19 (see chapters 6 and 7).

IS COVID-19 SIMPLY A MASS PANIC?

A panic is a sudden fear or terror which dominates thinking that can influence the behavior of groups. A panic can be an expression of fear or a hostile outburst of anger. When panics occur, individuals move away from group goals, and there is a collective retreat into a state of extreme "privatization." Privatization means individuals become more concerned with their safety and personal security than that of the group or society, whether the danger is physical, psychological, social, or financial. For example, mass shootings or building fires in confined spaces can result in panic as people present seek safety from harm. Panics shatter prior and basic understandings, social behaviors, and in some cases, the existing social order. With the capacity to share information and misinformation now available to individuals, groups, and organizations, ideas can easily be communicated to vast audiences. Differing views on whether COVID-19 is simply a mass panic and hence an overreaction or a real threat have surfaced. Skeptics of the pandemic have embraced the concept of panic. For instance, the book *The Great Covid Panic: What Happened, Why, and What to Do Next* (Frijters et al. 2021) illustrates this point.

Mass panics apply to larger groups and can be triggered by various threats, such as a fear of impending disasters, descriptions of violent crimes, stories of monsters, tales of unidentified flying objects (UFOs), terrorist attacks, and perceptions of weapons of mass destruction. Mass panic occurs when a large group of people share a mental state of anxiety or fear. Concerns about major threats to health, such as epidemics, outbreaks, plagues, and pandemics, can also generate mass panic. In the case of the pandemic, it was a fear of severe illness or death.

A classic case of a mass panic was how some Americans responded to the dramatic Orson Welles' *War of the Worlds* radio broadcast on Halloween in 1938. Although disclaimers were made before and during the performance, the broadcast was so realistic that some Americans did not realize it was fictional but responded as if it was. Cantril (1940) studied the mass panic resulting from the program. He concluded that people accepted the story of a violent invasion of earth by Martians because it conformed to their mental context, and people lacked information that would have contradicted the radio show. Plus, radio announcements that the show was only a dramatic story were ignored. He concluded that the lack of "critical ability" made radio listeners suggestible, leading them to wrong assumptions about the fictional Martian invasion.

Mass hysteria is a widespread, intense fear of and concern for a false or greatly exaggerated danger. Mass hysteria involves beliefs and perceptions that are false or at least gross distortions of reality. Moral panic is closely related to mass hysteria. A moral panic "refers to widespread concern over a perceived threat to the moral order that turns out to be false or greatly exaggerated" (Howard Community College 2016:n.p.). Often people become very concerned about a moral problem involving behaviors such as drug use, crime, or rampant sexual activity. Their high level of concern may not be justified or based on reality. An excellent example of moral panic was a concern that motivated the Prohibition movement in the early 20th century.

This movement was led primarily by rural Protestants who viewed drinking as a moral and social sin. They became fearful that American society was on a path of destruction unless alcohol was banned entirely. Other American moral panics include one over marijuana in the 1930s (see Goode and Ben-Yehuda 2009) and Latinx street gangs in the 1980s (Zatz 1987). A moral panic arises when an individual or group, frequently a minority or subculture, such as those possibly infected with COVID-19, is perceived as a threat to society.

Other mass panics, or as some scholars label them, mass or collective hysterias, have been documented that relate directly to perceived illness. Stahl and Lebedun (1974) studied how female co-workers were overcome with physical symptoms due to a perception that an invisible gas was present in their workplace that made them ill. According to Stahl and Lebedun, no evidence of gas was ever discovered, which suggested that the workers had imagined a gas. Some workers displayed medical symptoms of being ill due to a gas, although no gas existed. The power of suggestion and group contagion underlined the workers' symptoms, as no medical cause could be identified. Workers dissatisfied with work were more likely to have had medical symptoms. The findings suggested that the group's influence on the workers resulted in medical symptoms. In 2013, 93 female high school students rapidly developed various medical symptoms, such as abdominal pain, headache, chest pain, body aches, nausea, and fatigue after eating cake. After consuming the cake, a mass panic resulted in students' hospitalization. After a review, no organic explanation was found for the reported illnesses (Tardier et al. 2016). The only trigger appeared to be eating the cake, which the students said smelled different (for a discussion and other examples, see Boss 1997).

Regardless of the source of mass panic, all provide the basis for generalized beliefs. Miller (2014:108) wrote, "Collective behavior is based on generalized beliefs—simplistic and emotionally provoking explanations of an ambiguous situation created by structural strain." Generalized beliefs eliminate ambiguity by creating an object, such as the coronavirus, that is sure to harm or destroy anyone in its path. During a mass panic, prior social definitions, expectations, and relationships are upset by a sense of impending doom or concern for catastrophic consequences. Although these beliefs generate fear, they also provide social predictability and structure.

Mass panics are not always limited to group threats. For example, the run on household supplies during the earlier stages of the pandemic could be considered a mass panic. The fear of not having enough food, gasoline, cleaning supplies, and toilet paper motivated some to hoard these items. Sociologically, the sense of shared identity ("We are all in this together") may be diminished when others are perceived as competitors for necessities, such as toilet paper. Media images of empty shelves, weakened supply chains, and rumors can lead to panic buying. The definition of the situation becomes that everyone else is looking out for themselves. This results in others panicking and doing the same dysfunctional panic buying. Van Bavel, Baicker, Boggio, et al. (2021:462) observed, "They [panics] can foster the very individualism and competitiveness that turns sensible preparations into dysfunctional stockpiling and undermine the sense of collective purpose which facilitates people supporting one another during an emergency." Notions of sharing goods and services for the collective whole of the community become sacrificed for self-serving goals.

There are two polarized schools of thought regarding whether the pandemic is a justified mass panic (moral panic). One view is that COVID-19 is a serious public health threat that requires major efforts, such as lockdowns, mask-wearing, closures, vaccinations, and other measures to control its spread. This view stresses the risk of serious health consequences and the possibility of death for at-risk populations. People holding this perspective did not view America's response as an unjustified panic but rather as a necessary, albeit limited, response to a genuine danger.

In contrast are people who saw the pandemic as overblown and exaggerated. For some, COVID-19 was perceived as a non-serious threat and society overreacted (see chapter 7). Some authors capitalized on hysteria and characterized the pandemic as a massive hysterical response (see Siegel 2020) or a mass panic (Frijters et al. 2021). Skeptics and conspiracy theorists have downplayed the seriousness of the virus. For example, Siegel (2020) focused on the amount of fear generated by COVID-19. He observed that the fear generated by SARS (2003) was unjustified, as the predicted pandemics never materialized. In the same vein, he concluded, the news media exaggerated the threat of COVID-19. This definition of the situation was bolstered by the fact that some COVID-19-infected individuals had mild symptoms or were asymptomatic. Siegel and others view the fear of the pandemic as unjustified compared to the actual health risks and mortality rates. They see some of the responses to COVID-19 as unnecessary and damaging to individuals, their rights, and society. They believe the stress and strain of over-responding to COVID-19 significantly affected people's physical and mental health. They characterized measures to prevent COVID-19 as further evidence of mass hysteria or panic. Being a mass "hysteria," some opponents have suggested that government policies harm public health (Bagus et al. 2021).

Mass hysteria makes people convinced they have been or will be exposed to something dangerous. They believe the threat is real because someone said so or because of their own experiences. Bagus et al. (2021) noted that any perceived threat, whether real or imaginary, can cause collective anxiety. When this anxiety results in physical symptoms, it is considered an epidemic hysteria or mass psychogenic illness. They provide examples of mass hysterical behaviors. They wrote (2021:4):

> At least some anecdotal evidence points to the possibility of mass hysteria as manifested by the hoarding of toilet paper and other essentials, the masked driving of single persons in their cars, and people virtually not leaving their houses, not even for a walk, even though the risk of being infected outdoors with physical distancing is minuscule.

Those viewing the response to the pandemic as an overreaction and opposed to restrictions and mandates rest one of their arguments on the low mortality rates due to COVID-19. For example, the following CDC data makes the basic point that the chances of dying from COVID-19 are remote (see also discussion on COVID-19 mortality rates in chapter 1.).

COVID-19 SURVIVAL RATES BY AGE IN THE UNITED STATES

Age	*Survival Rate*
0–19 Years	99.997%
20–49 Years	99.98%
50–69 Years	99.5%
70+ Years	94.6%

Source: Centers for Disease Control and Prevention Planning Scenarios (2021), Updated March 2021. Note: The CDC changed the presentation of these 2019 data to a different format than the 2021 data, which presents deaths per million for various scenarios. The updated 2021 data does not show survival rates, so the reader has to reverse-calculate actual deaths per million by age to know the survivability rate. Conspiracy theorists might suggest this data presentation was a manipulation by the CDC.

Without question, the statistical odds of dying from COVID-19 are low, except for people with prior conditions or who are older. Undoubtedly, some people have undue strain because of COVID-19, and critics have commented on the health risks of overreacting to COVID-19. However, there are a few other statistics to consider. First, total deaths due to COVID-19 have been much higher than seasonal influenza deaths. In 2020, an estimated 20,000 Americans died from influenza (CDC 2022c). The number dying from influenza ranges close to this yearly and occasionally double depending on the strain, vaccination rates, and other factors. Keep in mind that influenza and COVID-19 deaths are underreported. Over the same span of years, the number of reported COVID-19-related deaths was 385,676 in 2020 and 463,210 in 2021. Compared to an average of 20,000 influenza deaths over these two years, the COVID-19 death ratio was 19 and 23 times greater than the flu.

A fundamental moral question is an "acceptable" number of deaths for any disease. Does a proper figure rest at 10,000; 100,000; 1,000,000; or higher? If a death touches an individual and a family, the acceptable number is likely close to being one. Finally, the long-term effects of COVID-19 are currently unknown and may play out over the life span of survivors as shorter life expectancies. On average, life expectancies during the pandemic have shortened, especially for minorities (see chapter 2).

Rothwell and Desai (2020) conducted a study of public perceptions of the severity of the pandemic and identified some of the economic consequences of overestimating the seriousness of the pandemic. As part of their study, they asked what percentage of people infected by COVID-19 required hospitalization. Only 18 percent guessed between 1 and 5 percent, which is the correct range. Another 35 percent said at least 50 percent of infections required hospitalization. They attribute overestimating to misinformation provided by the media. In addition, the researchers found that Democrats were more likely than Republicans to overestimate the seriousness of COVID-19. Republicans were more likely to give the correct estimate of hospitalizations than Democrats.

SELF-FULFILLING PROPHECY AND NOCEBO EFFECT

The concepts of self-fulfilling prophecy and the nocebo effect help interpret some social behaviors during the pandemic. Around 1948, the sociologist Robert K. Merton formulated the concept of "self-fulfilling prophecy." The concept is much older and originates from an observation put forth by W. I. Thomas that "if men [and women] define situations as real, they are real in their consequences." Self-fulfilling prophecies are evident in many ways with COVID-19. For example, when the public heard the prediction that there might be supply shortages of some items, such as hand sanitizers and COVID-19 tests, they tried to buy these items beyond their needs and thus created the predicted shortages. Such panic-driven buying became a self-fulfilling prophecy leading to actual shortages of the products. This was a self-fulfilling prophecy. In addition, hoarding items, such as food and hygiene products, further contributed to a self-fulfilling prophecy (Baddeley 2020).

The self-fulfilling prophecy can also frame American responses to the pandemic. Some Americans defined the pandemic as real. Its consequences have been real for them. For them, living with a real pandemic has changed the way they go about their lives. Social distancing, wearing masks, getting vaccinated, and otherwise complying with public health directives and recommendations. For those who define the pandemic as unreal, a hoax, or overblown, to the extent they could, they behaved differently, resisting public health restrictions and recommendations. These responses are consistent with the concept of the definition of the situation.

The nocebo effect is related to self-fulfilling prophecy (Bagus et al. 2021). The nocebo effect is different from the better-known placebo effect. The placebo effect is the concept that people's expectations influence their behaviors. Industrial psychologists and medical researchers have found that giving people attention and telling them what to expect can have positive outcomes. For example, during clinical trials of drugs, some experiment participants get the drug being tested, and others get a placebo (fake pill) that has no medical value. Then the placebo (fake) and real medication pill groups are compared to see if any benefits occur for both groups. In some cases, those who took the placebo improved because they believed they took the real medical pill. Some research subjects may report or display improved health, although the pill they took had no medical value. This is the placebo effect in that if people believe it will work, it does.

In contrast is the nocebo effect, when people become ill because they expect to become ill (see Colloca 2017). Bagus, Peña-Ramos, and Sánchez-Bayón (2021:4; see also Howick and Ongaro 2020) applied the nocebo effect to COVID-19 and the pandemic and commented:

> Due to the nocebo effect, the expectation of becoming ill can cause real symptoms in a self-fulfilling prophecy. In this way, a mass hysteria may develop when people believe they will become ill. Anxiety and fear contribute to this process. Indeed, during the Spanish flu in the wake of World War I, panic contributed to mass hysteria and deaths that otherwise would not have occurred because panic can have adverse health effects on ill persons. Once some people develop a hysteria, it can easily spread to others because fear and anxiety are contagious.

The nocebo effect is important for COVID-19 pandemic deniers or those convinced that the public health response to COVID-19 has been too restrictive and unnecessary. The nocebo effect is not due to a COVID-19 infection but individual perceptions and emotional overreactions to what they wrongfully believe is caused by COVID-19.

NOTE ON DISASTER RESPONSES

When disasters occur, there is a common belief that people panic, act in selfish ways, and may place others at risk. Without question, some people do act selfishly during disasters and emergencies. A considerable body of collective behavior research has been conducted on social responses to disasters, such as floods, hurricanes, earthquakes, fires, and other natural calamities. To this list could be added the pandemic (see Walby 2021, 2022). The vast volume of this research has concluded that disasters often bring out the best in people—many examples of altruism surface under challenging times. For example, in addition to neighbors helping neighbors with food banks, rental assistance, and support, medical care providers' altruistic and self-sacrificing acts demonstrated how people care for each other in challenging circumstances. Because disaster threats and experiences are shared, collective adversity can generate social solidarity. When people provide emotional, material, financial, physical, and other support for each other, new social bonds and relationships are created. Matthewman and Huppatz (2020:677) provided reasons for why people provide support during disasters and crises. They wrote:

> This outpouring of goodwill should not surprise us. First, disasters are essentially social phenomena. Threats and experiences of such are public and shared. Collective adversity creates social solidarity. This bonds people, providing the basis for physical and emotional support. We are all in this together. Second, collective action can be further encouraged as current power structures are nowhere near as robust as is commonly thought. The realisation that official assistance is seldom in the right place at the right time in sufficient numbers gives civil society a boost. Third, we are essentially social beings. We cannot exist alone. We are products of culture and collective labour. We are, to a degree unknown among any other species, remarkably altruistic.

Summarizing years of research on social responses to disasters, Marx and McAdam (1994:65) concluded, "Most disaster behavior can be seen as an effort at solving all the problems under atypical conditions. Individual responses to natural disasters are more likely to involve heightened rationality and altruism, rather than their opposites." With the COVID-19 pandemic, a shared identity and concern for others surfaced. This was most evident with the wearing of masks to protect the vulnerable. While masks offered the wearer some protection, masks were more beneficial to other people, particularly older people. Helping people get health care, housing, and food, helping shut-ins, or meeting other needs, several communities, their residents, and healthcare providers aided others. The national and local media presented many examples of neighbors and communities rising to help those impacted by the pandemic.

COLLECTIVE BEHAVIOR AS AROUSED EMOTION

Social disruption and uncertainty of the pandemic can give rise to emotional responses that may conflict with reality. There is an emotional component to COVID-19 that is similar to other pandemics. An enduring feature of collective behavior is that mobs, crowds, protests, social media, panics, and movements often have emotional components. For example, resistance to the 1918 influenza pandemic differed markedly from COVID-19. Most people complied with public health guidance in 1918. With a few exceptions, people wore masks and did not resist treatment. The infected were isolated (socially distanced) without much public resistance. There were anti-mask groups during the 1918 influenza pandemic, but for the most part, the vast majority feared the disease enough to comply with restrictions. With COVID-19, the emotions of some individuals appear to be polarized. That is, passion regarding restrictions, mandates, and vaccines have run high. Emotions play out in important ways, whether one conforms to or resists public health measures to control the pandemic.

Emotions often influence group and individual perceptions of risk and, sometimes, are more important than factual information (Van Bavel, Baicker, Boggio, et al. 2021). Making good health decisions depends on accurate perceptions of the costs and benefits of specific choices for oneself and society. Van Bavel et al. (2021) concluded that people with strong emotions might ignore important numerical information about the risk and scope of the problem, in this case, COVID-19. Within collective behavior, social scientists have acknowledged the role emotions can play. Miller (2014:11) summarized, "Clearly, there is a long-standing tradition which identifies collective behavior as a spontaneous social behavior directed by aroused and extreme emotion that distorts people"s normal critical abilities and exaggerates their normal likes, dislikes, and loyalties." For example, the role of emotions can be observed in the behaviors of people in crowds. Crowds can intensify people's attraction to particular objects and activities, such as for or against vaccinations. People do things in crowds they would not normally do. Crowds can distort people's critical abilities. People lose their inhibitions and sense of caution and act in ways they would not if they were alone. The emotions in crowds during the pandemic may exaggerate or underestimate the degree of the COVID-19 threat resulting in over- or under-reactions. These emotional reactions include prejudice, discrimination, social isolation, hampered interpersonal relations, and increased mental health issues.

To elaborate further, Brafman and Brafman's best-selling book *Sway* (2008) underscores the importance of emotions in decision-making. The central question addressed by the book is how emotions pull individuals and groups into irrational behaviors, sometimes with devastating consequences. They identify several cases, such as airline pilot judgments being hampered by emotional factors to make grievous errors resulting in significant loss of lives. Brafman and Brafman (2008:17) propose factors such as "loss aversion (our tendency to go great lengths to avoid possible losses), value attribution (our inclination to imbue a person or thing with certain qualities based on initial perceived value), and the diagnosis bias (our blindness to all evidence that contradicts our initial assessment of a person or situation)." Take aversion to loss as an example. During the Vietnam War, when it became clear the war was being lost, and the possibility of a victory was remote, the United States committed more troops to the losing effort. Similarly, the war in Afghanistan led to massive expenditures and the loss of troops in a bottomless pit. The avoidance of admitting defeat resulted in even more significant commitment and ultimately greater losses.

Brafman and Brafman (2008:30) also wrote of the persuasive pull of commitment, "We have all experienced a pervasive pull of commitment in some form or another; whether we have invested our time and money in a particular project report or our energy into a doomed relationship, it is difficult to let go even when things clearly aren't working."

The pull of commitment has played out on both sides of the pandemic. For those vested in COVID-19 prevention strategies, they were all in. Although inconvenient, most Americans wanted to be vaccinated and were willing to isolate and wear masks. Nevertheless, a minority of others resisted vaccinations and mask-wearing regardless of the proven benefits. Some resisters (around 25%) became unreachable despite public health efforts to increase the vaccinated numbers and undeniable proof that vaccines effectively reduced the risk of serious infections and, in some cases, death. They relied more on their emotions than facts to make personal health decisions.

Many of Brafman and Brafman's points on the role of emotions in decision-making (see chapter 4) apply to the pandemic. For example, take the effectiveness of hydroxychloroquine and ivermectin as treatments for COVID-19. Although the clinical proof of either's effectiveness was never established, some public figures and individuals continued to believe both drugs worked despite having no evidence. This is an example of people's emotions overpowering any evidence that contradicts their initial assessment of the situation, which in this case was two ineffective drugs. Emotions drove perceptions that both drugs had more medicinal value than they did. Finally, those pushing the use of both drugs for COVID-19 never publicly admitted defeat or their erroneous comments when contrary medical evidence was provided, which is consistent with what Brafman and Brafman suggested in their book.

Finally, Siegel (2020:217) made the following comment about emotions and tied it to world health:

> One thing we had not learned was to distinguish between emotion-driven responses and careful reasoning. We had never learned this and perhaps we can't. Perhaps our brains aren't programmed this way. We certainly have learned or should've learned that we are all in this together, we are part of the global health community.

COVID-19 AND CROWDS

Understanding crowds can help understand the pandemic. A crowd is an assembly of people who join with a shared purpose or intent and influence one another. Characteristics of crowds include that they can be distinguished from organizations, are temporary, are constantly developing and changing, and consist of a large number of people. Crowds can distort people's critical thinking. The sociologist Herbert Blumer identified five types of crowds: casual, conventional, expressive, protest, and acting. The motives of crowds differ, with some motivated by fear, joy, or anger. Of particular interest in understanding the pandemic are protest crowds. A protest crowd is a group of people gathered to protest a political, social, cultural, or economic issue (McPhail and Wohlstein 1983). Groups of people participating in marches, rallies, sit-ins, or demonstrations are examples of protest crowds. In addition, some crowds are diffuse and scattered across large distances. For example, the users of social media platforms could be considered a diffuse crowd.

Theories of collective behavior, in the case of crowds, generally fall into three schools of thought. The earliest theory is called the contagion theory. In 1896, Gustave LeBon proposed a contagion theory of collective behavior that held crowds have a hypnotic influence over their members. When this influence was combined with anonymity, irrational and emotional behavior in crowds would result. Today, LeBon's ideas have fallen out of favor and have not been supported by crowd research. It would be over a century and a half before modern communications and social media would shape the nature of crowds in ways unforeseen by LeBon. Social media platforms can accelerate dialogue and emotionality on any topic, including COVID-19. Today, the internet provides a sense of anonymity similar to what LeBon emphasized. Using the internet, individuals and groups of users can be very emotional and irrational, similar to LeBon's crowds of the late 19th century. Face-to-face participation is not necessary as it was in LeBon's time. Therefore, social contagion on the internet can and does occur.

Convergence theory suggests that crowd behavior is the product of similar-thinking individuals gathering together and is not an intrinsic characteristic of the crowd itself. The crowd's impact is less important than like-minded people gathering and reinforcing their views on issues. In the same way, emergent norm theory proposes that crowd behavior results from merging like-minded people, a sense of anonymity from being in a crowd, and shared emotions. With the pandemic, there have been clear patterns where like-minded individuals and groups have coalesced over rumors, myths, and conspiracy theories.

The phenomenon of homophily is related to the underlying concept of convergence. Homophily is the principle that contact between similar (like-minded) people occurs more often than among dissimilar people (McPherson et al. 2001). As a result, people form more lasting relationships with like-minded people. Homophily is a human tendency to form relationships (link up) with others in ways that confirm and reinforce rather than challenge their core values and beliefs. Tang and Liu (2010:20) described homophily as: " . . . we are more likely to connect to others sharing certain similarities with us, and similar people tend to become friends, leading to similar behavior between connected egos in a social network." Later they added, "In a connected environment, an individual's behaviors tend to be interdependent, influenced by the behaviors of friends. This naturally leads to behavior correlation between connected users." McPherson et al. (2001:415) wrote, "The result is that people's networks are homogeneous about many sociodemographic, behavioral, and intrapersonal characteristics." They added, "Homophily limits people's social worlds in a way that has powerful implications for the information they receive, the attitudes they form, and the interactions they experience."

A way to conceptualize homophily is to view it as an echo chamber where everyone interacting simply repeats and confirms what participants already believe. Communications reflect the shared opinions of the members of the group. Members of like-minded groups take cues from others on how to interpret and behave. Members validate and confirm rather than openly discuss or question ideas. The group treats falsehoods as truth if they reinforce pre-existing beliefs. Ideas come from central authorities that typically do not rebut conspiracy theories but support them if they conform to the group's shared beliefs. Notions of what is right or wrong spring from central authorities, such as podcasts, biased news commentators, politicians, and social media platforms. In the case of the pandemic, these biased sources of rumors, inaccurate information, and conspiracy theories echoed what audiences wanted to hear based on their pre-existing political beliefs. Commonly known is that repeated messages, over and over, become real in the minds of people. When repeated enough times, people come to believe the message.

Demographic characteristics, such as race, ethnicity, religion, age, level of education, gender, age cohort, social status, geographical proximity, and, increasingly, political orientation, all can be criteria for homophilous relations to form. These demographic factors were identified decades ago as status homophily, a gathering of people based on similar characteristics (Lazarsfeld and Merton 1954). These characteristics are often the same factors that stratify society. A second type, value homophily, is based on shared values. Value homophily shapes people's orientation toward society and the future. Social media firms' (Facebook, Twitter, etc.) use of algorithms to track user preferences helps ensure that newsfeeds match people's pre-existing beliefs and values (see Zinelonka 2021). In the case of COVID-19, political polarization has fueled value homophily regarding mandates and the role of government in addressing the pandemic. Whether supportive or opposed, camps of people received information regarding COVID-19 and policies that supported the pre-existing beliefs of like-minded people.

During the pandemic, virtual crowds have formed on social media platforms and the internet. Virtual crowds assume some features of traditional face-to-face crowds, such as critical thought going by the wayside and emotions running higher. Social media platforms and the internet have changed the nature of homophily and facilitated its expansion during the pandemic. Individuals now have greater freedom and capability to create or join like-minded groups or "crowds" with the same values and views (for discussion, see McPherson, Smith-Lovin, and Cook 2001). Being geographically close together is no longer a requirement for joining like-minded crowds. Virtual crowds can draw memberships of like-minded individuals from across the country. Unfortunately, these virtual crowds can intensify hatred, promote misinformation, and advance conspiracy theories, as witnessed during the pandemic.

COVID-19 SOCIAL MOVEMENTS

Social movements are large groups of individuals or organizations focusing on specific political or social issues. There have been several social movements in American history, including civil rights, abolitionism, women's suffrage, the Tea Party, Greenpeace, global warming, political reform, LGBTQ rights, the Moral Majority, ecology, consumer rights, gun violence, alt-right, Black Lives Matter, and Prohibition. Social movements are an integral part of present-day American society and all democracies. Social movements can involve people who are widespread geographically and typically do not interact personally. Nevertheless, members of social movements share certain beliefs, values, and perceptions. For example, social movements have been present during the pandemic, including pros and cons for vaccines, lockdowns, social distancing, and other public health mandates.

Turner and Killian (1957) viewed social movements as semi-rational responses to abnormal conditions. Events occur that upset the status quo in some unexpected way. Social movements typically have a sense of injustice. Social movements form to make a change when people sense something in society is not correct. When existing social institutions are viewed as unable to respond to unexpected crises (pandemics), social movements may develop when collective action is needed. Social movements are organized efforts by many people to bring about or hamper social, economic, political, or cultural change. Social movements may strive to restore or replace the pre-existing social order with an alternative. In the case of the pandemic, some social movements wanted to restore American society to what it was before the pandemic. They wanted to lift restrictions and mandates. They do not have to be formally organized to be considered social movements, but some are. In some cases, social movements may form broad alliances with other social movements that share common purposes.

There are several ways to classify types of social movements. Perlstadt used a typology that classifies types of social movements into four categories based on the degree of change (limited or radical) desired and the focus on the individual/group or society. Perlstadt (2016:1049) described reformative social movements as advocating "for limited social change but seek to affect that change across an entire society. The change may be progressive toward new social relationships or institutions or retrogressively attempting to restore the *status quo ante*." Using Perlstadt's typology, the anti-mandate and mandate social movements seem best described as reformative. Both want to transform society on a limited basis, either returning to an America without mandates and restrictions or having mandates and restrictions to protect society by adjusting to a new way of life.

Social scientists have proposed that certain factors promote the development of social movements. However, these factors differ by what approach is used. From a structural strain perspective, Marx and McAdam (1994:78–81) identified factors that lead to the formation and development of social movements. These can be directly applied to the social movements observed during the pandemic. These include:

1. Structural conduciveness as people come to believe their society has problems. Examples from the pandemic include inequitable health care, the spread of COVID-19, the economic disruption from pandemic restrictions, and so forth.
2. Structural strain as people experience deprivation. With the pandemic, everyday life in America was disrupted, and Americans were deprived

of many social relationships, from going to work, attending school, or maintaining personal friendships. All of these changes for many Americans had an element of personal deprivation and sacrifice.

3. Solutions to problems people are experiencing are proposed and disseminated. During the pandemic, alternatives emerged, such as defying mandates and restrictions, seeking alternative treatments, or simply resisting.
4. Discontent often requires a specific event to turn it into a social movement. In the pandemic, several events served as catalysts ranging from misinformation from social media and the White House to later presidential policies mandating vaccines for large employers. In addition, proof of vaccination cards was a catalyst for some people, as were lockdowns of businesses and schools.

Certain conditions are more likely to give rise to social movements. For example, social movements arise out of social unrest and aroused emotions. Perlstadt (2016:1048) noted, "Social movements often arise in sudden changes and social unrest, becoming a source of spiritual and political empowerment." In times of social unrest, people are apprehensive, insecure, easily annoyed, have short attention spans, and are psychologically unstable. The social unrest in the United States can be witnessed by political polarization, an increasing gap between higher- and lower-income Americans, and strained foreign relations with traditional allies. In addition, obvious racist events, such as white supremacist protests, police shootings of Black Americans, and agitators in the media promoting controversy over facts, are evidence of social unrest. For COVID-19, it was a perfect storm. The preexisting social unrest provided yet another stage for discontent and unrest to flourish. Social movements for both compliance with and opposition to pandemic prevention efforts would quickly surface. In addition to these factors, others were present, such as people having free time to devote to favorite or important causes (Miller 2014).

During the pandemic, social media provided ample opportunities for those involved in social movements to further their causes. As a result, a few movements surfaced, such as the trucker convoys, but they were short-lived as the pandemic waned. Additionally, if a social movement is quickly and powerfully repressed, it may disappear. In the democratic United States, repression of pandemic-related social movements never occurred as in other countries, such as China. American society is dynamic and open to the freedom of expression, in some cases but not in others, and hence provides a context for dissent and compliance, both of which can mobilize people into social movements.

THEORIES OF SOCIAL MOVEMENTS

Social scientists have developed theories about social movements (see Miller 2014). One is deprivation theory which suggests that social movements appear when people believe they are deprived of specific goods or resources. Similarly, a mass-society theory proposes that social movements result from the marginalization of groups of people. When people, such as minority ethnic groups, believe they are marginalized (excluded) from mainstream society, they may form social movements.

Some social scientists suggest that resources are critical to why social movements occur. They place resources at the center of the formation and success of social movements. Labeled resource mobilization theory, it views knowledge, money, media, labor, solidarity, legitimacy, and internal and external support from a powerful elite as examples of resources.

Structural-strain theory proposes that social movements emerge due to structural conduciveness, structural strain, growth and spread of a solution, precipitating factors, lack of social control, and mobilization. Structural-strain theory can explain many of the political and socioeconomic conditions that have led to strain and, thus, the formation of social movements (see also chapters 1 and 8).

Finally, cultural theory stresses the importance of culture. This theory emphasizes the critical role of injustice in movement formation, stating that successful movements must create a strong sense of injustice to mobilize people to join social movements. It emphasizes the role a sense of injustice plays in social movement formation.

Evidence for any one or a combination of these theories can be found in the pandemic. For example, deprivation theory would explain why some groups, such as business owners, have organized and protested COVID-19 lockdowns. There is little doubt that lockdowns, social distancing, and other restrictions hampered many American businesses. The mass-society theory would point to how many people have been marginalized from mainstream everyday activities, such as attending school, shopping, or running a business. As a result, they may feel that they need to be heard by public health and government officials. Evidence for resource mobilization theory could lie in the support the government, non-profits, and drug companies have given to pro-vaccination social or public health movements (campaigns). Parents protesting school closures likely had concerns about how such measures negatively impacted their children and families.

Social movements use several tactics to achieve their objectives. First, they strategically use protests, social media statements, convoys, occupations of buildings, blockades, boycotts, marches, propaganda, and demonstrations to promote social change. Some of these efforts target populations of people to gain support or new members. In addition, these activities can draw attention to the issues and purposes of the social movement. Finally, public relations and marketing are a component of social movement events.

Some social movements endure and evolve into formal organizations and are labeled social movement organizations. Miller (2014:56) defined a social movement organization as "a complex and often formal organization that attempts to implement the goals of the social movement." For example, Robert F. Kennedy Jr.'s Children's Health Defense organization is an excellent example of a social movement organization that promotes anti-vaccination efforts. So, in contrast would be the Advertising Council's (Ad Council) social movement organization that has promoted COVID-19 vaccinations.

CONCLUDING OBSERVATIONS

Social stress occurs when there are no explicit norms or shared expectations, the effectiveness of norms has been undermined, or a social organization is lacking, ill-defined, or disrupted (see Lang and Lang 1961). As previously noted, recent political events, post-truth politics, polarization, mass shootings, substance abuse (opiates) on a grand scale, a widening gap between the upper- and lower-income groups, debates over immigration, climate change, inflation, a sense that some Americans act as if they are above the law, and other trends all contributed to gaps in the social structure (society). For example, political protocols and civility, once adhered to in Washington, DC, have been abandoned. Traditions, such as the civility in Congress and American society, the peaceful transition of power, and other traditional processes, are now uncommon. American politics is post-truth politics. Areas of discretion, once bounded by customs, conventions, norms, and laws, are more likely to be ignored or challenged. Internal divisions regarding American social life that center around perspectives on politics, religion, personal freedom, what is best for society, and how to treat others, among others, need to be more clearly defined than in the past. These and other factors create gaps filled by collective behaviors, such as protests, social movements, and rumors. Negative preexisting factors that divide Americans surfaced during the pandemic. Delanty (2021b:12) summarized, "Other responses to disease have revealed cultural pathologies, such as, for example, stigmatization, scapegoating, mass hysteria, and conspiracy theories." This is the situation with the pandemic.

All societies, including America, place social demands on individuals that are only sometimes followed. When individuals cannot meet these demands, alienation can occur. People become estranged from these social demands to the point where they are viewed as no longer valid or meaningful. Instead, social demands are viewed as being hostile and unjustified. When alienated individuals become aware that others share their perspectives, they may join like-minded groups to respond to social demands by non-conforming or actively resisting. For example, resistance to federal COVID-19 mandates and recommendations has led some to protest and form groups opposed to public health and government directives.

Several social science theories and concepts are valuable in understanding the social aspects of the COVID-19 pandemic. The stage for collective behaviors, such as rumors, protests, crowds, mass panic, conspiracy theories, social movements, and others, was set before the pandemic started. Social unrest, polarization, marginalization of groups, uncertainty stemming from COVID-19, and other factors fueled informal collective responses. Collective behavior concepts, such as that of rumor, find multiple examples in the context of the pandemic. Others, such as self-fulfilling prophecy and crowd formation, also can be observed throughout the pandemic. The point is that many lenses and concepts can be used to interpret pandemic social behavior. In the following chapters, many of these concepts and theories will be valuable tools for making sense of the pandemic.

Chapter 5

COVID-19 Social Behaviors and Trends

> "If you're thinking that the side effects from the shot are worse than the COVID,
>
> or that you can't just take a chance, you are just dead wrong."
>
> President Joseph Biden (June 2, 2021 White House Briefing)

SOCIAL CONSTRUCTION OF REALITY AND SOCIAL UNCERTAINTY OF COVID-19

Social scientists have proposed for decades that the amount of uncertainty is an important dimension for understanding social behavior and societies. Societies with high uncertainty tend to be those where members feel uncomfortable and social unrest is more likely to be present. People, in general, feel more comfortable when their lives are somewhat stable and predictable. Most people prefer routine over chaos, the familiar over unfamiliarity, and structure over disorder. When societies become disrupted, chaotic, and socially disorganized, social norms (rules that guide behavior) change, as do the daily patterns of social life. Without question, the COVID-19 pandemic has resulted in disruptions in everyday life, social disorder, chaos, and uneasiness. These have led to confusion and emotional and immediate responses as people have tried to adjust to pandemic living.

The COVID-19 pandemic removed a degree of control in American lives. For many Americans, the pandemic created chaos and social disorder. Some people believed that some pandemic developments were not controlled by anything. Pandemic restrictions and new social norms for public spaces, such as required mask-wearing and social distancing, impacted relationships and social activities. Ordinary activities were disrupted, such as going to a grocery store, meeting with friends, going to work, religious gatherings, traveling, dining out, and meeting in groups. These daily social behaviors operated under a new set of norms that limited the freedom and control many Americans had enjoyed.

People like to have some degree of control over their lives. Americans exercise control by making their own life decisions, such as where they live, what they do in their free time, whom they associate with, and how they live their lives. Americans sometimes label the ability to control their lives as freedom of choice. American freedom of choice includes the ability to have differing opinions and the opportunity to share those opinions. The latter is addressed in the United States Bill of Rights, referencing the pursuit of happiness, freedom of speech, and other provisions. During the pandemic, Americans have lost some of these individual freedoms in the interest of the greater good. COVID-19 mandates and restrictions are inconvenient and an imposition on lifestyles, personal liberties, and social relations. Ferreira, José Sá, Martins, and Serpa (2020:10) proposed that such restrictions and mandates had profound implications beyond public health and medical controlling of the pandemic. They noted that questions about individual freedom and human rights are raised but acknowledged that these measures were important to control the disease. They wrote (Ferreira et al. 2020:9):

> Another significant impact of this crisis is on the operating conditions of democracy. The response to the pandemic raises the restriction of freedom of movement, containment of activities, and the strengthening of the countries' executive powers. In some countries, the strategy of governments has been to annul democratic order, suspend the functioning of parliaments and attempt to govern by decree and trivialize exceptional symbolic resources—e.g., the use of the armed forces to control public order. The world is witnessing the consolidation of some features of technocratic authoritarianism, which is very present in China, namely the attraction of the electronic means of citizens' permanent surveillance—surveillance of contact networks and surveillance of infected people, among others.

Others have reached similar conclusions, such as Bagus, Peña-Ramos, and Sánchez-Bayón (2021), and Siegel (2020). In their view, violating fundamental human rights by imposing lockdowns, curfews, masks, social distancing, and closures of businesses may be unnecessary and detrimental to overall public health. Whether the restrictions are considered necessary or excessive, the enduring question is how to balance the "demands for individual autonomy with the community's need for safety" (Delanty 2021a:10).

The current social response to the COVID-19 pandemic did not occur in a historical vacuum. Various social factors have influenced the uncertainty of the pandemic and reactions to it. Instead, the social responses to the pandemic were shaped by social trends in the preceding decades. These trends include the loss of trust in institutions like government, science, and medicine, reduced critical thinking skills, non-reliance on facts, and a lack of responsibility and accountability for misinformation. The biological nature of the COVID-19 virus also has contributed to uncertainty.

UNCERTAINTY RESULTING FROM THE COVID-19 VIRUS

Human health responses to COVID-19 dramatically differ from mild reactions to death. Individuals, groups, and communities have varied susceptibility, immunity, and symptoms (see McNeill 1976: chapter 1). Some of these individual differences are due to hereditary, preexisting conditions, immune systems, and past exposures to invading organisms. Human populations constantly evolve to cope with infections by microorganisms, but some viruses also evolve. Although scientists have studied coronaviruses for years, the continually changing biological characteristics of the COVID-19 virus make it challenging to understand, predict, and plan for. Like other coronaviruses, the COVID-19 virus mutates into new variants and subvariants, each with differing characteristics. Medical experts knew that COVID-19 mutations were likely, but no one foresaw the impact of the Delta and Omicron variants.

From the beginning, world governments were challenged by the threat of COVID-19, and little was known about the virus and how it was spread (Offe 2021). In addition, there were no proven treatments or vaccines. Consequently, the general public had to rely on information from various sources, such as neighbors, social media platforms, news media, and the internet. They also relied on personal experiences with prior viruses, such as H1N1 and seasonal flu, and medical providers who needed to become more familiar with this new type of coronavirus. Many medical scientists and practitioners used seasonal flu to model estimates of and respond to COVID-19 (Benjamin et al. 2020).

Some countries in Asia took a proactive strategy while others in the developed West, such as the United States, and the World Health Organization moved slower. The pattern for Western countries with prior disease outbreaks was to help contain them locally and regionally in the areas of origin before reaching the developed West. This strategy had worked well for the SARS (2003), MERS (2012), and Ebola (2018–2020) virus outbreaks that were essentially limited to their regions of origin in Asia and Africa. Using major restrictions to contain COVID-19 worked well in some countries, such as

New Zealand and Taiwan, which embraced such measures and closed their borders. Public compliance was high in these countries with strong governmental mandates, such as lockdowns, border control, and mask-wearing.

COVID-19 poses a challenge unique from other pandemics because infections are only sometimes apparent, unlike other diseases. When individuals are infected and thus contagious, it is not always obvious to others. In comparison, individuals having smallpox, measles, chicken pox, or mumps display visible symptoms that let others know they are ill. This is only sometimes the case in the early stages of COVID-19. Some individuals are asymptomatic and show no signs of being contagious to others when they are. In addition, there is randomness with COVID-19 because of predicting how infected individuals will respond. Complicating matters is that some of the symptoms of COVID-19 are the same as influenza, common colds, allergies, and other commonplace illnesses. In addition, as noted in chapter 1, the COVID-19 virus is a moving target. The virus and its characteristics have changed, making it challenging to identify and control.

The uncertainty surrounding COVID-19 is important because the virus changes. Efforts to understand and control it have needed to change, sometimes unpredictably. This unpredictability leads to anxiety, as people want fixed and definitive answers. For example, business owners have been frustrated with local lockdowns and mask-wearing fluctuations. Secondly, a degree of uncertainty in everyday social interactions can result in tension, especially among strangers. This tension is elevated when individuals openly resist and defy COVID-19 restrictions, such as wearing masks in public. A degree of stress also exists when it comes to vaccination status. Without proof, judging whether another person has been vaccinated is difficult.

INDIVIDUALISM VERSUS THE COMMON GOOD

Globally, socio-cultural responses to the pandemic have varied. Zinn (2021) observed that during the pandemic's early stages, many democratic societies in Europe and the United States debated the topics of restrictions on civil rights and privacy concerns. These countries were reluctant to limit people's behaviors and movements. Although technologies were available to monitor and track the spread of COVID-19, these tools were rejected as a threat to democracy and individual freedom. However, in China and other Asian countries, many of these tools were implemented to control the pandemic successfully. Zinn believed the role of culture was influential in implementing restrictive but successful prevention measures. Some cultures, such as those in Asia, were more accustomed to complying with government directives and wearing face masks.

Others have echoed Zinn's assessment of the importance of culture. Van Bavel, Baicker, Boggio, et al. (2021) noted that Western and North American cultures embrace individualism in contrast to other cultures with a more substantial commitment to collective entities, such as the nation, tribe, and family. They (2021:463) outlined some critical cultural factors that applied to Asian countries during the pandemic:

> First, the priority given to obligations and duties in Asian societies may motivate individuals to remain committed to social norms while suppressing personal desires. Second, Asians may more readily recognize unobservable situational influences on viral infection, like herd immunity. Third, social norms and conventions in North America and much of Western Europe tend to positively value the expressivity of the self (for example, kissing, hugging, and direct argumentation) relative to Asia. This is another reason why interpersonal virus transmission could be more likely in independent cultures than in interdependent cultures. Another related dimension of cultural variance is a society's "tightness" vs. "looseness." Research has found that tight cultures, such as those of Singapore, Japan, and China, have strict social norms and punishments for deviance, while loose cultures, such as the US, Italy, and Brazil, have weaker social norms and are more permissive.

In the United States, individuals and groups both have rights. A group holds collective rights due to shared membership. Group rights have been used to infringe upon and facilitate individual rights. During the pandemic, public health restrictions have impinged on individual rights by stressing the rights of the collective whole. Both rights are foundational in the debate over COVID-19 mandates and restrictions. Although there has been self-sacrifice, most Americans have complied with pandemic mandates and restrictions and getting vaccinated. They have sacrificed personal freedoms for the safety of themselves and others. They have made the greater good a higher priority than their interests. For example, by 2022, over 70 percent of Americans had been vaccinated. Medical experts have consistently noted that vaccinations are the best control of COVID-19. The more people vaccinated, the greater the odds of eliminating or at least controlling it, and the negative impact reduced. However, others have held fast to their resistance to vaccinations and other preventative measures. To some, the balance between individual choice and the benefit of the greater good tips in favor of the individual. An American cultural value is the freedom of choice. Americans pride themselves on the value of individualism and freedom of choice. They prefer to choose whether to be vaccinated or to follow restrictive mandates. Individualism, coupled with a distrust of and resistance to authority, forms some basis for opposition to pandemic control measures. Early in the pandemic, conservative commentator David Brooks (2020:n.p.) shared the following perspective on the issue:

> Aside from a few protesters and a depraved president, most of us have understood that we need to suspend the old individualistic American creed. Amid a complex epidemiological disaster, to be anti-authority is to be ignorant. Amid a contagion, to act as if you are self-sufficient is just selfish.

Notably, crises and emergencies, such as the pandemic, are not favorable to democratic processes and individual rights (Walby 2021). During the pandemic, COVID-19 infections spread so rapidly across the globe that elected officials and their appointees had little time to make policy decisions following democratic principles. To do so would have resulted in potentially higher infection and death rates. Time was of the essence. As Delanty (2021b:15) argues, democratic government "requires time for deliberation, but pandemics and other catastrophes require rapid action that can produce long-term unanticipated consequences." Democratic processes do not adjust well to the rapid decision-making pandemics and crises require. Public officials need to make quick decisions based on limited information. It is not efficient or possible to thoroughly evaluate every decision. Authorities and subject matter experts make decisions that may not represent the public's or elected officials' wishes.

The American emphasis on individualism has been present in its culture long before the pandemic. American examples of the expression of individualism have been numerous over the decades. One example of individualism can be witnessed in the counterculture of the 1960s and 1970s. During these decades, the youth counterculture stressed the values of self-determination, individual freedom of lifestyle, choice, and a distrust of authority.

The counterculture movement of the 1960s and 1970s rejected mores, values, and norms of mainstream society. Most hippies came from White middle-class backgrounds. They rebelled against many aspects of their experiences, such as having traditional careers and materialism. They challenged some central values of the "American Way of Life." Most hippies were not involved in politics, but some were active in the anti–Vietnam War effort. They constructed a lifestyle that was marginalized from mainstream society, and in this vein, some experimented with communal living and holistic medicine. They promoted nonviolence, love, openness, and tolerance compared to middle-class lifestyle restrictions. They lived for today, and doing their own thing was a way of life free from unnecessary restrictions, such as those imposed by government or business. They were nonconformists in many ways, such as in music, clothing, appearance, and values. These rebellious ideas and lifestyles would carry on to future generations.

Some counterculture movement values and norms may have impacted American cultural responses to COVID-19. Alternative lifestyles and cultures were interwoven into the movement. For some in the movement, naturalism in diet and lifestyle was important. Natural foods and self-administered health care, such as herbal teas and treatments, became more prominent. The hippie counterculture introduced the *Whole Earth Catalog* and other naturalistic ideas about life. One of the mottos of the counterculture movement was "Do your own thing."

Nevertheless, more important was the counterculture push to question authority and the status quo. In general, counterculture adherents (hippies) did not automatically buy into conventional lifestyles but created their subculture that questioned authority. The counterculture movement, the Vietnam War, environmental issues, and world peace were important causes worthy of protests. The government became looked upon with suspicion and could not be trusted. Personal choice and liberty, and the questioning of the government's intrusion into the lives of individuals, all became key perspectives that would surface and be institutionalized by the counterculture lifestyle.

The 1960s and 1970s counterculture values and perspectives surfaced during the pandemic. Those individuals in opposition to restrictions or mandates, the lack of choice, doing one's own thing, and rejecting authority may have philosophical roots in the counterculture of the hippies. The positions and values held by those in opposition to public health dictates and government interventions would sound remarkably familiar to those of the counterculture movement. The freedom of self-determination and questioning of authority would underpin some individual and group resistance to controlling COVID-19. For example, in reacting to COVID-19 mask requirements for schoolchildren, some parents would say it is a matter of parental choice on what is best for their children and not the government's. They would not realize that the foundation for their autonomy and choice is partly in the counterculture movements of their parents or grandparents formulated in the 1960s and 1970s.

Americans like to selectively apply individual liberty to those causes that reflect their values. For example, the Second Amendment is seen by some Americans as a personal right to bear arms. Likewise, some pro–gun rights individuals seek to limit a woman's right over her body regarding abortion. Individual choice and freedom are a mixed bag for many Americans, depending on what choice or freedom is being considered. This point was witnessed with the pandemic.

EROSION OF TRUST IN INSTITUTIONS

The questioning of authority and distrust of government and institutions would underpin some of the social responses to COVID-19. An institution is a set of beliefs, practices, rules, positions, and organizations that cluster around a particular function or need. Examples of institutions include the family, education, economy, and government. Hand in hand with the counterculture movement of the 1960s and 1970s was a general alienation from authority and declining trust in institutions.

Survey data have found that Americans' trust in science, government, and medicine has declined over the past decades. Trust and reliance on institutional knowledge have become less valued, trusted, or respected. Family, religion, education, government, and medical institutions do not carry the same influence that they did for prior generations. Alienation from authority is the unwillingness to accept guidance from institutions, such as the government or the scientific community. One form of this alienation is moral indignation, which need not be directly vented on the authority, but may be diverted to substitute targets. For example, institutions such as the CDC, public health agencies, and pharmaceutical companies, and Dr. Fauci became targets of alienated groups. The conspiracy website InfoWars was critical of Dr. Fauci's leadership, competence, and decision-making (Zielonka 2021).

Evidence suggests that public distrust of institutions preexisted the pandemic. For example, two linked surveys were conducted by Priniski and Holyoak in 2020, early in the pandemic. The surveys focused on beliefs about the severity of COVID-19 and related topics. They found that distrust of Democratic politicians and medical scientists existed before the pandemic, and additional factors that emerged following the first wave were linked to what they labeled "auxiliary beliefs." Examples of auxiliary beliefs during the pandemic are abundant (see chapters 6 and 7). Skepticism about the severity of COVID-19 increased over time, as did anti-science attitudes and distrust of prominent medical organizations.

It should be noted that American institutions have earned some of this public distrust. Major examples include the history of the Catholic Church covering up cases of child sexual maltreatment. Pharmaceutical companies were not disclosing the dangers of but promoting the use of opiates. The eugenics movement by pseudo-scientists in the 1930s justified racism and classism and the tobacco industry was reluctant to acknowledge the health risks of cigarette smoking. Law enforcement agencies failing to disclose or address officer misconduct. Countless denials of the environmental damage resulting from resource extraction and manufacturing. All of these and others have promoted a public distrust of institutions. To this list could be added all of the conspiracy theories that have flooded American society.

TRUST IN SCIENCE

Science uses facts (evidence) that are replicable, confirmed, and validated by others, such as experts in the field (peer-reviewed). The scientific method is objective and does not rely on predetermined outcomes but reports on what the evidence and not opinion indicates. Science relies on methods that provide substantial evidence (proof) that something is true and accurate. The goal of the scientific method is to find the objective truth. Once a statement or fact has been scientifically validated, the research findings can be trusted. Over the centuries, the evolution of science and scientific findings have brought about significant social progress.

In contrast, these are subjective opinions that rely on personal beliefs, superstitions, predetermined outcomes, political agendas, or emotions. Any group or individual can communicate ideas, beliefs, claims, or evidence that may or may not be accurate. Some statements or assertions are less about facts and evidence and more about the motives, such as political appeal, values, or beliefs. Some Americans (individuals and groups) have abandoned science because they do not understand how it differs from biased opinions or does not support their views or motives. Science may or may not support political objectives or provide popular answers to controversial issues. Although science has brought value to societies and human progress, national surveys report that trust in science has decreased over time, and some groups are inclined not to believe science or its findings. Ironically, much of the distrust in science is facilitated by scientific-technological advances, such as smartphones, social media, et cetera.

The decline of confidence and trust in science can be attributed to several factors. One factor is the decline in governmental support for science. Science has been under recent political and financial attacks. Recently, some elected officials have discredited science when it has reached conclusions that do not conform to or support political positions. One way to sanction science is to publicly contradict it, label it "fake," or rely on pseudoscience, which does not adhere to scientific methods. Take climate change as an example. Evidence is abundant that climate change is altering weather patterns across the globe. Nevertheless, some elected officials have denied this scientific evidence and declared it a "hoax" because it does not conform with their political agendas. They employ denialist strategies to downplay what the world can observe directly.

Recent federal reductions in financial support for science reflect a shift in thinking and policy. Since the beginning of the 20th century, many Americans have viewed science as crucial to social progress. This was particularly true during the years following the end of World War II and the Cold War. When the Russians launched Sputnik 1 on October 4, 1957, many Americans were concerned that the United States was losing the scientific race to space. The concern about falling behind the Soviet Union led to the establishment of the National Aeronautics and Space Administration (NASA). On September 12, 1962, President Kennedy challenged the United States to land a man on the moon before 1970. On July 20, 1969, Apollo 11 would successfully land two men on the moon's surface. Americans' trust in science and appreciation of science seemed to be at a high point, but today this trust has declined for some Americans.

Some have credited former president Trump, as a national leader, with bad American science. They contend that the president had undermined science and scientific institutions. For example, *Nature* magazine published a timeline regarding former president Trump's actions related to science (Tollerson 2020). In 2017, the president attempted to cut funding for the National Institutes of Health and banned key scientists from serving on advisory boards. Re-establishing scientific integrity in agencies where government scientists have been sidelined and censored by political appointees will not be easy, says Andrew Rosenberg, who heads the Center for Science and Democracy at the Union of Concerned Scientists, an advocacy group based in Cambridge, Massachusetts. The center has documented more than 150 attacks on science under president Trump's tenure. "Under Trump, political appointees have the authority to override science whenever they want if it does not conform to their political agenda," Rosenberg said. "You can reverse that, but you have to do it intentionally and directly" (cited by Tollerson 2020).

In recent years, scholars have tried to understand the trend toward rejecting science, which has been likened to a war. Sabin (2022) reviewed an assessment of the trend of dismissing science undertaken by Aviva Philipp-Muller and her associates. Sabin cited Philipp-Muller:

> "If you come to conclusions through gut instincts or listening to people that do not know about a topic, you can come to believe just about anything," she says. "Sometimes it can be dangerous for society when people believe wrong things. We have seen this in real-time, as some people have rejected COVID-19 vaccines not for scientific reasons but through nonscientific means." (Sabin 2022:n.p.)

Sabin (2022:n.p.) summarized what Aviva Philipp-Muller and her co-authors identified as four primary reasons why people reject science:

- People refuse to believe the messenger—If the people providing scientific information, such as Fox News or CNN, are viewed as not credible,

biased, lack expertise, or have agendas, their scientific messaging may be rejected.
- Pride creates prejudice—People who build their identities on labels or associate with social groups may dismiss any information that threatens or challenges that identity. For example, people belonging to a group whose identity focuses on anti-government or anti-science will oppose both if they believe their views are underrepresented or are being exploited.
- It is hard to beat long-held beliefs—People find it difficult to let go of them. When information and evidence go against long-held beliefs, people tend to reject or ignore that information. The easiest path for them is to reject contradictory information. As noted elsewhere, people do not put much energy into updating information but fall back on previous beliefs. For example, some people continue to believe COVID-19 is spread by food or that MMR vaccines cause autism in children.
- Science does not always match how people learn—Scientific literature is often difficult for laypeople to understand. If information about COVID-19 is presented in too technical ways, many people will not understand it and are more likely to reject it. The old concept of "You can get statistics to prove anything" runs similarly. When information gets too technical, people tend not to value what it means.

FOLLOW THE SCIENCE DEBATE

"Follow the science" (or facts) has been a famous slogan during the pandemic. Government and public health officials have used it to support pandemic health responses, such as mask-wearing, lockdowns, and vaccines. Other countries like Great Britain have also taken this approach (Walby 2021). Research and scientific facts should guide decisions and public health policies during the pandemic. Policymakers have used this slogan to defend COVID-19 policies and practices. Walby (2021:29) observed, "The government position was that 'the science' supported the policy to reduce COVID and to learn to live with it, while the public health position was that the policy should be used to more vigorously suppress and even eliminate COVID."

While some authorities have embraced science and adopted the phrase "follow the science" or "follow the facts," others have criticized this approach. The problem is that sometimes science may be misleading (wrong), and unthinkingly following science eliminates dialogue and questioning. One commentator observed that society may be experiencing a near reversal of the Age of Enlightenment (see Larson 2020). Centuries ago, science was viewed as an escape from religious dogma, and now science has become a dogma in its own right. Some authorities contend that medical research on COVID-19 and corresponding vaccines has been inadequate and rushed. Some argue that scientific findings and recommendations have not been thoroughly reviewed, and contrary evidence has been repressed or censored if it contradicts government public health policies (Paul and Haddad 2023). They characterize the scientific community and the public as unthinkingly following science without reasonable questioning.

Russell and Patterson (2021) have argued that many of the policies regarding COVID-19 mask-wearing and school closings have been promulgated by "elites" who quickly dismissed counterarguments suggesting the benefit of these measures was questionable. They indicated that elites are motivated by personal gain and profit and convince the public to follow the science without having an appropriate discussion. Russell and Patterson suggested that following the science has evolved into a general response to populist objections, questions, and skepticism. Following the science, in their view, has locked public health officials into confrontations with a changing virus and fatigued public. Russell and Patterson (2021:n.p.) summarized their point of view:

> The simple, elite explanation for all our problems during the pandemic has been that the public failed to trust the experts and didn't "follow the science." This, they argue, is the result of tolerating too much skepticism, which is an ordinary feature of scientific debate. Instead, elites have openly embraced the notion that the public is better served by exaggeration, downplaying uncertainty, or even deception (such as in official estimates of herd immunity).

Evidence shows that unquestioning trust in science can lead to unwarranted faith in pseudoscience. The Annenberg Public Policy Center (2021b) reported that a recent study found that people who trust science are likelier to share false claims containing scientific references than those who do not. This pattern impacts public information on COVID-19. For example, COVID-19 vaccines have been characterized as having pollutants and dangerous ingredients by pseudoscientific sources. People who typically trust science have believed these claims based on what they believe to be scientific evidence when they (claims) are not. Put differently, people who trust science can be fooled by what they think is science.

O'Brien, Palmer, and Albarracin (2021) conducted a study of four samples of between 382 and 605 participants with varied degrees of trust in science to assess the validity of four studies. They found that for people who did not trust science, the presence of scientific content in any of the four studies did not significantly affect their confidence. However, people with higher trust in science were likelier to believe and share the studies. In a related research phase, people with critical mindsets were less likely to believe in pseudoscientific research, regardless of whether it sounded scientific. The Annenberg Public Policy Center (2021b:n.p.) cited one of the principal researchers of the study as commenting:

> People need to understand how science operates and arrives at its conclusions. People can be taught what sources of information to trust and how to validate that information. It is not just a case of trusting science, but being more critical and understanding how to double-check what information is really about.

The COVID-19 pandemic and the politicization of prevention measures, such as vaccination and mask-wearing, have highlighted the need for people to accept and trust science (Annenberg Public Policy Center 2021b). However, caution must be exercised because some research may appear scientific but is not.

Likewise, some scientists have reported being demonized for challenging scientific COVID-19 research findings. In a published opinion, associate professor of medicine Vinay Prasad and former dean of Harvard Medical School Jeffery S. Flier (2020) expressed concern that professional colleagues should not be demonized if they question scientific findings. Instead, they argued that having "vigorous" academic debate over research during the pandemic is even more critical. They characterized the current climate as one where research disagreements are attributed to political motives or ignorance. Instead, they call for a willingness to listen and consider ideas that initially may be wrong. They (Prasad and Flier 2020:n.p.), referring to COVID-19, research wrote:

> These critical decisions should be influenced by scientific insights independent of political philosophies and party affiliations. They must be freely debated in the academic world without insult or malice to those with differing views. Examining and disclosing conflicts of interest and salient biases is essential, but if none are apparent or demonstrated, the temptation to speculate about malignant motivations must be resisted.

Graso, Henwood, Aquino, Dolan, and Chen (2022) studied beliefs (faith) in COVID-19 science. In three studies involving 743 adults, they assessed respondents' views regarding COVID-19 science. They found how an individual's strong belief in science influenced their distrust of unmasked individuals and more robust support for more intensive pandemic mitigation mandates. They labeled this pandemic mitigation authoritarianism. Graso et al. contend that some respondents believed that public health experts are the only ones capable of handling the pandemic. Those believing firmly in COVID-19 science even thought unsupported claims still had merit, such as that wearing masks outdoors had medical benefits. They also found that both conservatives and liberals miscalculated the risk of COVID-19. Conservatives underestimated and Democrats overestimated the risks of COVID-19.

Finally, Zinn (2021) noted a danger in viewing science as a cure for all problems, including those in medical science. Although seeing science as a solution for all of the world's problems is appealing and provides a sense of progress, it can also be misleading, and societies may place too much trust in science. Zinn commented that a view of science as reliable, morally neutral, and always aiding social good is not always accurate. She argues that real science is based on humans with biases and whims. Zinn (2021:605) wrote, "The application of scientific discoveries to challenging healthcare problems is even more complex and even more likely to be waylaid by political needs, special interests, and incompetence."

Scientific knowledge cannot, as she noted, "replace responsibility for political decisions since science lacks the political compass and legitimacy" (Zinn 2021:605). Public health decisions, such as those for COVID-19, cannot solely be based on science. A political aspect of such decisions sometimes runs contrary to science. Politicians who defer to science (follow the science) when making tough pandemic policy decisions at the end of the day share some responsibility for those decisions. Good science that has been thoroughly vetted is necessary for good pandemic responses. The danger is when political considerations override solid science recommendations (see chapter 6).

NATIONAL SURVEYS ON PUBLIC TRUST AND VIEWS OF SCIENCE

What do national surveys indicate on public trust in science? A Pew Research Center survey of 10,260 adults conducted in November of 2021 found that most Americans (65 percent) believe science has had a positive effect on society, 28 percent say a mixed effect, and 7 percent say mostly a negative one (Spencer and Funk 2022). According to the study, when U.S. adults think about science, they are most often focused on medical and health science and developments in treating diseases.

According to a different Pew Research Center survey of 14,497 U.S. adults conducted in December 2021, 29 percent of the adults indicated they had a great deal of confidence in medical scientists to act in the best interests of the public, which was down from 40 percent in November 2020 (Kennedy et al. 2022). According to the center, this reflects a shift in American attitudes toward medical and general scientists. The survey found that public confidence in other groups, such as the military, law enforcement, and public school principals, had also declined. However, the majority of those surveyed had a "fair amount" of confidence in medical scientists (78%) and scientists (77%). The survey found low confidence in journalists, elected officials, and business leaders. Sixty percent said they had little to no confidence in journalists and business leaders to act in the public interest. Confidence in elected officials was even lower. Seventy-six percent said they did not have too much or no confidence that elected officials acted in the public's best interest.

A significant survey result was that differences in trusting medical scientists hinged on political affiliation. In short, Democrats were more likely than Republicans to trust that scientists act in the public's best interests. Nine in ten Democratic and Democratic-leaning adults had a great deal or a fair amount of confidence in medical scientists working in the public interest. In contrast, Republican and Republican-leaning adults had lower levels of trust in medical scientists, and this trust had steadily declined. Only 15 percent had great confidence in medical scientists, down from 31 percent in an earlier April 2020 survey. Thirty-four percent of this group indicated little to no confidence in medical scientists acting in the public interest. This was a threefold increase since the outbreak of COVID-19. A similar downward trend in trusting general scientists was found.

An Associated Press article echoes these recent survey findings. It noted that American trust in science is deeply polarized according to political affiliation. Borenstein and Fingerhut (2022:n.p.) summarized a recent survey that found that Republicans' faith in science and medicine is falling, while Democrats relied more on it during the pandemic. Overall, 48 percent of Americans said they had "a great deal" of confidence in the scientific community. Regarding political party, 64 percent of Democrats said they had "a great deal" of confidence compared with about half as many Republicans, at 34 percent. This gap was much smaller in 2018, when 51 percent of Democrats and 42 percent of Republicans had high confidence in the scientific community. The survey also found a growing gap in confidence in medicine, driven primarily by increasing confidence among Democrats. Forty-five percent of Democrats said they had a great deal of confidence in medicine, compared with 34 percent of Republicans.

The survey data suggest that a portion of Republicans and Democrats are following the cues of their leaders when thinking about science. Borenstein and Fingerhut's (2022:n.p.) data concluded this is the case. They cite Professor Marshall Shepard of the University of Georgia, who commented, "We live at a time when people would rather put urine or cleaning chemicals in their body than scientifically vetted vaccines." The professor added, "That is a clear convergence of fear, lack of critical thinking, confirmation bias, and political tribalism." They also include a comment from the president of the National Academy of Sciences, Marcia McNutt, who noted, "Scientists and policymakers tend to be conservative—not politically but in terms of being cautious and wary of risk—pushing safety, masks, and vaccines while Republicans as a group value individual liberty," McNutt said. She added, "So no wonder that Republicans are less supportive of the scientifically conservative decisions in the face of uncertainty."

Some of the decline in public trust can be attributed to unquestioned loyalty to political parties. However, differing views on science are not limited to one's political allegiance. When looking at racial and ethnic groups, a Pew Research Center national survey found that trust in medical scientists has slightly declined for White, Black, and Hispanic (Latinx) adults since April 2020 (Kennedy et al. 2022). However, confidence in medical scientists plays out differently between Democrats and Republicans when racial and ethnic groups are considered. A higher percentage of White Democratic and Democratic-leaning adults (52%) were more likely to have a great deal of confidence in medical scientists than Hispanic (36%) and Black (30%) adults. In contrast, among Republican and Republican-leaning Whites, lower confidence levels were reported among all three racial and ethnic groups. Regarding educational level, 95 percent of Democratic and Democratic-leaning adults with college educations had at least a fair amount of confidence in medical scientists compared with college-educated Republican and Republican-leaning adults at 73 percent.

A word of caution is needed regarding the issue of public trust in science. Science is critical for the survival of society, especially when addressing crises such as pandemics. With science, human progress continues. Action must be taken to increase the public's understanding of what science is, what it is not, and how to use it to sensibly make sound decisions and policies. To the extent possible, policies should be based on scientific information and not on conjecture, misinformation, or otherwise biased sources. O'Brien, Palmer, and Albarracin (2021:11–12) proposed a middle ground for approaching science and concluded:

> Although cynicism of science could have disastrous impacts, our results suggest that advocacy for trusting science must go beyond scientific labels, to focus on specific issues, critical evaluation, and the presence of consensus among several scientists. . . . Fostering trust in the "healthy skepticism" inherent to the scientific process may also be a critical element of protecting against misinformation. . . . Empowering people with knowledge about the scientific validation process and the motivation to be critical and curious may give audiences the resources they need to dismiss fringe but dangerous pseudoscience.

TRUST IN GOVERNMENT

The level of public trust and confidence in government institutions is an essential pandemic dimension. The level of trust in government is driven by its performance, events that were either covered up or violated the public trust, political affiliation, and consistency of messaging. In addition, rumors and the perception of government conspiracies impact trust. For instance, conspiracy theories regarding the government have been common for decades. Examples of conspiracy theories include the government's role in covering up unidentified flying objects (UFOs), stolen elections, efforts at mind control, surveillance of ordinary citizens, secret wars, and CIA plots to assassinate President Kennedy. Like all conspiracy theories and rumors, these and others take on a life of their own and, at some level, cause a portion of the public distrust of the government (see chapter 7).

American trust in government has historically been high, but over recent decades has waned. According to the National Election Study, public trust in the federal government to do the right thing was relatively high during the Eisenhower (73%), Kennedy (77%), and Johnson (77% to 62%) administrations but fell to 36 percent at the end of the Nixon administration (Pew Research Center 2021). Public trust in the federal government began a downward trend in the 1960s and continued in the 1970s. The Vietnam War, Watergate, the Iran-Contra Affair, and the economy did little to improve public trust in government. Trust continued to decline during the Ford (34%) and Carter (28%) administrations.

In 1994, the Contract with America helped Republicans gain control of the U.S. House of Representatives. The Contract with America (CWA) promised tax cuts, term limits, and a balanced budget amendment to the U.S. Constitution and made other commitments. The CWA was developed by Representative Newt Gingrich and Republican Party Chair Richard K. Armey without much input from moderate Republicans and no input from Democrats. With the majority of the House in line, the political agenda of the CWA leaders became dominant. The approach of shutting down the government through the budget process became a tool to force legislation through Congress. For example, the federal government was shut down temporarily in 1995 to force budgetary cuts. Compromise, dialogue, and other traditional congressional procedures and civility were abandoned. The CWA reflected dissatisfaction with government programs and policies. While distrust in the federal government cannot solely be attributed to these political moves, little was done to enhance the public's trust in the government.

President George W. Bush's administration initially scored a trust in government rating of 49 percent, but that percentage declined to 24 percent at the end of his term. An increase in public trust followed the terrorist attack on the World Trade Center on 9/11, but that spike decreased soon after. After 2007, public trust in the government never exceeded 30 percent. In 2010, the Republicans regained control of the house and, under the influence of the Tea Party, worked to block any legislation to limit Democratic President Barack Obama to be a one-term president. Unfortunately, none of these efforts improved public trust in government.

Since the 1970s, trust in government has been higher among the members of the party that controls the White House (Pew Research Center 2021). "Trust in government doing the 'right thing' has been strongly correlated with party preferences," and fueling public distrust of the party in power is a common political strategy (Offe 2021:39). Also, the level of trust is influenced by ethnic and racial group memberships. According to a Pew Research Center survey, Black Americans' trust in government was substantially higher in 2021 than in 2020 (15% then, 37% now), while views among White and Hispanic adults have seen less change during the pandemic. As was the case under the Obama and Clinton administrations, Black and Hispanic adults now express more trust in the government to do the right thing than White adults. Asian Americans' trust in government is substantially higher than White Americans.' During the Republican presidencies of Reagan, G. W. Bush, and Trump, White Americans were substantially more likely than Black Americans to express trust in the federal government (Pew Research Center 2021).

It is important to note that once government proclamations and communications are made public, it is easier for officials to admit errors. It is better to let the mistakes ride until people forget. For example, bold unsubstantiated claims were made about Barack Obama's citizenship. Known as the "birther conspiracy," the allegations were found to be untrue. Nevertheless, the false rumor persisted for months without any consequences. The same pattern was observed with the declaration that the 2020 election was "stolen." Multiple reviews, audits, and court decisions have found no evidence that the election was stolen, but some held unchangeable public opinions by then. Some never publicly acknowledged what the facts revealed. Once proclamations are made, they take on a public life of their own and become "facts," whether true or false.

Nevertheless, some claims erode public trust in institutions. If statements are restated repeatedly, they take on a reality of their own. People need time or energy to confirm repeated claims. It is far easier to assume that their sources and information are accurate. In the case of COVID-19, some Americans reached a comfort level of trusting and relying on uninformed opinions over public health and government information.

INCONSISTENT GOVERNMENT POLICIES AND MESSAGING REGARDING COVID-19

COVID-19 will continue in 2023 and the foreseeable future, posing challenges and issues to public health and government that undermine public trust (Shear et al. 2022). When considering the pandemic, some distrust and lack of confidence in the government can be traced to inconsistent government messaging about COVID-19 and how best to respond to the coronavirus. While much of the communications and guidance regarding COVID-19 remained consistent, other messages have been reversed. For instance, the early government COVID-19 guidance recommended wiping down surfaces, mail, and groceries to prevent the disease from spreading. As more was understood about COVID-19, the value of these preventative measures came into question. In addition, the CDC issued unclear guidance regarding the number of days an infected person should stay in quarantine (see Wachter 2022). There have been other reversals of official positions and policies regarding COVID-19, such as the usefulness of masks, the length of time vaccines are effective, which medicines work, lockdowns, social distancing, means of transmission, and school closures or openings.

Additional examples of inconsistent messaging from government agencies include the CDC publishing new testing guidance released in September 2020. However, political appointees with no medical training at the CDC's parent agency, the U.S. Department of Health and Human Services, had published them without proper scientific review (*Nature* 2020). Another example was when the government inadvertently misled the public by implying that COVID-19 vaccines would prevent the vaccinated from getting the coronavirus. However, in July 2021, it became clear that some people became infected despite being vaccinated. These infections would be less severe but still occur. Almost immediately, opponents of the vaccine claimed that the vaccines were ineffective and, thus, had no value.

In addition, government messaging regarding the seriousness of the pandemic has fluctuated, partially due to changes in the virus and scientific knowledge. For example, early in the pandemic, scientists predicted that under the worst-case scenario, as many as 500,000 Americans could die from COVID-19, but by May 2022, over one million had died. This estimate would need to be revised as more people died from COVID-19. President Biden's administration withdrew its workplace vaccination rule for large employers following a United States Supreme Court 6 to 3 ruling that the Occupational Safety and Health Administration had no authority to require workers to be vaccinated or tested weekly. This and other public health orders have varied throughout the pandemic.

Consequently, employers were and are subject to a patchwork quilt of federal, state, and local laws on COVID-19 workplace safety. These messages undermine the public trust in the government and its guidance when found to be inaccurate. For example, restaurant and bar owners have had to close, then were allowed to reopen only to be locked again with upticks in COVID-19 infection rates. As a result, it became difficult for some businesses to recruit and retain staff, keep customers, and maintain any financial viability.

For the CDC, extensive commentary by President Trump on the pandemic and interference with its COVID-19 and public health messaging by the Trump White House helped erode public trust in the agency. From the many White House pandemic updates, it became clear that CDC messaging was being controlled and, in some cases, hampered by the White House (Pollard and Davis 2021; Weiland 2021). Lewis (2021) observed that early in the pandemic, the Centers for Disease Control and Prevention informed the media that the threat to the American public was low but eventually warned that disruptions to daily life could be "severe." The agency was quickly silenced, and President Trump placed himself at the forefront of daily briefings on the disease. The president became the government's primary conduit for COVID-19 updates through his briefings. The CDC and Food and Drug Administration became supplanted and suppressed. This limiting of what the federal health officials could share made it difficult for the CDC and FDA to communicate accurate and fact-based information to the public. Lewis noted that, under President Biden's administration, federal government science and health agencies have been given renewed respect and independence; however, rebuilding public trust in these agencies will take some time.

Other non-governmental agencies, such as the World Health Organization (WHO), also have sent mixed messages. On March 28, 2020, the WHO announced on its website that COVID-19 was not airborne. Instead, the WHO believed that COVID-19 was primarily spread through droplets when a person sneezed, coughed, or talked. Early in the pandemic medical authorities and government agencies thought COVID-19 was spread mainly by direct contact with large droplets from a cough or sneeze and not smaller droplets called aerosols that linger in the air. Considering this, officials emphasized wiping surfaces, washing hands, and using hand sanitizers. These are reasonable public health measures when addressing many diseases but ineffective in preventing COVID-19.

Later it was discovered that COVID-19 was spread mainly by tiny airborne droplets (aerosols) and seldom transmitted from surfaces. Wearing high-quality masks and proper ventilation proved to be more effective ways of preventing the spread of the coronavirus. This led to confusion and reduced public trust and confidence in the WHO. It took two years for the WHO to correct its error on October 20, 2020 (Lewis 2022). Some reasons for such a long delay in correcting the error were related to competing theories of spreading viruses, institutional momentum (tradition), and the problem of rescinding proclaimed "facts." In addition, critics would label this error as the "hygiene theater" because managers of businesses and public spaces continued to unnecessarily emphasize and dramatically over-rely on unwarranted hygienic scrubs and extensive cleaning (for discussion, see Lewis 2021).

NATIONAL SURVEYS REGARDING GOVERNMENT PANDEMIC RESPONSE

National surveys have addressed the issue of the changing messages regarding the pandemic. One study by the Pew Research Center surveyed 10,348 American adults (Funk and Gramlich 2021). The researchers asked respondents for their reactions to changing public health guidance around some aspects of the pandemic, including information about how the virus spreads and the effectiveness of face masks. Three-quarters or more of unvaccinated Americans expressed adverse reactions to the changing guidance, such as saying it made them wonder if public health officials were holding back vital information (78%). They also indicated that changing messages made them less confident in public health officials' recommendations (75%). Again, the respondent's vaccination status mattered when expressing confidence in public health guidance. Consistent with the Funk and Gramlich study, another later Pew Research Center study by Tyson and Funk (2022:n.p.) found that 60 percent of Americans reported being confused by public health officials' messages regarding how to slow the spread of COVID-19. This represented a 7 percent increase in adults indicating they were confused from the earlier study. Other evaluations of how government officials responded to the pandemic also decreased.

The University of Pennsylvania's Annenberg Public Policy Center (2022) surveyed adults nationally in January 2022. The survey results revealed that after waves of COVID-19, new variants of the virus, delays in understanding the virus, and confusion over shifting government policies and messages, Americans reported a decline in confidence in the Centers for Disease Control and Prevention (CDC). This decline in confidence occurred for respondents regardless of political allegiance—Democrats, Republicans, and independents. The center found that public confidence in the CDC in providing trustworthy information on the prevention and treatment of COVID-19 declined from 77 percent in November 2021 to 72 percent in January 2022 (Annenberg Public Policy Center 2022).

In addition to messaging, surveys have explored public attitudes toward the government's handling of the pandemic. For example, Funk, Tyson, Pasquini, and Spencer (2022) reported on a survey of 10,282 adults conducted from May 2 to 8, 2022. The study focused on attitudes toward the government's handling of the pandemic. Respondents felt the government did not prioritize the educational needs of K–12 students. Fewer than half thought the government had given the right amount of support for quality of life, economic activity, and protection of public health. Respondents indicated that face masks and vaccines are somewhat effective in limiting the spread of COVID-19.

Funk et al. (2022:n.p.) found, "Regarding the central goal of protecting public health, Americans have decidedly mixed views: 43 percent said the country has given about the right amount of priority to protecting public health." In comparison, 34 percent said this had received too little priority, and 21 percent said it had received too much. The mixed pattern should come as no surprise, as Americans are divided on what they believe is the appropriate role of government in everyday lives. Funk et al. (2022) further elaborated that Republicans thought the country had not focused enough on business concerns and respecting individual choices. In contrast, Democrats focused on efforts to protect public health and limit the risk to vulnerable adults. In general, Democrats felt protecting public health was not prioritized enough, while Republicans believed it had received too much priority.

TRUST IN MEDICAL RESEARCH AND PUBLIC HEALTH

Public trust in medical providers has been another important survey topic during the pandemic. During pandemics, people generally assume that physicians "are in a better position than politicians" to make health-related decisions (Zielonka 2021:59). This is the pattern even though Zielonka (2021) observed that physicians do not always agree and can be influenced by economic and political pressures. Nevertheless, national surveys consistently have found that most Americans trust their physicians and medical providers but report less trust in the public health and medical systems.

Public distrust in medicine and public health has surfaced throughout American history (see chapter 3). For example, enslaved African Americans often did not trust White doctors in the antebellum South for good reasons (Covey 2007). In 1894–1895, public health officials in Milwaukee, Wisconsin, were seen as threats to the community during a smallpox outbreak. According to Randall (2019:5), armed Polish American women patrolled Milwaukee's streets with knives and bats to combat health inspectors who they feared would confiscate their property in the name of controlling smallpox. Public distrust of public health also surfaced during the 1918 influenza pandemic in San Francisco and other American cities (see chapter 3).

Nevertheless, national surveys have found that most American adults trust their primary care doctors. For example, the Annenberg Public Policy Center (2022) surveyed adult Americans nationally to determine their trust and confidence in their physicians. Regarding COVID-19, the center found that 82 percent of respondents were confident their primary healthcare provider was providing trustworthy information about the coronavirus, with a slight increase in the percentage saying they needed to be more confident. The same survey found that most (74%) believed the Food and Drug Administration provided trustworthy information. This percentage compares to 72 percent confidence in the CDC. Confidence in Dr. Fauci, the most prominent national expert, was at 65 percent and had declined by 6 percent since April 2021. Thirty-five percent indicated they needed more confidence in Dr. Fauci providing trustworthy information on COVID-19. The decline in confidence for Dr. Fauci represents an example of scapegoating, as he has had to deliver complex messages about the pandemic that the public needed but did not want to hear. Dr. Fauci has been the messenger of both good and bad news.

If the survey results are accurate, most Americans trust their medical providers, the Food and Drug Administration, the CDC, and the lead spokesperson Dr. Fauci. Van Bavel, Baicker, Boggio, et al. (2021:465) concluded, "It is important to note that alternative surveys of Americans suggest higher levels of confidence in medical providers. American trust in medical doctors remains high compared to public health officials."

A November 2021 Annenberg Public Policy Center (2021a) survey of 1,672 American adults asked about public trust in medical providers. The study found that an individual's primary healthcare provider was the most trusted source of information about preventing and treating COVID-19. However, the survey found varied levels of trust for different information sources:

- Primary health care provider: 85 percent are confident their primary health care provider was providing trustworthy information about COVID-19.
- Food and Drug Administration: 76 percent are confident that the FDA, which authorized emergency use of COVID-19 vaccines in the U.S., provided trustworthy information on COVID-19.
- Centers for Disease Control and Prevention: 77 percent are confident the CDC was providing trustworthy information on COVID-19.
- Dr. Anthony Fauci: 67 percent are confident that Dr. Fauci, director of the U.S. National Institute of Allergy and Infectious Diseases (NIAID), provided trustworthy advice on COVID-19.

According to a Pew Research Center study, differing ratings of public health officials are an example of intensifying partisan differences that have formed throughout the COVID-19 pandemic (Funk et al. 2022). Democratic and Democratic-leaning adults were far more likely than Republican and Republican-leaning adults (72% vs. 29%) to indicate that public health officials, such as those at the CDC, have done an excellent or good job responding to the coronavirus outbreak. In the early stages of the outbreak, most Republicans and Democrats gave public health officials positive ratings. Sharply lower assessments among Republicans have driven the overall decline in ratings for public health officials.

The erosion of trust in public health officials and medical personnel by nearly 25 percent of American adults can have severe consequences for relying on and using public health interventions. Untrusting people are more likely to ignore their own health needs and those of others. To build trust, valid and reliable information needs to flow from public health officials, medical personnel, and in the case of pandemics and epidemics, political leaders at the local and national levels (Organization for Economic Co-operation and Development 2020). In addition, misinformation needs to be addressed and rebuked to minimize the negative consequences to public health.

In summary, while most Americans appear to trust and have confidence in scientists (science), medical scientists, medical providers, and government agencies to act in the public interest, this trust and confidence has declined since the beginning of the pandemic and is trending downward. An earlier Annenberg Public Policy Center survey conducted in June 2021 found that an individual's primary healthcare provider was the most trusted source of information for treating and preventing COVID-19 (Annenberg Public Policy Center 2021c). In this regard, political affiliation matters, with Democratic and Democratic-leaning adults trusting medical and general scientists more than their Republican counterparts. America's pandemic polarization is not about science; however, it is about what is done with science and when we exchange individual freedoms for collective safety. This gap between the two political orientations appears to be widening. Race and ethnicity also accounted for some differences in levels of confidence and trust (see chapter 6). Similar findings were reported by a Pew Research Center study conducted in April 2020. The study found that Black adults were more hesitant than White adults to trust medical scientists, embrace experimental medical treatments, and sign up for a potential vaccine to combat the illness (Gramlich and Funk 2020).

THE DEGRADATION OF THE NEWS

In the first decades of the 21st century, how Americans were informed dramatically changed. There used to be journalistic standards for reporting and the news, but they have corroded over time. For decades the flow of mass communications and news was predominantly a one-way process originating from professional media organizations that flowed to mass audiences. Traditional media organizations, such as national and local television news programs, newspapers, and radio, were the predominant sources for the news. The news was transmitted through formal institutional (traditional) channels. Miller (2014) described institutional channels as being well organized, having a stable set of rules and staff serving in clearly defined roles, and relying on well-established procedures that can be followed by interchangeable personnel. He added, "Within most institutional channels, there are fixed standards of acceptable news, procedures for obtaining news, prescribed routes of transmission, verification procedures for obtaining news, and codes of reliable conduct" (Miller 2014:114). These traditional news sources involve editors, journalists, and advertisers deciding what good news is. Journalists and editors are professionally trained and have historically adhered to fixed professional standards of what is news, including truthful reporting of facts. A system of checks and balances characterizes traditional news media and what it reports and helps ensure that news is accurate and factual. With these traditional news sources, the public presumes the news is factual and honest; for traditional news to be identified as a spreader of falsehoods would distract from their credibility and ability to inform opinion in the future.

Social media platform news fundamentally differs from traditional news sources (e.g., Bullock and Korinek 2022). For instance, social media relies on audience or consumer-generated content for a portion of its material. In contrast, consumers and audiences of traditional media news reporting do not contribute to the news' nature or content. Social media news sources' content is seldom fact-checked and may not even be informative. No formal system of checks and balances ensures that social media posts are factual, although some platforms try to police their content for accuracy. Social media platforms prompt audiences and users to engage by sensationalizing information and reinforcing pre-existing biases. With social media, anyone can be a source of "facts and truths" and to be more outrageous is to be the most effective in reaching audiences. The more extreme the claim or content, the more likely it is to accomplish the goal of maximizing engagement. In short, social media platforms state and confirm what users believe or want to believe. Recommendation systems drive social media, that is, whatever information promotes maximum user engagement. The more users are involved in a social media platform, the more the platform caters to content that further engages the users. This increases the political polarization witnessed in American society, as users tend to engage with social media platforms that reaffirm their beliefs and emotions.

With social media, audiences can communicate back to the originator and others by providing feedback. This feedback may or may not necessarily be objective and contain accurate information. Social media blogs and posts are a source of misinformation and accurate information. The reader needs to learn what is factual or made-up. The same can be said of biased news sources. It is known that readers can and do embrace statements and feedback and sometimes carry it forward as being factual. Similar to rumor generation, comments and feedback gets repeated over and over without any mechanism for verification or checks on reliability. Social media affords the originator a degree of anonymity and lack of accountability for misinformation and false statements that harm individuals or groups. This has occurred with COVID-19 and during the pandemic (see chapter 7).

During the pandemic, trolls have put misinformation and rumors on social media that distort the facts. A troll is a lay term for individuals who intentionally put false information on social media platforms. Trolls publish inflammatory, hateful, or outlandish claims and comments on the web that provoke people into responses, confirming or opposing. The difference between rumor and traditional news lies more in the degree of anonymity than accuracy. Under conditions of increasing anonymity, responsibility for information or misinformation is diminished. Originators and spreaders of information (rumors) are not held accountable for what hearsay they transmit.

Turning to the effect of drama and radical claims in the news, drama and extremism draw and engage audiences and are good for the media business. There is money to be made in drama and extremism. If an influential public figure can convince an audience to think what they state is a fact, then some people tend to believe them despite the facts. If a public figure or group repeatedly says that anything that disagrees with them is "fake news," audiences increasingly turn to them for the news. It is easier to accuse credible media of being biased (fake news) when it does not present information that confirms beliefs and political policies. After all, no one wants to rely on "fake news." Audiences tend to see them as credible and do not take the time or energy to fact-check their information. Bullock and Korinek (2022:n.p.) observed:

> There is a willingness to overlook facts and rely on beliefs and biases to confirm perspectives. The current polarized political climate has locked individuals into mindsets that hamper the ability to process information that might be correct or incorrect. Anytime information is presented that does not conform to emotions, beliefs, or political objectives, it is now customary to declare it "fake news."

> It can be declared fake news to raise doubts without presenting any facts to the contrary.

With social media and biased news sources, much of the believability is in the style of the presentation and who is presenting more so than the facts. Marshall McLuhan (1967) observed in his book *The Medium is the Massage: An Inventory of Effects* that the manner of information delivery is more important than the actual content. He wrote long before the advent of the internet and social media. However, his observation still seems appropriate. The immediacy of information on the internet is valued because it is convenient, accessible, and widely dispersed. Surveys find that younger generations tend to draw their news from primary and sometimes inaccurate social media sources simply because of the format (medium) rather than the accuracy of the content. K. Eric Drexler (cited by Bullock and Korinek 2022:n.p.) summed up the current situation with social media:

> Social media today is degraded by the influence of [misinformed] and unsourced content, a problem caused (in part) by the cost of finding good information and citing sources and (in part) by fact-indifferent actors with other agendas. Well-informed replies are relatively costly and scarce, but mob noise and bot spew are abundant.

National survey data suggest that trust in traditional news sources is waning. Kaiser Family Foundation researchers Hamel, Lopes, Kirzinger, Sparks, Stokes, and Brodie (2021) found that no single news source had the trust of most adult Americans. Almost half of American adults trusted what they saw on networks and local television. Trust was lower for other news outlets. Where people get their news influences their responses to the pandemic—case in point: unvaccinated adults distrusted traditional news sources about COVID-19 more than vaccinated adults.

Regarding information, the type of news source used matters, according to survey data. The media source affects users' confidence in official government information about COVID-19. A November 2021 Annenberg Public Policy Center (2021a) survey of 1,672 American adults found that heavy social media users did not have significantly lower confidence in health authorities than the overall sample. However, the level of confidence did differ by news source. The center's survey reported that individuals' confidence varied by information source:

- Very conservative sources such as Newsmax, One America News (OAN), Gateway Pundit, Parler, or Telegram: 46 percent had confidence in Dr. Fauci, 50 percent in the CDC, 54 percent in the FDA, and 86 percent in their primary health care provider.

- Conservative media sources such as Fox News, Mark Levin, or Breitbart: 47 percent had confidence in Dr. Fauci, 59 percent in the CDC, 64 percent in the FDA, and 90 percent in their primary health care provider.
- Social media such as Facebook, Twitter, Instagram, or YouTube: 70 percent expressed confidence in Dr. Fauci, 75 percent in the CDC, 72 percent in the FDA, and 89 percent in their primary health care provider.
- Mainstream broadcast/print media such as CBS News, NBC News, ABC News, the Associated Press, or the news pages of *The Wall Street Journal* or *The New York Times*: 87 percent expressed confidence in Dr. Fauci, 91 percent in the CDC, 90 percent in the FDA, and 95 percent in their primary health care provider.

The survey concluded that very conservative sources of information tend to have less confidence in the government. In addition, if Americans' information diet is based mainly on partisan social media sources, then erroneous perceptions of the risk of COVID-19 can be either under or overestimated (Rothwell and Desai 2020). Regardless of the source, primary care providers consistently have the highest confidence level.

THE DECLINE IN CRITICAL THINKING SKILLS

Individuals who lack critical thinking skills are more susceptible to collective acts, such as cultism, radicalized beliefs, rumors, misinformation, and risky behaviors. The social climate during the pandemic has been one where rumors and misinformation about COVID-19 have been ample (see chapters 1 and 7). The relationship between critical thinking skills and rumor is essential. Buckner (1975) proposed that there are three orientations toward rumors. The first is a critical set. This occurs when a person is knowledgeable about the subject matter of the rumor. A second orientation is when the individual knows what to expect from the experience. The person is suspicious of rumors that do not sound plausible. The third orientation is the person with stable interaction systems that provide a sense of credibility and reliability when it comes to information. These are useful in critical thinking and assessing the truth in rumors.

Some individuals are uncritical thinkers when it comes to rumors. Rumors usually serve the psychological needs of those who create or pass them on to others. If a rumor fills the needs of individuals, they will more likely accept it as fact. Rumors are accepted from almost any source, including friends, strangers, overheard conversations, emails from strangers, and social media platforms. Rumors thrive among those without prior knowledge of a topic such as COVID-19. Those lacking critical thinking skills and prior knowledge are more easily persuaded to believe rumors. When people know little to nothing about a topic, critical standards (thinking) are temporarily lowered until more reliable and valid information is available. Until then, they are more suggestible and open to rumors. Miller (2014:117) summarized, "The loss of critical ability, coupled with increased suggestibility, makes it more likely that people will act on the information from anonymous sources." According to Klapp (1972:116):

> Likely rumor participants include the uneducated. Increasing levels of education tend to insulate people from the gullible acceptance of rumors. Other likely participants include those with pent-up hatred, aggression, or other tensions. Spreading rumors allows for expressing feelings that would otherwise be held in check.

THE PANDEMIC HAS HIGHLIGHTED INEQUALITY AND RACISM

Social inequity is a central pattern in much of the COVID-19 pandemic commentary and research (Maestripieri 2021; Pickersgill 2020). The pandemic has raised racial and geographic discrimination, social class differences, and health inequity. The social class differences in America that were present before were highlighted during the pandemic. Preexisting differences among groups became more apparent, particularly among the different socioeconomic classes and minority groups, and geographical locations. Most studies have found that lower-income groups were more dramatically and negatively impacted by COVID-19.

Sociologists, policymakers, and elected officials have highlighted existing racial inequities regarding access to COVID-19 vaccinations (Joseph 2021; Reich 2021). It is a combination of systemic inequality and individual choice. Several scholars have acknowledged that inequities are abundant in the healthcare system (see Joseph 2021). It is also accurate that individual choice and cultural factors also are important.

During the pandemic, inequality has surfaced in a variety of ways. Americans have not had equal access to healthcare resources. In addition, inequality plays out in the risk of severe COVID-19 infection and death rates (see chapter 2). This also influences the ability of some groups to adopt preventive measures to slow the spread of the disease. Within the context of the pandemic, individuals without health insurance found it challenging to obtain needed health care. Low-wage earners could not take time off work to get vaccinated. Some undocumented workers avoided vaccinations and health care for fear of being deported, incarcerated, or losing employment. Those in institutional settings, such as prisons, homeless shelters, refugee facilities, and detention centers, could not socially isolate or distance themselves from others. Homeless living on the streets could not correctly socially distance or access sanitary items. Those dependent on public transportation were crowded into buses, subways, and trains with little chance of social distancing.

A specific example of inequality during the pandemic was the early distribution of a limited number of vaccines. Because of a general shortage of vaccines and high demand, distribution criteria would need to be established. The Advisory Committee on Immunization Practices (ACIP) guides vaccines' safe use and distribution. The committee knew initially that the vaccine demand would exceed the supply and developed distribution criteria. According to Reich (2021:6), the committee set two primary goals for vaccine distribution, "prevention of morbidity and mortality" and "preservation of societal functioning." For the first goal, priority was given to the most at risk of severe illness or death, such as older residents living in congregate settings. The second goal led to initial vaccinations of health care and then essential workers. Reich noted that the distribution policies were "unsurprisingly inequitable" due to many factors, such as race, ethnicity, place of residence, homelessness, and occupation. The prioritization of vaccinations also varied across states and localities. For example, rural area residents had less access to vaccines than urban dwellers. Public distrust of the vaccine distribution criteria grew as a sense of unfairness developed.

The COVID-19 pandemic is not the first instance of inequality surfacing during a pandemic or epidemic. Racial and class differences were highlighted when the bubonic plague broke out in Honolulu and San Francisco, and later in Los Angeles, in the late 19th and early 20th centuries. Racist and classist attitudes toward people of Chinese ancestry blossomed into segregation, disruption, attacks, and restrictions during the bubonic plague in these cities. San Francisco officials ordered walls built around Chinatown and Chinese Americans quarantined, which led to a general disruption of the city's commerce. In San Francisco, public health officials and police intrusively entered Chinese-American-owned businesses and homes looking for plague cases. Once the plague was acknowledged, city officials sought to downplay the disease to minimize its impact on commerce. Officials suppressed rumors about the plague, whether true or not, because the plague was terrible for business. These reactions sound remarkably similar to those of COVID-19 in some circles that promote the idea that contracting the virus is no worse than the flu. Like COVID-19, the plague in San Francisco would become politicized by elected officials seeking to minimize the extent of the plague and those seeking to relieve the restrictions placed on the Chinese American community. It would take a group of wealthy Chinese American business leaders to politically force the lifting of restrictions on the Chinese American community.

There has been a pattern of associating diseases with foreigners. For example, the English labeled syphilis the "French Disease," the French labeled it the "Spanish Disease," and the Spanish the "Italian Disease," and so on. This same pattern was observed during the 1889–1890 influenza pandemic, which was named the "Russian Flu," and the Russians labeled it the "Chinese Catarrh," the Germans named it the "Russian Pest," and the Italians the "German Disease." For the 1918 flu pandemic, the French press initially called it the "American flu" but later named it the "Spanish flu." In the spring of 1918, British soldiers called it "Flanders flu," and German soldiers called it the "Flandern-Fieber (Flemish fever)," named after a battlefield where soldiers in WWI on both sides caught the flu. There are other examples from other countries, but the Spanish Flu seemed to be the most common because, as some modern historians have observed, the 1918 influenza was first publicly announced in Spain.

A similar pattern emerged for COVID-19. A degree of racism and ethnocentricity was observed during the COVID-19 pandemic. In the case of COVID-19, President Trump referred to COVID-19 as "Kung Flu" and the "Asian Flu." His unstated intent was to blame the Chinese for creating and accidentally or purposely releasing the coronavirus (see Van Bavel, Baicker, Boggio, et al. 2021:462).

There is an element of truth to the attribution of COVID-19 to China, as authorities agree that the virus first appeared in that country. However, COVID-19's origin has been debated since it was first identified. Some scientists have speculated it originated in Wuhan, China, in a wet market, escaped from a laboratory there, or originated from natural sources, specifically bats. Regardless, American leaders blamed China. As might be expected, the Chinese government denied being the origin and stopped sharing COVID-19 information. Within days of the first COVID-19 cases, the Chinese quickly attributed the source of the virus to the United States. The linking of COVID-19 to the Chinese was only one dimension of racism, as federal policies were quickly put in place prohibiting travel to the United States from certain Muslim countries and restricting border access (immigration) of some foreigners, specifically from Central and South American countries.

In America, a consequence was racially motivated attacks on anyone with East Asian ancestry. The origins of the virus being identified as Chinese and politically charged statements resulted in displays and acts of prejudice, such as Sinophobia (racism targeting Chinese people or those of Chinese ancestry) and xenophobia, a fear or hatred of anyone viewed as foreign or culturally different (strange). Social media and politically biased news sources and the press worsened acts of racism. In the United States and worldwide, East Asians became a catalyst for violent attacks. Reports of physical attacks on ethnic Asian people in predominantly White countries, including the United States, increased (Van Bavel, Baicker, Boggio, et al. 2021).

Early in the pandemic, Tsai, Phua, Pan, and Yang (2020) explored the relationship between the perceived threat of COVID-19 and Chinese (Asian) and Asian Americans. Politicized claims that Chinese and Americans of Asian ancestry spread COVID-19 had led to over 2,000 reports of anti-Asian racial and hate crime incidents. This number would grow over the pandemic. Tsai et al. compared exposure to traditional news, social media use, and biased news sources to determine how each source cultivated prejudice and trust in Asians and Asian Americans. They surveyed 430 American adults in May 2020. Their results suggested that conservative ideology, personal infection history, frequency of intergroup contact, traditional news exposure, and trust in social media emerged as positive predictors of prejudice against Asians and Asian Americans. Likewise, adults who relied on left-leaning news or more objective news sources showed less prejudice toward Asian people.

In summary, as sociologist Geoffrey Pleyers (2020:3) wrote, "The COVID-19 pandemic exacerbates social inequalities and reveals the social structures, notably in terms of class, race, and gender." In the United States, minorities and lower-income groups were and continue to be much more affected by COVID-19. The same is true for other countries. Ferreira, José Sá, Martins, and Serpa (2020:9) concluded, "The pandemic crisis has led to the worsening of social inequalities in the global context, between countries and within countries; the most disadvantaged and vulnerable ones are increasingly disadvantaged and vulnerable."

CONCLUDING OBSERVATIONS

Social behavior during the pandemic did not occur in a historical vacuum. Some social responses to the pandemic have roots in American history, the socioeconomic and political context in which the pandemic arose, and the biological nature of COVID-19. A climate of social unrest, erosion of trust in science and government, and the politicization of the pandemic have led some to embrace acceptance of some public health measures to control COVID-19 and others to distrust, question, and even adamantly oppose these measures. At the pandemic's beginning, American society was characterized by social strain, unrest, political polarization, and uncertainty, creating ideal conditions for collective action. As a result, Americans were motivated to either buy into or resist COVID-19 public health policies and strategies.

American trust in traditional institutions has eroded over recent decades. Science has come under attack, as has medical research, traditional news, and government. These institutions, sometimes for justifiable reasons, have seen a decline in public support and trust. While most Americans continue to trust these institutions, not all Americans do. Instead, these Americans turn to alternative sources of information, such as social media platforms. For Americans, discerning biased opinions from facts has proven challenging, as biased news and social media personalities have polluted the air with misinformation and falsehoods. Social media platforms are not inherently wrong but can mislead and are not as subject to the exact adherence to the facts as traditional news sources and institutions. This can be problematic when it comes to public health efforts.

The collective behavior concept of mass conversion is a valuable tool for framing what has occurred regarding trust in American society. Mass conversion is a complete change in fundamental values that becomes relatively permanent. Mass conversion is a process of changing social norms, a change in a way of life, or a change in a fundamental perspective. A typical example of a mass conversion is when a group converts to a new religious set of beliefs. The distrust in science and medicine for some Americans represented a mass conversion, albeit a gradual one, from valuing and having faith in science to not trusting either. National political leadership in recent years helped expedite this decline in trust. For some individuals, there never was much trust in medicine or science, but for others, their political viewpoint increasingly drove their distrust.

Besides these conditions, social media and politically biased news media shaped public opinions and behaviors during the pandemic. Marx and McAdam (1994) observed that cable television and social media provide adequate resources to mobilize social movements and behaviors. This was the situation with the pandemic, as both fueled public compliance and resistance groups.

During the pandemic, skeptics questioned traditional news sources based not on reporting factual news but on whether they conformed to political views. When COVID-19 facts were reported that did not conform to or support political agendas, they were contradicted, suppressed, characterized as exaggerated, or dismissed as "fake." This pattern was and is familiar to news about COVID-19 and the pandemic. As would be expected, not knowing this, some Americans lacking critical thinking skills turned to emotions and political allegiances to determine how they should respond to the pandemic. Calvillo, Ross, Garcia, Smelter, and Rutchick (2020) found this to be the case and how the perceptions of the COVID-19 threat and susceptibility to fake news were influenced by political ideology.

The United States is transitioning into a non-factual society in some sectors, such as science and politics (see chapter 6). In their 2018 book *Truth Decay*, Kavanagh and Rich noted the diminished role of facts and analysis (critical thinking) in American society. Today, rather than rely on facts, there is a greater tendency by some individuals and groups to dismiss anything that does not conform to one's views as "fake news." This is not a new approach to communications and societies. Sociologists and psychologists have known for years that people tend to associate with others who share their beliefs, views, and interests. Multiple non-factual sources of misinformation and politically motivated ideas have shaped our responses during the pandemic and our perceptions of society. The enhanced power of mass and social media, coupled with the right to free speech, promotes the spread of misinformation but also the ability to more easily correct misinformation.

An important but neglected aspect of the pandemic has been the key role played by ignorance. Most scholars should pay more attention to ignorance's key role in pandemic policymaking. Paul and Haddad (2023) are an exception who explored the role of ignorance during different stages of the pandemic. They provided multiple examples of how different types of ignorance shaped pandemic policies. For example, they observed that decision-makers "turned a blind eye" to prior experiences with past epidemics that have found that such events often cross national boundaries (Paul and Haddad 2023:226). Instead, decision-makers implemented policies that were nationalistic and focused on isolation. They identified inconsistent data and data collection across regions, especially regarding vaccinations, as contributing to ignorance about COVID-19. Poor data resulted in public, medical, and decision-maker uncertainty about the pandemic. Pharmaceutical companies failed to share information about their research findings, which contributed to ignorance about COVID-19. Corporate trade secrets and patents hampered vaccine development and distribution. Paul and Haddad (2023:230) summarized how different forms of ignorance affected pandemic policies when they wrote:

> Ignorance assumes different forms, some of them more strategic and intentional than others, but all of them doing political work at different stages of the policy process. As we have seen, these may occur in the form of turning a blind eye to historical lessons, or bracketing out alternative forms of knowledge in an over-reliance on quantitative knowledge, actively concealing and delaying knowledge, or in simply not sharing knowledge in the case of vaccine development.

Finally, a dimension of the pandemic has been the erosion of truth in American society. In a report prepared by the Rand Corporation, Kavanagh and Rich (2018) made the case that truth in American society has deteriorated, a trend that they label truth decay, which is very applicable to some of the aforementioned social behaviors and trends during the pandemic. For example, they wrote (2018:ix):

> In national political and civil discourse, disagreement over facts appears greater than ever. Opinions are crowding out and overwhelming facts in the media, and Americans are placing less faith in institutions that were once trusted sources of information. This shift from facts and data in political debate and policy decisions has far-reaching implications: It erodes civil discourse; weakens key institutions; and imposes economic, diplomatic, and cultural costs.

Kavanagh and Rich viewed truth decay as the result of four basic trends: increasing disagreement about facts and analytical interpretations of facts and data; a blurring of the line between opinion and fact; the increasing relative volume, and resulting influence, of opinion and personal experience over fact; and declining trust in formerly respected sources of factual information.

Chapter 6

Political Tribalism and the Politicization of COVID-19

"I pass my days in a state of exasperation. First, with the fools who do not want any of the things that ought to be done, and second, with the equally obnoxious fools who insist upon so much that they cannot get anything done."

Theodore Roosevelt, *Letter to his son Kermit,* January 17, 1903

"This dog will not hunt this time. We are not buying it. States have already prepared for this for the midterm elections when the Democrats try and pull the same thing they did in 2020."

[Referring to the latest increased wave of COVID-19 sub-variant BA.5 infections.]

Unknown Blogger 2022

"Your vaccines are only moneymakers for big pharma that the politicians make money on."

Unknown Blogger 2022

THE POLITICIZATION OF COVID-19 COMPARED TO OTHER PANDEMICS

In the beginning, the intense political polarization in America took a back seat to American concern over the pandemic. Conflicts between political parties waned and medical expertise took center stage. However, Zielonka (2021:66) observed, "With the passage of time, political battles resurfaced, and medical arguments were pushed aside." Unlike prior societal responses to epidemics and pandemics, COVID-19 became more politicized than past pandemics. Siegel (2020:viii) wrote, "Any attempt to put this pandemic in proper medical context was immediately overcome by politics."

Pandemics and epidemics always seem to have a political aspect. For example, the Black Plague outbreak in San Francisco had several political dimensions. In 1918, the American military and politicians ignored the influenza pandemic because the country needed troops to fight in WWI. Regarding HIV/AIDS, Democrats and Republicans had different degrees of commitment to the battle against the disease. However, the politicization of COVID-19 set the bar high, as some members of both parties aligned themselves as seeing COVID-19 as a real danger and others viewing it as overblown and, in some cases, a hoax. Unlike any previous pandemic, Americans made medical decisions based on political allegiance, a perspective that would have been unthinkable during other pandemics. America's political polarization led to antagonism among groups and a decline in the boundaries of political decency (see Vandenberghe and Verán 2021:171).

The stage for politicizing COVID-19 was set years before the pandemic. The polarization of the traditional two-party system started with both parties shifting to appease the far-left or far-right interests. Miller (2014:511) insightfully wrote:

> The Democratic and Republican parties of the United States have sought to accommodate and assimilate more marginal political groups from both the left and right. Marginal groups have also sought to have their concerns addressed through the agendas of the two major political parties. In 1994, many disaffected groups entered electoral politics by way of H. Ross Perot's Reform Party of the United States of America.

This point is illustrated by the emergence of the right-leaning Tea Party, which focused on libertarian ideals of small government, limited taxes, and little governmental intrusion into Americans' individual, family, and economic life (see also discussion on the Contract with America in chapter 5). While the Tea Party was less prominent in American politics by the pandemic's beginning, some of its ideas persisted. Social issues, such as gun control, abortion, school curriculums, birth control, public assistance, and police reform, served as deal-breaker issues and interest groups and individuals would take sides with whatever party embraced the positions of left- or right-leaning groups.

The pattern of politicization and polarization of the COVID-19 pandemic is not unique to American politics. The United States was not the only country politicizing the coronavirus; other countries have shown similar patterns. Flores et al. (2022) found that at least seven countries displayed evidence of politicizing the pandemic. Their survey of 13,000 respondents from seven countries found that responses to COVID-19 depended on who proposed them. Respondents generally wanted to know which political side offered the policy before responding. There was a strong dislike for any policy viewed as coming from the opposing side. Respondents were more likely to support or comply with policies that had bipartisan or nonpartisan scientistic support. Respondents, whether liberal or conservative, supported policies if they originated from their political party and not those from the other party. They reported that the public took cues from political elites (leaders), which often polarized public attitudes toward COVID-19 policies. Flores et al. (2022:1) summarized:

> Liberal and conservative respondents supported policies proposed by ingroup politicians and parties more than the same policies from outgroup politicians and parties. In addition, respondents disliked, distrusted, and felt cold towards outgroup political elites, whereas they liked, trusted, and felt warm towards both ingroup political elites and non-partisan experts.

Since the virus was first identified, the Chinese government also has politicized the pandemic and treated it in secrecy. For the Chinese, political polarization is not the issue but the motives of other countries. According to Maxmen (2022), in China, the pandemic is a politically sensitive topic. The Chinese attempted to cover up the outbreak from the beginning (Zinn 2021). The Chinese government instructed researchers and health officials to censor all information regarding COVID-19. Those disobeying government directives would be held accountable. Finally, within days of the outbreak in Wuhan, China, the Chinese government politicized COVID-19 by accusing the United States of developing and releasing the virus.

Returning to the United States, the normlessness of congressional leaders experienced over the last decades has been a model for American behavior. The traditional norms for congressional behavior have been abandoned for posturing and conflict. Congressional paralysis and challenging legislation that might benefit American society have become the norm. The age when dealmakers in Congress could bring sides together and reach workable solutions was long gone. Regardless of party affiliation, name-calling and posturing on any issue became the rule of the day. The nation entered what some characterize as a post-truth society where facts are dismissed as "fake" and falsehoods promoted if they support political objectives. Party affiliation now matters more than the content of bills, appointments, and policies (for discussion, see Lempert 2022).

It increasingly became embedded in American politics that compromise, cooperation, and moderation were signs of political weakness. Issues increasingly separated elected officials along party lines. Consequently, COVID-19 and its restrictions became grounds for political posturing and collective action for some extreme Americans and their elected officials. The pandemic and what the government requested or mandated became a politically charged and divisive issue for some extremist individuals and groups.

Nevertheless, congressional Republicans and Democrats sponsored bills designed to alleviate the pandemic and ease the economic stress of Americans. Both houses of Congress did take collaborative budgetary and policy measures to address the pandemic. Congressional and executive branch members did attempt to address COVID-19 by passing major budget packages designed to encourage the development of vaccines, distribute medical supplies, and minimize the economic impact of the pandemic on Americans. For example, the CARES Act allocated $500 billion to large corporations and banks, and other financial institutions, which was leveraged for trillions of additional dollars with little oversight to offset the economic impacts of the pandemic (for a discussion, see Chomsky and Waterstone 2021:240–241). Adults were given a one-time payment of $1,200 and $500 per child. Unemployment checks were also increased by $600 per week. President Trump and the White House did establish task forces and groups at the federal level to address COVID-19 and supported the budget initiatives directed at the pandemic.

Congress also responded to COVID-19 by conducting multiple House and Senate hearings. In 2021, 32 hearings addressed the topic of vaccines and, specifically, vaccine rollout, their distribution, and vaccine hesitancy (Nayak and Reynolds 2022). Vaccine development and effectiveness were discussed in 13 of the hearings. Fifteen of the hearings covered the subject of vaccine hesitancy, misinformation, and barriers to success. Vaccine distribution was discussed in 27 hearings, with vaccine access of minority groups being a topic.

However, balancing the economic needs of society and avoiding a major recession while managing restrictions that negatively affected the economy served as a political flashpoint (see Funk, Tyson, Pasquini, and Spencer 2022). Most people agreed that forced lockdowns, restrictions of public spaces, social distancing, school closures, mask-wearing, travel restrictions, and mandatory quarantines negatively impacted the economy. The travel, entertainment, restaurant, and transportation sectors were hit particularly hard. Absenteeism due to COVID-19 illness also affected the economy. However, some sectors of the economy did benefit, such as medical and cleaning suppliers and pharmaceutical companies. Some elected officials took public stances that weighed public health interventions against economic impacts. For example, Matthewman and Huppatz (2020:679) cited the lieutenant governor of Texas, Dan Patrick, commenting that he would rather die than have public health interventions interfere with the economy. He also urged workers to return to work and let older people fend for themselves.

When thinking about the pandemic, it is crucial to understand how groups influence understandings, perceptions, and behaviors. The old saying "birds of a feather flock together" rings valid for social and political relationships. People tend to associate with similar people who share common beliefs and interests. Sociologists labeled this behavioral pattern homophily (see Chapter 4). The concept of homophily applies to political affiliation and allegiance. Americans tend to form their opinions and craft their behaviors from groups and people who generally reaffirm their beliefs and behaviors. Many obtain political information from confirming sources, such as liberal, conservative, or radically charged sources. During the pandemic, evidence of homophily was abundant (see chapters 4 and 5).

Another point is the critical role political ideology played in the pandemic. Political ideologies are beliefs that mobilize people for action. Ideologies are rhetorical tools used in the struggle for public opinion on whether to gain support for or against opposing ideas. Ideologies support actions and positions taken, such as determining the appropriate role of government during the pandemic. Ideologies help adherents make sense of the world but can be frustrating, confusing, and needing direction. Political ideologies served to guide many of the responses to COVID-19.

A useful concept is that of Eric Hoffer, the true believer, which seems applicable to those individuals on either side of the political divide who either unquestionably buy into pandemic policies or entirely oppose them regardless of the evidence. They are true believers holding to their particular ideology irrespective of what the facts indicate. During the pandemic, some true believers were terrified of COVID-19 and eagerly sought vaccinations. Likewise, true believers at the opposite extreme opposed vaccination and believed the pandemic was overblown.

THE ROLE OF POPULISM IN THE PANDEMIC

One of the important political aspects of the pandemic is populism. According to the *Encyclopedia Britannica*, populism is a "political program or movement that champions, or claims to champion, the common person, usually by favourable contrast with a real or perceived elite or establishment" (Munro 2023:n.p.). Furthermore, Munro (2023:n.p.) stated, "Populism usually combines elements of the left and the right, opposing large business and financial interests but also frequently being hostile to established liberal, socialist, and labour parties."

In the United States, the Democratic and Republican parties are often criticized by populists. Populists complain about organizations or groups that interfere with the relationship between the common person and government or political leadership. Populists generally oppose big government and those groups they view as elites. There are links between populism and some of the COVID-19 conspiracy theories. To populists on the right, when bad things happen, suspicion and conspiracy theories surface. In a context of fear and suspicion, Offe (2021:34) observed, "As this logic is also widely employed by the populist right, there seems to be a 'natural' affinity between populism and emotions of suspecting dark forces being held responsible for the corona health crisis." Thus it is no surprise that populist politicians linked the Chinese and "elites," such as Bill Gates, to dark conspiracies (left- and right-leaning). They became targets in many conspiracy theories advanced by far-left and -right populists (see chapters 5 and 7).

Far-right populists believe that migration needs to be controlled or stopped, globalization has destroyed and is destroying local communities and corresponding economies, and global elites do not care what happens to common people (Turner 2021:154). Far-right adherents believe personal health is mostly a private matter and the free market is better suited to make decisions and provide healthcare than government agencies (Zielonka 2021:70–71). For example, right-wingers linked the spread of COVID-19 to border crossings and foreigners and resisted public health mandates.

According to Innerarity (2021:96), "There are three things that populist leaders hate whose value is increased by this type of crisis [pandemic]: expert knowledge, institutions, and the global community." Several examples of populist hatred of these three have emerged during the pandemic. For instance, Innerarity observed that "former President Trump rejected science and reduced the agency's budget responsible for overseeing responses to the pandemic." In addition, he downplayed Covid-19 by announcing it was similar to seasonal flu. He denied the risks associated with Covid-19 (Paul and Haddad 2023).

Regarding the global community and institutions, he discredited the World Health Organization (WHO) and federal agencies responding to the pandemic. He attempted to withdraw American support from the WHO. These efforts reflect some of the basic tenets of populism.

Populism has attacked science, scientists, and facts. Furthermore, far-right populist stress on nationalism and isolationism surfaced. The "America First" concept implied isolationism and nationalism and emerged with the distribution of medical supplies and limiting international travel. These actions were taken from the far-right populist playbook.

Ironically, populists' embracing the values of fervent nationalism and isolation is occurring at a time when worldwide pandemics are more likely to occur. Pandemics do not respect national boundaries, and isolation of populations is virtually impossible. Delanty (2021b:3) observed, "It is now widely recognized epidemics must be located in the global context; contagion, by its nature, is not confined by national boundaries or borders." Complicating matters even more, humans are changing the global environment in ways, such as climate warming, deforestation, population growth, and pollution, that favor the evolution and spread of new diseases. Turner (2021:139) said, "As our natural environment is further corrupted, we can expect more global plagues. In short, we are not in a post-bubonic plague era and, as with influenza, we may never be entirely free from Covid-19 outbreaks."

On the far left, populists believe health policies are public matters and should not be up to the individual to decide. To left-wingers, an important goal of healthcare is to provide equal access to all people (Zielonka 2021). Thus, during the pandemic, they focused on equal access to vaccines and healthcare for underserved populations (rural, people of color, older people, etc.) and favored mandates. However, some left-leaning populists also felt uncomfortable with orders, such as mandatory vaccines, because they represented government intrusion into their lives. They distrusted the "elites," such as the leaders of "big pharma." They accused the elites of financially profiting from the pandemic.

PRESIDENTIAL LEADERSHIP AND THE COVID-19 PANDEMIC

Social scientists have studied and documented leadership's important role in influencing social behavior. Some believe the White House, specifically President Donald Trump's leadership and policies, exacerbated the COVID-19 pandemic (Offe 2021:26). Others have concluded that his leadership and policies minimized what they believed was an unnecessary overreaction and panic. As the nation's leader, statements made by the president were highly influential for some Americans.

Regardless of which view is taken, what can be documented is what the president publicly stated about COVID-19 and the pandemic. Texas Democratic congressman Lloyd Doggett (2022) and Kiely, Robertson, Rieder, and Gore (2020) have published timelines of President Trump's COVID-19 comments (actual quotes) and the dates they were publicly stated. With limited medical information, the president was compelled to comment on the coronavirus. The following are samples of the comments that helped shape some Americans' understanding of COVID-19 and the pandemic.

TIMELINE OF PRESIDENT TRUMP'S PUBLIC STATEMENTS ON COVID-19 JANUARY 22, 2020, TO JANUARY 20, 2021

- January 22, 2020 – "We have it totally under control. It is one person coming from China. It is going to be just fine."
- February 2, 2020 – "We pretty much shut it down coming in from China."
- February 10, 2020 – "I think the virus is going to be—it's going to be fine." President Trump told supporters at a rally that when the weather warmed up, the coronavirus would "miraculously go away."
- February 24, 2020 – "The coronavirus is very much under control in the USA . . . the stock market starting to look very good to me!"
- February 25, 2020 – "CDC and my administration are doing a great job of handling the coronavirus."
- February 26, 2020 - At a press conference, he told reporters, "This is like the flu."
- February 27, 2020 – "It's going to disappear. One day, it's like a miracle, it will disappear."
- March 4, 2020 – "If we have thousands or hundreds of thousands of people that get better just by, you know, sitting around and even going to work—some of them go to work, but they get better."
- March 6, 2020 – "You have to be calm. It'll go away."
- March 6, 2020 – "I like this stuff. I really get it. People are surprised that I understand it. Every one of these doctors said, 'How do you know so much about this?' Maybe I have a natural ability. Maybe I should've done that instead of running for President." (Referring to COVID-19 and its treatments.)
- March 10, 2020 – "Just stay calm. It will go away."
- March 19, 2020 – "I intended 'to always play it down.' I still like playing it down because I don't want to create a panic." (President Trump excerpt from a taped interview with Bob Woodward made public on September 9, 2020.)
- March 31, 2020 – " . . . it's not the flu. It's vicious."
- April 7, 2020 – "You are not going to die from this pill. Period. I really think it's a good thing to try." (Referring to Hydroxychloroquine, an unapproved treatment for COVID-19).
- April 23, 2020 – "I see the disinfectant that knocks it out in a minute, one minute. And is there a way we can do something like that by injection inside or almost a cleaning? As you say, it gets in the lungs, it does a tremendous number on the lungs, so it would be interesting to check

that." (Referring to using a household cleaner containing bleach to combat COVID-19.)

- April 23, 2020 – "So, supposing we hit the body with a tremendous, whether it's ultraviolet or just very powerful light, and I think you said, that hasn't been checked out but you're going to test it. And then I said, supposing you brought the light inside the body, which you can either do through the skin or some other way." (Proposing a possible treatment for COVID-19 infections.)
- May 9, 2020. – "This is going to go away without a vaccine."
- May 14, 2020 – "Don't forget, we have more cases than anybody in the world. But why? Because we do more testing."
- June 23, 2020 – "Cases are going up in the United States because we are testing far more than any other country, and over-expanding. With smaller testing we would show fewer cases!"
- July 21, 2020 – "You will never hear this on the fake news concerning the China virus, but by comparison to most other countries, who are suffering greatly, we are doing very well—we have done things that few other countries could have done."
- August 5, 2020 – "If you look at children, children are almost—and I would almost say definitely—but almost immune from the disease."
- September 10, 2020 – "This is nobody's fault but China."
- October 5, 2020 – "Don't be afraid of Covid-19."
- October 12, 2020 – "I went through it. Now, they say I'm immune. I can feel—I feel so powerful."
- October 8, 2020 – "Covid, Covid, Covid is the united chant of the fake news lamestream media. They will talk about nothing else until November 4, when the election will be (hopefully) over. Then the talk will be how low the death rate is, plenty of hospital rooms, and many tests of young people."
- November 3, 2020 - The U.S. presidential election occurs, with response to the COVID-19 pandemic response being one of the issues most debated.

The following is an analysis of the messaging of the president's comments regarding COVID-19 covering January 2020 to January 20, 2021. As the nation's leader, the president's comments are important to the masses. The Office of the President has assumed public credibility and trust for many citizens regardless of who holds the presidency. The analysis focuses on themes repeated in the president's public comments. All presidents have been known to politicize their statements. Possible motives behind the comments are suggested. With some of the president's remarks, there is an element of truth, which is often the case with rumors.

Table 6.1. Summary Analysis of President Trump's Public Comments about COVID-19

Message	*Dates of Presidential Public Comments in 2020 (unless otherwise noted)*
One of the messages is that of optimism regarding COVID-19. In a nutshell, everything will be just fine, and we should not worry. It's no big deal. COVID-19 is mild.	Feb. 10, 25, 26, Mar. 2, 4, 5, 7, 11, Apr. 6, 7, 22, May 5, June 23, 25, July 1, 7, Sept. 10, 23, Oct. 5, 10, 22, and 27.
The current administration is doing a great job addressing COVID-19.	Feb. 25, 28, Mar. 6, 8, 12, 14, 27, Apr. 5, 9, 13, May 6, July 21, Aug. 3, 5, 31, Sept. 10, 21, Oct. 11, 15, Dec. 8, 22, and Jan. 3, 2021.
There needs to be more testing or testing readily available. There are plenty of tests. Testing is overrated. The United States has lots of cases because of more testing, and as a nation, we overdo testing, and thus more COVID-19 is detected.	Feb. 26, Mar. 6, 9, 30, May 14, 19, 20, 23, July 19, Aug. 3, Oct. 30, and Nov. 2.
The press is not giving the administration due credit for its successes with COVID-19. The president is not getting the credit he deserves. Some of the press coverage exaggerates COVID-19. There is fake news about COVID-19.	Mar. 17, 20, May 16, June 25, July 21, Sept. 21, Oct. 24, 26, 27, 28, and Jan. 3, 2021.
COVID-19 will disappear like a miracle. It will go away.	Feb. 27, Mar. 10, 11, Apr. 29, May 8, 9, June 15, 17, 18, and Aug. 5.
COVID-19 vaccines are here or close. There is a conspiracy to delay the vaccine until after the election. COVID-19 will go away without a vaccine.	Feb. 25, May 9, 15, July 27, Aug. 22, Sept. 4, 10, 16, 28, and Nov. 9.
Schools and the workplace should reopen because lockdowns are not needed and impact the economy.	Mar. 24, 25, Apr. 15, 23, July 8, Aug. 3, and Sept. 21.
Alternative medical solutions or miracle cures such as Hydroxychloroquine are available and effective.	Feb. 10, Mar. 2, Apr. 7, 23, Aug. 22, and Oct. 12.
The coronavirus is under control.	Jan. 22, Feb. 24, Mar. 15, May 11, and Aug. 3.
The problems with managing COVID-19 are due to Democrat governors and states.	Mar. 26, 27, Apr. 1, 2, May 5, and Sept. 16.
COVID-19 is more deadly and serious than the flu. It is very contagious.	Feb. 7, Mar. 15, 29, 31, and May 5.

Message	Dates of Presidential Public Comments in 2020 (unless otherwise noted)
China is doing a good job. China is the source of the coronavirus. It is China's fault the world is experiencing a pandemic.	Jan. 22, 24, Feb. 2, Sept. 10, and Oct. 26.
People should stay calm and relax. The virus should be played down to avoid a mass panic.	Mar. 6, 10, 15, 19, and 30.
The president understands and has insights about the coronavirus that others, including medically trained people, do not. Strong White House leadership has mitigated the negative impacts of the virus.	Mar. 6, 17, Apr. 26, and Oct. 12.
Cases are going down not up. We have low numbers.	Feb. 26, May 11, and Aug. 4.
American death rates due to COVID-19 are low compared to other countries.	June 25, July 19, and Oct. 15.
Do nothing but weather out COVID-19.	May 15 and July 19.

There are additional President Trump messages, such as that people are tired of mandates and restrictions (Apr. 3 and Oct. 19), that mandates represent a prison state (Nov. 1 and 2), and that the coronavirus will be rough and deadly (May 5). To supporters of the president, many of these messages are comforting, reassuring, and what they wanted to hear. For example, it is not unreasonable for a president of any nation to want constituents not to panic and stay calm. Winston Churchill and President Franklin Roosevelt certainly conveyed a message of calmness during WWII. A panic results in social unrest and upheaval, as normal social and business relationships are disrupted. Only some sitting leaders want disruption under their watch.

Furthermore, in the prominent position of president of the United States, citizens mostly want assurances that everything is under control and strong leadership is guiding the government. The alternative is uncertainty and disorder, and collective behavior theorists (chapter 4) suggest people do not feel comfortable when social unrest exists. The goal of controlling Americans' responses to the pandemic proved challenging for Presidents Trump and Biden. Turner (2021:152) noted that factors in the United States make it difficult for any president to maintain consistent control over the pandemic. Turner wrote, "These include federalism, individualism, business interests, fake news, the second amendment, and populist hostility to government overreach."

Understandably, regardless of political party, any government administration will want to address a major pandemic quickly. In this regard, elected officials have options, such as denying a pandemic and hoping it will quickly run its course and there will be a return to normalcy. They can also directly address pandemics by supplying resources for research and development and rollouts of medical solutions. In this vein, it is common for administrations to fall into the trap of unbridled optimism (see Arnold-Foster 2021). For example, President Trump labeled the COVID-19 vaccine development and rollout "Operation Warp Speed." What could be faster than a "warp speed" response? The president announced that vaccines would be developed by the end of 2020. This optimism would later be tempered by the reality of bureaucratic red tape, production delays, distribution challenges, and public vaccine hesitancy. Following the announcement of Warp Speed, behind-the-scenes movements were made to further restrict pandemic messaging by moving the collection of COVID-19 data away from the CDC.

Critics would point out that the president's mixed messages demonstrate incompetence, ignorance, or avoidance of the facts (for a fact check of some of the president's comments, see Kiely, Robertson, Rieder, and Gore 2020; Paz 2020). Paz (2020) concluded that the president's statements were lies. Public comments about COVID-19 differed from what the president thought privately or what the facts indicated. For example, infection and mortality rates have consistently been higher in the United States than in any other developed country. Critics have concluded that many of the president's comments were propaganda and catered more toward his political base than reality. Had the president acknowledged the problem sooner, they contend, much of the harm caused by the pandemic could have been averted. Collective behaviorists would suggest that these and other statements reflect features common to propaganda and the manipulation of information to serve one's purpose.

Tollerson (2020) was not surprised by the president's defiance and accused him of lying and undermining efforts to control the coronavirus. Tollerson wrote, "Trump has belittled masks and social-distancing requirements while encouraging people to protest against lockdown rules to stop disease transmission. His administration undermined, suppressed, and censored government scientists working to study the virus and reduce its harm." In addition, the White House politicized the Centers for Disease Control and Prevention and the Food and Drug Administration and provided ill-advised health guidance, such as untested cures for the virus.

During 2020, people came out for political rallies during the pandemic, not wearing masks or practicing social distancing in defiance of recommended COVID-19 health guidelines. For example, President Trump and attendees ignored public health guidelines at a Henderson, Nevada, rally on

September 13, 2020. Attendees flaunted the restrictions and dared local health officials to stop the rally. Following the rally, White House staff experienced a COVID-19 outbreak. The president also eventually caught COVID-19 and was hospitalized for three days. On October 5, 2020, when he was discharged, he promised, "The vaccines are coming momentarily." His repeated claims that a vaccine would be approved before Election Day had politicized the subject.

Regardless of whether one supports or opposes the president and official public health policies, the following conclusions can be drawn. Sometimes, the official messaging regarding COVID-19 could have been more consistent, but was only sometimes factual or medically sound, politically charged, and unrealistically optimistic. Collective behaviorists have suggested that the public will take away whatever messages it is predisposed toward. People hear what they want, and when they hear it from leaders sharing their views, the messaging becomes even more powerful. Most people do not take the extra step of fact-checking comments and statements but take them at face value, especially when it is what they want to hear and is coming from their leader.

The social isolation occurring during the pandemic contributed to political polarization. Over time, the two polarized political factions increasingly relied on their respective political camps for information on the nature of the pandemic. For example, Van Bavel et al. (2021:464) observed that:

> One issue with polarization during a pandemic is that it might lead different population segments to arrive at different conclusions about the threat in the situation and appropriate actions. In addition, partisans may receive other news because individuals can self-select polarized news sources or partisan "echo chambers" or communicate in ways associated with less cross-partisan information sharing. Nevertheless, in-person political interactions can provide more opportunities for cross-partisan communication (that produces a shared understanding). Decreasing in-person contact due to Covid-19 may reduce cross-partisan interactions and information sharing.

Put differently, because of social isolation, people increasingly relied on information sources aligned with their political views rather than interacting with others who might hold different opinions. Ultimately, the echo chamber concept applies because their ideas became increasingly insular. Biased news sources contributed to insular views on COVID-19. Research on where people get their news has been revealing. For example, research by Hamel, Lopes, Kirzinger, Sparks, Stokes, and Brodie (2021:n.p.) supports this observation:

As well documented (in particular by the Pew Research Center), the U.S. media environment has become increasingly polarized in recent years, with Democrats and Republicans placing trust in completely different news sources. This is true when it comes to trust in COVID-19 information as well. Majorities of Democrats say they trust information about COVID-19 from network news (72%), local TV news (66%), CNN (65%), MSNBC (56%), and NPR (51%), while a majority of independents or Republicans trusts none of these sources. Republicans' most trusted sources of COVID-19 information are Fox News (49%), followed by smaller shares who trust local TV news (34%), network news (25%), and Newsmax (22%).

THE HEALTH CONSEQUENCES OF POLITICAL ALLEGIANCE

Researchers have surveyed American adults on COVID-19 topics, such as belief in the seriousness of the disease and attitudes toward vaccinations or other preventative measures. Regarding political affiliation and perceptions of the severity of the disease, a Kaiser Family Foundation study (Kirzinger et al. 2021) reported that vaccinated Republicans were somewhat less likely than unvaccinated Republicans to say the seriousness of the pandemic has been exaggerated in the news (88% vs. 54% respectively). Both groups contrast with vaccinated Democrats, most of whom indicated the news was generally correct (56%) or underestimated the seriousness of the pandemic (31%). An overwhelming majority of unvaccinated Republicans (96%) and a somewhat smaller but still substantial majority of vaccinated Republicans (73%) said getting vaccinated against COVID-19 was a personal choice. In comparison, a large majority of vaccinated Democrats (81%) saw it as everyone's responsibility to protect the health of others. Moreover, while vaccinated Republicans were about twice as likely as unvaccinated Republicans to worry that they will personally get sick from COVID-19 (25% vs. 11%), the share that was worried was still substantially less than it was among vaccinated Democrats (46%).

The dimension of individual choice is essential for understanding the politicization of the pandemic. A Pew Research Center study investigated the role of government and the restriction of individual choice. Funk, Tyson, Pasquini, and Spencer's (2022) survey of 10,282 Americans found that most Republicans said the country had done too little during the outbreak regarding respecting individuals' choices (69%). A smaller percentage of Democrats expressed this view. Democrats were roughly as likely to have said that too much priority has been given to respecting individuals' choices compared with too little (33% and 28%, respectively).

Some research has focused on political allegiance's role in determining whether people have resisted vaccinations. Researchers have conducted surveys exploring whether political allegiance influences vaccination rates. One study, a Pew Research Center survey of American adults, examined the relationship between Americans' sources for COVID-19 news and vaccination status (Jurkowitz and Mitchell 2021). A question about COVID-19 news sources was asked on April 20–26, 2020, and whether Americans received at least one vaccine for COVID-19 was asked on August 23–29, 2021. A total of 6,686 U.S. adults completed both surveys.

The survey found that Americans who relied on President Trump and the White House for information on COVID-19 were least likely to have been vaccinated. At the time of the study, 59 percent of respondents who relied mainly on President Trump for guidance indicated they had received at least one dose of the vaccine, and 38 percent had not. Adults depending on family and friends, online forums, or local newsletters for news broke down to 58 percent having at least one vaccine and 38 percent not. Jurkowitz and Mitchell (2021) found that the most highly vaccinated groups were adults who, in April 2020, relied most on national news outlets, public health organizations, and officials for COVID-19 news; 83 percent and 82 percent, respectively.

A different study by the Kaiser Family Foundation found that political affiliation played a role in determining vaccination status (Kirzinger et al. 2021). The survey found a strong relationship between partisan identification and how individuals perceived and experienced the pandemic. While most people surveyed were vaccinated regardless of political party, political partisanship still mattered for some individuals. Republicans made up an increasing proportion of those unvaccinated. The researchers found that political partisanship was a stronger predictor of vaccination status than demographic factors, such as education, race, age, and insurance. Another researcher reached a similar conclusion. Reich (2021:7) wrote, "Political identity and affiliation appear to matter, with those who identify as Republican consistently expressing the lowest desire for a vaccine."

In addition, the Kaiser Family Foundation's study revealed that those respondents living in rural communities expressed lower interest in getting vaccinations (Kirzinger et al. 2021). The study found that young adults who were told they were unlikely to be seriously affected by COVID-19 showed low interest levels. The survey discovered that some essential workers (i.e., nurses, grocery workers, and police, among others) were unwilling to be among the first to be inoculated, despite the job risks they faced. The finding regarding vaccinations and partisanship had surfaced in previous Kaiser Family Foundation studies for other COVID-19 control efforts, such as wearing masks and social distancing. Unvaccinated Republicans tended to be younger, less educated, and living in rural areas than vaccinated Republicans. Throughout the pandemic, individuals were drawing on cultural information to make pandemic decisions that they felt were personally relevant.

In a similar vein, a Pew Research Center study found that political affiliation influenced confidence in the effectiveness of vaccines. Pew researchers Funk, Tyson, Pasquini, and Spencer (2022) surveyed 10,282 adults and found that partisan gaps over the effectiveness of vaccines were the widest they had observed. Specifically, 75 percent of Democrats said COVID-19 vaccines had been highly or significantly effective at limiting the spread of the coronavirus; 16 percent said they have been somewhat effective, and only 9 percent described them as not too or not at all effective. In contrast, Republicans had a more skeptical view of vaccine effectiveness. A larger share of Republicans said vaccines were not too or not at all effective at limiting the spread of COVID-19 than said they have been extremely or very effective (39% vs. 32%). Twenty-nine percent of Republicans said vaccines were somewhat effective.

Vaccine resistance (see chapter 8) cannot be attributed solely to political allegiance. Referring to the history of vaccination resistance, McNamara (2021) cited the director of the Institute for Research on Women and Gender at the University of Michigan, Dr. Anna Kirkland, as stating:

> There are a lot of parallels—many of the same arguments. Some of the differences now are the stark political alignments by the party that we see under COVID-19, which were there in some ways before but became very prominently organized by the party. However, those are only differences in degree because there has long been an anti-government backing of anti-vaccine sentiments.

Former president Trump learned how entrenched this vaccine-hesitant constituency was. He was booed at a political rally in Alabama on August 21, 2021, after he recommended his supporters get the vaccine. He stated:

> Everything that we did, and then we developed three vaccines in three months, in nine months. Moreover, I'll tell you, it was three days less, three days less than nine months. Furthermore, it's great. And you know what? I believe totally in your freedoms, I do. But you got to do what you have to do, but I recommend, take the vaccines. I did it. It's good. Take the vaccines, but you got . . . No, that's okay. That's all right. You got your freedoms. But I happened to take the vaccine. If it doesn't work, you'll be the first to know, okay. I'll call up Alabama and say, "Hey, you know what?" But it is working. But you do have your freedoms. You have to keep; you have to maintain that. And you got to get your kids back to school. And the mask issue is interesting because Fauci said, "Masks are bad," and now he's a radical masker." (Transcript of Donald Trump speech at a Cullman, Alabama, rally August 21, 2021)

DEATH RATES AND POLITICAL ALLEGIANCE

Death rates are an important indicator of how COVID-19 impacts populations. Various demographic factors, prior health history (preexisting conditions), access to health care, residence, age, and race were described in chapter 2 as playing a role in COVID-19 infection and death rates. In addition, researchers have studied if political allegiance influenced COVID-19 death rates. At the beginning of the pandemic (first wave), death rates per 100,000 population were higher in Democratic-leaning cities. Fundamental factors accounting for this pattern include higher population density and, thus, person-to-person contacts (exposure) in cities. Urban areas have more travelers, which can spread the disease to others. The risk of infection is lower in less populated rural areas. Another initial factor was the inadequate medical capacity to address COVID-19 patients. Urban residents could do little besides isolate, social distance, wear masks, and hope they could avoid infection. Once medical experts knew more about COVID-19, how it was transmitted, and vaccines became available, death rates shifted to Republican-leaning rural areas and cities. In Republican-dominated rural areas, access to vaccines was limited, and residents saw less need for vaccinations. Support for these patterns, and specifically the role of political partisanship, can be found in survey data. For example, a Pew Research Center (Jones 2022:n.p.) study reported:

> Partisan differences in COVID-19 death rates expanded dramatically after the availability of vaccines increased. Unvaccinated people are at far higher risk of death and hospitalization from COVID-19, according to the Centers for Disease Control and Prevention, and vaccination decisions are strongly associated with [political] partisanship. Among the large majority of counties for which reliable vaccination data exists, counties that supported Trump at higher margins have substantially lower vaccination rates than those that supported Biden at higher margins.

Later, during the third wave of COVID-19 infections, the death rate for Americans living in counties that supported Trump was 170 percent higher than that of counties that heavily supported Biden by the highest margins (Jones 2022:n.p.). When vaccines became more widely available, differences between Democratic and Republican counties became even more significant with the spread of the Delta variant during the summer and fall of 2021. According to the Pew Research Center study, COVID-19 death rates were four times higher in heavy pro-Trump than in heavy pro-Biden counties during the fourth pandemic wave. These differences narrowed when Omicron began its spread, but death rates remained 180 percent higher in the pro-Trump counties throughout the late 2021 and early 2022 months. In addition, death rates have been higher throughout the pandemic in pro-Trump counties, at 326 per 100,000 population, compared to pro-Biden counties, at 258 per 100,000 population (Jones 2022). While party affiliation does not fully account for COVID-19 death rates, it does appear to explain some of the differences observed between the two political groups.

Other studies and experts have reached similar conclusions. For example, in a National Public Radio broadcast, Wood and Brumfiel (2021) reported that since May of 2021, those in counties that voted for Trump during the last election were three times more likely to die from COVID-19 than those voting for Biden. They attributed this difference to misinformation and political polarization. They compared the deaths per 100,000 people in approximately 3,000 communities when vaccinations had become readily available. Those counties voting 60 percent or higher for Trump had 2.73 times the death rate from COVID-19 than those that went for Biden.

Columbia University scholars looked into what if the United States had taken earlier preventive measures against the coronavirus (Pei et al. 2020). They developed a model of what would have happened if the nation had taken steps, such as shutting down two weeks earlier. In a published paper, they estimated that 35,000 lives could have been saved. Their model was published before new virus variants like Delta and Omicron surfaced. President Trump would label Columbia University a political hit job by a very liberal institution (Tollerson 2020).

ELIMINATIONIST MOVEMENT AND COVID-19

The politically extreme far right has played a vital role in the pandemic (see shapter 5 for an overview of the role of social media, the news, and COVID-19). The term "eliminationist" describes the malignant influence of right-wing hate talk on the American conservative movement. It helps understand some of the extreme right-wing thinking about the pandemic. Much of the pandemic rhetoric comes from para-fascist right-wing groups. David Neiwert (2009) has documented persistent ideas and rhetoric that promote eliminating opposition groups. This hate rhetoric has influenced the right-wing conservative movement and made it not genuinely conservative but potentially dangerous to democracy (for a discussion, see Finkel, Ball, Cikara, et al. 2020). Neiwert proposed that the traditional conservative movement has stood aside and emboldened groups on the far right's extreme fringes. In the case of the United States, the election of President Barack Obama fueled right-wing extremists. In contrast, the election of President Donald Trump emboldened them to strengthen their political resolve. Later, the election of President Joseph Biden sparked some to challenge the election results, and threats of domestic terrorism increased.

In recent years eliminationist rhetoric has become more common in the United States. According to Miller (2014:103), "Eliminationist rhetoric is hate rhetoric, and some rumors are stated through the use of eliminationist rhetoric." Miller (2014:103) wrote, "Hateful rants and rumors about liberals, gays, Muslims, Teabaggers, Occupy Wall Street, Democrats, Republicans, government, unions, and illegal immigrants abound." Thus, any government COVID-19 restriction or mandate would be resisted based on the core values of the eliminationist movement. Eliminationist rhetoric depicts targeted groups as evil and dangerous and advocates the elimination of these groups by violent or civil means. In the case of COVID-19, eliminationist rhetoric targeted people of Asian ancestry, whether American or not. Former President Trump's comments about "Kung Flu" and accusing China of being the source of the pandemic moved some predisposed individuals to attack Americans of Asian ancestry. These Asian Americans became scapegoats, a typical pattern for understanding and responding to mass contagions. It also targeted public health agencies, the federal government, and spokespersons as needing to be overthrown or eliminated.

ROLE OF GOVERNMENT IN THE PANDEMIC

The role of government in providing public health services, research, guidance, and directives to the American public has spurred debate and controversy. One study by Parker, Horowitz, and Minkin (2021) surveyed 9,676 American adults in October 2021 to better understand American views on where they prefer to live and the impact of COVID-19 on local communities. Part of their survey asked them to rate federal, state, and local governments' handling of the pandemic. American views of the federal government's response to the pandemic were mixed. Most Americans did not rate any level of government as doing an excellent job addressing the pandemic. However, respondents did rate local governments as doing a better job than the federal government. Findings indicated that 38 percent of Americans gave their state and 39 percent gave county governments excellent to good ratings for COVID-19 responses. These ratings are compared to 29 percent for the federal government.

In contrast, 39 percent thought the government at all levels was doing a poor or very poor job, and 32 percent indicated an average job. Parker et al. found that Republicans were particularly damaging in their views of how the federal government has handled the pandemic, with 65 percent saying it has done a poor or very poor job, compared with 18 percent of Democrats.

With differing political opinions about the government's role, some respondents would likely view anything the government does at any level as either poor or good.

Additionally, Parker et al. (2021) found that most (77%) Americans believed the pandemic had driven people further apart, and only 8 percent thought it had brought people together. The pandemic, in the opinion of most Americans, regardless of party, has added to the country's polarization but not necessarily in their local communities. According to the survey, demographic groups held different opinions on the pandemic's divisiveness. White adults (83%), four-year college graduates (83%), and upper-income adults (84%) were among the most likely to have said the pandemic had driven people apart at the national level. Republicans (81%) were more likely than Democrats (75%) to express this view. This latter percentage represents a slight difference of 6 percent, so opinions were generally shared regardless of party affiliation.

Political partisanship surfaced in other ways during the pandemic. Beyond public health functions, another role of government is that of social safety net. The Pew Research Center surveyed a national random sample of 10,334 U.S. adults in January 2021 to learn how American financial outlooks and personal finances had changed during the pandemic (Horowitz et al. 2021). Horowitz et al. found that Americans disagreed on who should ensure people could meet their basic economic needs during the pandemic. Less than half (43%) said the federal government should have the most significant responsibility. Fewer (12%) indicated local governments and even less (6%) thought charity should have the most significant responsibility. Again, party lines mattered when forming these opinions. Sixty-one percent of Democrats and Democratic-leaners said the federal government should primarily ensure people can meet their basic economic needs during the COVID-19 pandemic, compared with 28 percent of Republicans and Republican-leaning adults. In contrast, 51 percent of Republicans compared to 18 percent of Democrats said people themselves or their families should have this responsibility. These findings are consistent with traditional Republican and Democratic views on the role of government and economic security.

Political affiliation has led to scapegoating of Asian American and immigrant populations (for discussion, see chapters 1 and 2). The politicization of COVID-19 also led to scapegoating of key national spokespersons at the federal level. For example, Dr. Fauci has been the subject of scapegoating along political lines. Dr. Fauci has had a distinguished career in understanding and addressing viruses. Dr. Fauci was appointed the National Institute of Allergy and Infectious Diseases (NIAID) director in 1984. He has overseen research on infectious diseases like HIV/AIDS, zika, malaria, tuberculosis, and Ebola. He is internationally known for his contributions to studying and treating

HIV and other diseases. He had advised seven presidents, including Obama, Trump, and Biden. Despite a stellar reputation in the field, Dr. Fauci has been targeted and scapegoated since the beginning of the pandemic.

Reasons why he has been targeted and been a scapegoat is that he has been the bearer of pandemic news that people do not want to hear, such as that the infection rates will increase, death rates will be high, masks should be worn, vaccinations should be taken, and so forth. In addition, he is a spokesperson of the federal government and thus was politically opposed for being a national government member. Political affiliation drives the propensity to scapegoat him. As a scapegoat, he has been publicly ridiculed, threatened, and put at risk by radicalized individuals and groups. However, survey data indicates that support for Dr. Fauci has been high among self-identified Democrats and those who lean Democratic. That support eroded gradually, from 92 percent in April 2021 to 88 percent in January 2022, a notable change. Among self-identified Republicans and those who lean Republican, confidence in Dr. Fauci was much lower to start—47 percent in April 2021—and dropped significantly to 36 percent in January 2022 (Annenberg Public Policy Center 2022).

The Annenberg Public Policy Center (2022) found that heavy users of conservative and radical right-wing social media sites and similar news and media sources expressed less confidence in Dr. Fauci, the Centers for Disease Control and Prevention (CDC), and the federal Food and Drug Administration (FDA) when compared to others who relied on traditional news sources for information. This is an example of scapegoating the messenger. Dr. Fauci carried the CDC shield into the pandemic battle. He was simply the vessel for carrying the message but true to scapegoating, he was a convenient target for blame. Put differently, opponents quickly blamed the messenger and held him accountable for all statements. This standard of accountability was not applied to the president and White House for misleading information about the pandemic. The Annenberg Public Policy Center (2022:n.p.) observed:

> Fauci has been the target of attacks in conservative media outlets for many months, and as noted in our November survey released on one night in November, a Fox News viewer would have seen Fauci likened to the Nazi doctor Josef Mengele and the Italian fascist dictator Benito Mussolini. The CDC likewise has been the focus of attacks in conservative media over its vaccination and masking guidance. Most recently, in January [2022], it was hit by accusations in conservative media that it "lied" about the extent of Covid-19 casualties, based in part on a deceptively edited video clip of CDC Director Rochelle Walensky.

CONCLUDING OBSERVATIONS

Early in the pandemic public health recommendations were welcomed by most Americans. However, some Americans resisted as the pandemic persisted, and personal, economic, and social impacts were felt. Hurt (2022) noted that responses to public health restrictions and mandates became increasingly partisan, aggravated by the ideological divide promoted by news sources and social media. Over the pandemic, COVID-19 and social responses to it increasingly became politicized, creating a perfect storm for the coronavirus to spread and thrive. It is no accident that the United States had one of the highest COVID-19 death rates of any industrialized country. Political posturing, tribalism, and polarization explain some of these patterns.

Much research has concluded that political ideology influences people's beliefs, attitudes, and misconceptions about COVID-19 (Calvillo et al. 2020). In America and elsewhere, liberals have been more likely than conservatives to recognize the severe health risks of contracting the virus (Priniski and Holyoak 2022). Politicizing COVID-19, political polarization, and adherence to political ideologies have ensured that COVID-19 will persist in the United States. In addition, the political polarization of the pandemic has affected the interpretation of facts. Rothwell and Desai (2020:n.p.) summarized, "Republicans consistently underestimate risks, while Democrats consistently overestimate them."

People rely on rumors for communication when institutional channels are broken down. A similar situation exists when totalitarian governments shut down the media in times of political crisis. The pandemic was a political crisis because it disrupted much of American society and everyday operations. With COVID-19, federal medical experts were essentially censored because their messages regarding COVID-19 were inconsistent with the administration's political views. Examples of this were apparent during the periodic White House press conferences (daily briefings) on COVID-19, where inaccurate presidential messages were non-verbally negatively reacted to by medical experts in the background. The pandemic did not stop politicians from abusing information and facts. Zielonka (2021:68) characterized President Trump's daily briefings as "the most vivid manifestation of this." No one present could contradict the president; the federal government's medical experts had to navigate misinformation.

Van Bavel, Baicker, Boggio, et al. (2021:464) described two types of political polarization that directly apply to the COVID-19 pandemic. They wrote:

> One cultural barrier for coordinated action within countries is political polarization. Polarization among citizens comes in two varieties. "Attitudinal polarization" concerns partisans taking extreme opposing issue positions, whereas

> "affective polarization" refers to partisans disliking and distrusting those from the opposing party(ies). Affective polarization has political consequences, such as decreasing trust, privileging partisan labels over policy information and believing false information, that can undermine social and economic relationships and impair public health.

In short, examples are numerous attitudinal polarized groups accepting or rejecting information regarding COVID-19 solely based on political sources. Attitudinal polarization is a form of uncritical patriotism. That is, adherence to either side of the polarization allegiance interferes with their critical thinking and acceptance or rejection of policies (for a discussion on uncritical patriotism, see Rieger 2022). The same can be said for affective polarization, as themes of trust and distrust of policies color the noise about government COVID-19 policies. Affective polarization can be found in much of the pandemic and vaccine misinformation abundantly available on social media platforms and politicized news sources (see chapter 5). The problem is that the current political climate has locked groups into polarized mindsets, which makes it harder for them to distinguish between factual information and misinformation. Americans live in a post-truth political environment where political groups do not adhere to the facts or are not inclined to be honest (see Delanty 2021b). Some originators of misinformation have fed the social media rumor mill intending to manipulate public opinion and, thus, behavior.

Early in the pandemic, Vinay Prasad and Jeffery S. Flier (2020:n.p.) warned of the risks of politicizing science and policy when they wrote:

> Society faces a risk even more toxic and deadly than Covid-19: that the conduct of science becomes indistinguishable from politics. The tensions between the two policy poles of rapidly and systematically reopening society versus maximizing sheltering in place and social isolation must not be reduced to Republican and Democratic talking points, even as many media outlets promote such simplistic narratives.

Commenting on the pandemic, Chomsky and Waterstone's (2021:343) description of American social responses to the pandemic encapsulates some of what can be extracted from this chapter:

> Finally, we want to note some important linkages between the pandemic and social reactions. On the right, predictably, we have seen numerous examples of authoritarian regimes around the globe utilizing the pandemic as a cover for repression, added surveillance, and curtailing of civil liberties. In the US, as we write, those most anxious to open up the country and get back to business as usual or straight-up combinations of financial insecurity, boredom, impatience, and distrust of government provoke flouting of stay-at-home orders, thereby

> putting the protesters themselves and others at increased risk. Politicians and several US states are responding to and encouraging these demands. However, unfortunately, they are either contemplating or opening their states back up prematurely before the necessary conditions and safeguards are in place.

Politics did not always align with medical science and practice during the pandemic. Elected officials at the national and local levels took public positions that directly contradicted what medical experts were stating. This pattern was not unique to the United States, as observed in other advanced economy countries (Silver and Connaughton 2022). Elected officials' agendas and timelines did not match those of medical research. In the case of the pandemic, medical scientists did not reach conclusions fast enough to satisfy some elected officials' promises and agendas. Specifically, medical researchers did not rush clinical trials of treatments or vaccines. However, vaccine development was exceptionally rapid and safe even within strict scientific rigor. Vaccine researchers were caught in a "Catch 22" and were either accused of moving too fast in testing vaccines or too slow. The slow development and testing of vaccines were linked to a conspiracy theory that unnecessary delays were being managed to influence the upcoming national elections by making President Trump look bad. Complicating matters was that some national elected officials, groups, and individuals spread non-scientific misinformation that promoted a sense of control and mastery over the virus (see chapter 5). In direct opposition to national political leadership, medical scientists did not support elected officials' claims for alternative and unsupported treatments.

Consequently, some national elected officials, specifically the president and White House administration, dismissed, discredited, publicly mocked, and even censored what national medical experts reported. This approach to the pandemic had a political cost. Turner (2021:152) concluded:

> In the months leading up to the November election, Trump has lost support over his management (or mismanagement) of the Covid crisis and trailed behind Joe Biden. Trump's views on masks, lockdowns, vaccinations, the WHO, the severity of the crisis, its origins, and the importance of social distancing have been inconsistent. Nevertheless, his version of political theology continues to win support from his base, but his political credibility has been compromised by his unpredictable responses to the policies that are necessary to bring the pandemic under control.

Finally, unbending solid political allegiance has had notable health consequences for those on the far right who have consistently opposed public health directives, vaccines, and other public health measures. On average, those opposing vaccines and other public health preventative measures have had more serious COVID-19 infections, longer hospitalizations, and higher death rates. Someone, often taxpayers, ultimately pays for these expensive occurrences. Liberals and conservatives both directly and indirectly help pay the social and financial costs of resistance to efforts to control COVID-19. Both pay through higher taxes for federal health care, cost shifting by health care providers to those who can pay, and higher health care insurance premiums.

Chapter 7

COVID-19 Rumors, Myths, and Conspiracy Theories

"When in doubt, tell the truth.
It will confound your enemies and astound your friends."

Attributed to Mark Twain

COVID-19 CONFUSION

Rumors, misinformation, and conspiracy theories are abundant in American society. Some have coined the excessive COVID-19 and pandemic misinformation as an "infodemic." An infodemic is a blast of information about a problem, in this case COVID-19, that is false, often misleading, expands rapidly, and makes a solution more difficult to achieve. The COVID-19 infodemic seems to have generated more than a fair share of misinformation, rumors, and conspiracy theories than American society has experienced recently. There are many reasons why this is the case. Generally, in the absence of information and understanding, there is a human tendency to fill in knowledge gaps by creating true and false information. Initially, there was little public information about COVID-19, but data from various sources expanded as the pandemic spread. Americans sought whatever information they could obtain on COVID-19. This hunger for knowledge was fueled by people's need to know how to respond to COVID-19 and whether it should be feared. Whenever a new situation, such as COVID-19, requires immediate action, people will not always wait for absolutely verified information (Lang and Lang 1961). In the absence of factual information, some people tend to rely on unverified or rogue sources.

Today, the challenge for Americans is not the need for more information but instead filtering out what is true from what is false. Americans have been flooded with misinformation, rumors, and conspiracy theories regarding the pandemic. These distorted sources have influenced Americans' choices and behaviors during the pandemic. They have made important health decisions on getting vaccinated, wearing masks, using unproven drugs, and social distancing. Most people would not rely on a plumber or Uber driver to perform surgery and would think the idea unsafe. However, some of these people might depend on medical advice from a medically untrained stranger on the internet or a neighbor about COVID-19, the risks of vaccines, or how to treat COVID-19 using unproven remedies. How can misinformation, rumors, dangerous advice, and conspiracy theories about COVID-19 be possible in modern American society?

One explanation is the uncertainty of having a new crisis, in this case, the pandemic. People seek quick information and solutions to crises, such as public health problems. They scan their environment for risks, explanations, solutions (remedies), and courses of action. Dingwall, Hoffman, and Staniland (2013:168) wrote:

> Emerging diseases disturb our assumptions of a known universe of risk. A new hazard disrupts our established strategies for managing our everyday lives. What appears irrational may be a locally rational response to uncertainty or at least an attempt to use locally available resources to re-establish sufficient certainty for practical action.

Whether right or wrong, information creates a sense of certainty on which people base their behaviors. If this information is misleading or false, the behaviors may result in unnecessary health risks, irrational fears, justifiable concerns, and stress.

COVID-19 MISINFORMATION AND DISINFORMATION

Information about COVID-19 can be intentionally and unintentionally inaccurate. Unfortunately, individuals, private organizations, politicians, interest groups, and government agencies have spread false information for profit to avoid responsibility, scapegoat others, avoid criticism, advance political goals, sow distrust, disrupt society, and undercut opposing groups. The ability to spread misinformation has never been more effortless due to new mechanisms of communication, such as social media, politically biased news sources, Facebook, Twitter, TikTok, and other media platforms (see chapter 5). All of these have changed the ways factual information and misinformation are shared. As a result, groups and individuals can expand their reach and influence in unimaginable ways.

When information is intentionally manipulated, distorted, fabricated, misinterpreted, or otherwise changed from fact, it is labeled misinformation or disinformation. Misinformation about the pandemic has been propagated by celebrities, politicians, and other prominent public figures (see chapters 5 and 6). For example, Green Bay Packers quarterback Aaron Rodgers made public claims about COVID-19 that have been fact-checked and found to be inaccurate (Robertson et al. 2021). Washington Wizards basketball player Bradley Beal also made misleading comments about COVID-19, as did Florida governor Ron DeSantis that, when fact-checked, proved to be false.

Reasons behind spreading misinformation and disinformation vary and may include financial gain, political posturing, desire to appear knowledgeable, personal beliefs, influence, fraud, and to exert control or power over others. For example, the financial exploitation of people in crisis can be a reason. In times of disasters, crises, and pandemics, people tend to be more vulnerable to financial exploitation. Fraudulent claims about COVID-19 treatments and prevention have been abundant. Numerous commercial scams involving disinformation have surfaced during the pandemic regarding at-home tests, COVID-19 preventatives, and miracle cures (Federal Communications Commission 2021). In addition, scammers have conducted bogus surveys on vaccines to steal personal information (Tresseler 2021).

SURVEYS ON THE EXTENT OF MISINFORMATION

National surveys have tried to determine the nature of COVID-19 misinformation, regardless of its form (rumor, conspiracy, etc.), present in American society. Researchers have studied what factors have led some Americans to believe this misinformation. For example, the Reuters Institute for the Study of Journalism sampled 225 pieces of COVID-19 misinformation dating from January to March 2020 (Brennen et al. 2020). The study found that most (59%) misinformation involved reconfiguration, a process when true information is spun, recontextualized, reworked, or twisted. The study reported that 12 percent of the misinformation was fabricated. Most false claims originated from ordinary people. However, people at the top had the most media engagements and, thus, the broadest public influence. Most (88%) of the false claims appeared on social media platforms, 9 percent on television, 8 percent on news outlets, and 7 percent on other websites. The most influential sources of the misinformation were from the top echelon of society, including celebrities, politicians, and prominent figures. The largest category of misinformation (39%) was misleading or false claims about the actions or policies of public authorities, such as the government.

A study by Kaiser Family Foundation researchers Hamel, Lopes, Kirzinger, Sparks, Stokes, and Brodie (2021) summarized key findings of their vaccine monitor research on COVID-19 misinformation. The research team relied on multiple data sources, including an extensive survey of adults. They concluded that the slow pace of information from researchers, social media, and the polarization of news sources created conditions where it was easy for ambiguous information, misinterpretation, and deliberate misinformation (disinformation) to spread. Critical to their findings was that 78 percent of adults said they had heard at least one of eight false statements about COVID-19 and thought it was true or were unsure. Some adults surveyed believed or were uncertain about at least four false statements. In addition, the researchers found a correlation between vaccination status and political affiliation with belief in false statements, with Republicans, more than Democrats or vaccinated adults, tending to believe or be unsure about misinformation (false statements).

SOURCES OF MISINFORMATION AND DISINFORMATION

Sources of COVID-19 information, misinformation, and disinformation are numerous. The focus here is on misinformation and disinformation. One of the major sources of information is family members, neighbors, friends, co-workers, and others who have routine social interactions. In everyday life, human beings communicate and share factual and non-factual information. Interpretations and misinterpretations have generated much misinformation about COVID-19 and the pandemic through daily social interactions. Individuals hear and pass on facts and falsehoods without always knowing whether the information is true or false. This is the familiar pattern of John telling Betty, Betty telling Chris, Chris telling Kelly, and so forth. Each time information is shared, something changes in the message (see chapter 4). For example, people have shared considerable informal information about COVID-19 symptoms, treatments, and where and how they caught the disease. During the pandemic, social scientists have not paid much attention to everyday interactions and their role in spreading information and misinformation about COVID-19.

TRADITIONAL OR INSTITUTIONAL NEWS SOURCES

A notable amount of COVID-19 information is transmitted through formal institutional or traditional channels, including most national television networks and national publications. These outlets are well organized, have rules, clearly defined procedures, and professional personnel dedicated to publishing or presenting known facts. They have fixed definitions of what is good news, designated routes of transmission, verification procedures for factual content (checks and balances), and established codes of professional conduct (see chapter 5 for more detail). Those involved with reporting the news are held accountable for what they say and how they report it. Professional reputations are at stake, and reporters, researchers, editors, and presenters can lose their jobs and careers for misconduct, such as knowingly reporting misinformation (lies and falsehoods). This is the institutional model for news reporting.

In recent years, this has changed for some news organizations. Today, some right- and left-leaning news media appear to operate with more relaxed procedures and standards for news reporting. They have a different concept of a newsworthy story and very loose criteria for verifying information (Miller 2014). There is less accountability and a tendency to slant information. Furthermore, the news may be manufactured or interpreted to suit viewers' prejudices and perspectives or the owner's objectives. For some national media outlets, the lines between the news, opinion, and propaganda have been blurred.

Some news sources have distorted their reports about COVID-19 to conform to political viewpoints. For example, right-leaning Fox News has run news stories and broadcast opinions that the pandemic is a hoax; the animal de-wormer ivermectin is effective in treating COVID-19; the pandemic is overstated and a politically motivated response by Democrats; promoted the use of hydroxychloroquine as a treatment; and death totals from COVID-19 were overstated and people actually would have died anyway from pre-existing conditions. In addition, when vaccines became available, Fox News repeatedly questioned the effectiveness of the vaccines. For some viewers, their trust in Fox News for information on COVID-19 influenced their taking fewer cautionary measures and more risks related to COVID-19 (Ash et al. 2020; Zhao et al. 2020).

In addition, a tactic used by those motivated to spread COVID-19 misinformation and disinformation is to discredit credible journalists and institutionalized (traditional) news outlets. The objective is to erode public trust in factual news sources (see chapter 5). When sources of information are not trusted because they have been discredited by political leadership, the door opens for spreading misinformation and disinformation. The expression "fake news" is frequently used by political pundits to undercut more accurate sources of information about COVID-19.

SOCIAL MEDIA MESSAGING ABOUT COVID-19

Social media platforms play a more significant role in shaping messaging than they have in the past (see chapter 5). Because some people rely on social media for their news, their coverage of events and topics carries increased significance. Informal social media networks, such as blogs, email groups, and the like, provide excellent venues for the spread of information, misinformation, and disinformation on COVID-19. Social networks on the internet have more capacity for users to spread COVID-19 rumors and conspiracy theories than face-to-face interactions, which are physically limited.

The ability to use smartphones to make live videos has also changed how information and events are communicated. Public spaces are now open to any number of potential videos taken by amateur reporters using their smartphones. Unlike institutionalized news organizations, these amateur reporters are different. They outnumber professional journalists and news reporters, are often first at the event, and are not delayed by editorial fact-checking (controls). Their videos usually spread over the internet much quicker than professional media. Sometimes, amateur videos inform traditional news sources and officials of important events. A case in point is the videos of police misconduct in the George Floyd and Rodney King cases. The same technology enables individuals to record COVID-19 protests, deaths, and closed businesses and share them online. Thanks to technology, it is now possible and common to see major newsworthy events happen as they occur (in real time). This is true for protests over COVID-19 mandates. What would be a local protest over a school board's decision to require or not require masks or close or open schools now can play out in local and national media. The public awareness of such pandemic events has been broadened to a wider audience.

The costs of communicating and protesting policies are low compared to what they were a couple of decades ago. E-mails, text messages, tweets, Instagrams, photos, images, and other electronic communication methods have lowered the costs for protest groups and social movements. In addition, such tools are more immediate than traditional mail, ads, hard copy brochures, and posters. They have become the preferred way for collective groups to communicate and reinforce their activities.

Social media platforms such as Facebook, Twitter, Digg, YouTube, Flickr, TikTok, and MySpace have played a vital communications role during the pandemic. Tang and Liu (2010:19) wrote, "Moreover, online social networks tend to be noisier than those in the physical world because it is much easier for users to connect online. Some users have thousands of online friends, whereas this is hardly true in reality." The use and reliance on social media can shed light on collective behavioral responses to the pandemic.

Social media have played positive and negative roles in providing information about COVID-19. Social media has a reputation for spreading misinformation about COVID-19. However, medical professionals have been sharing tweets that are medically sound and factual (Villasenor 2022). In a positive vein, Robinson (2021) reported that nurses shared valuable information on how to care for COVID-19 patients on social media platforms. Yale University's medRxiv Twitter site provides medical research papers before peer review. This opens up draft research to broader commentary by the scientific and medical community (Villasenor 2022). For example, Dr. Bob Wachter of the University of California, San Francisco's Department of Medicine has shared factual figures on the number of asymptomatic COVID-19 cases. Other medical experts and agencies have used Twitter to provide fact-based information on COVID-19. The problem is that some users do not always know which sites can be trusted.

Podcasts are a source of COVID-19 information available on the internet. Some podcasts, such as those by professional public health experts, medical schools, and government agencies, provide factual information about COVID-19. However, misinformation about COVID-19 has also been available via several podcasts, including some on the Spotify platform. For example, the far-right media personality Joe Rogan has made podcasts on the pandemic available on Spotify that have been inaccurate and misleading. According to news sources, he has commented on using the untested drug ivermectin to treat COVID-19. In response, some recording artists withdrew their music from Spotify and called for more stringent policies regarding the platform's content. In addition, a *New York Times* report noted that COVID-19 misinformation, such as that presented on December 31, 2021, on the Joe Rogan podcast, drew criticism from medical experts for advancing falsehoods (Petri 2022). Another example was a TikTok video that suggested COVID-19 was the same as a common cold. The post had more than 4 million views (Spencer 2021a). The video was posted by a group that advocated against public health measures.

An important question is to what degree people rely on podcasts for information on COVID-19. One national survey found that podcasts differed from the platform most Americans used to get their news. In a 2021 Pew Research Center survey of 11,178 adults, Walker (2022) found that 23 percent of Americans sometimes got their news from podcasts. Seven percent said they often get their news from podcasts, and 56 percent reported never getting it from a podcast platform. Younger adults, more than older, got their news from podcasts. Minor differences among racial and ethnic groups and affiliated political groups were found. Using the same survey but focusing on social media, Mitchell and Liedke (2021) found that 30 percent of respondents said they got some and 18 percent a lot of their information about COVID-19 vaccines on social media. Only 6 percent indicated that social media was the most important way to get information about COVID-19. They found that younger Americans and women are more likely than older adults and men to get COVID-19 news on social media.

COVID-19 RUMORS AND MYTHS

The pandemic has been a new experience with many unknowns for Americans. Americans have wanted answers on how serious COVID-19 is; what works to prevent it; whether they are going to die if they catch it; when they can get back to everyday lives; are restrictive measures always necessary and effective; what are the real risks of infection; and, when will a cure be available. Virtually all would agree that whatever the answers are to these questions, the sooner the pandemic ends, the better.

As noted earlier, COVID-19 and its variants and subvariants are a moving target that provides fertile ground for rumors and myths to be advanced. People want information and answers, and rumors and myths offer solutions. The problem is knowing when they are factual or not. Myths are stories and a product of imagination or emotion. Rumors and myths usually have some limited basis in fact, but over time take on a surreal larger-than-life meaning. Researchers and commentators have used rumors and myths interchangeably during the pandemic without clear distinction.

There is no shortage of myths and false rumors about COVID-19 and vaccines. Some Americans and groups have promoted rumors and myths, such as that COVID-19 vaccines cause erectile dysfunction; mouthwash prevents the disease; vaccines can be detoxed by bathing with borax; migrants are responsible for surges in COVID-19 cases; airplane crashes are linked to vaccinated pilots; and mask-wearing causes facial deformities. In light of these and other rumors and myths, several organizations have worked to debunk false rumors, myths, and misinformation about COVID-19. According to the CDC (2021) and faculty at Johns Hopkins Medical School (Maragakis and Kelen 2021), some myths and inaccurate rumors about COVID-19 and COVID-19 vaccines contradict the facts.

VACCINE MYTHS OR FALSE RUMORS

- Myth: The ingredients in COVID-19 vaccines are dangerous. Fact: COVID-19 vaccines do not contain ingredients like preservatives, tissues (like aborted fetal cells), antibiotics, food proteins, medicines, latex, or metals.
- Myth: A person's natural immunity from being sick with COVID-19 is better than their immunity from COVID-19 vaccination. Fact: Getting a COVID-19 vaccination is a safer and more dependable way to build immunity to COVID-19 than getting sick with COVID-19. The vaccine provides a more predictable immune response than an infection.
- Myth: COVID-19 vaccines cause variants. Fact: COVID-19 vaccines do not create or cause variants of the virus that causes COVID-19. Instead, COVID-19 vaccines help prevent new variants from emerging.
- Myth: COVID-19 vaccines contain microchips. Fact: COVID-19 vaccines do not contain microchips. Vaccines are developed to fight against disease and are not administered to track individuals' movements.
- Myth: Receiving a COVID-19 vaccine can make you magnetic. Fact: Receiving a COVID-19 vaccine will not make a person magnetic, including at the site of the vaccination, which usually is the arm. All COVID-19 vaccines are free from metals.
- Myth: COVID-19 vaccines can alter a person's DNA. Fact: COVID-19 vaccines do not change or interact with DNA in any way.
- Myth: A COVID-19 vaccine can make a person sick with COVID-19. Fact: Because none of the authorized COVID-19 vaccines in the United States contain the live virus that causes COVID-19, the vaccine cannot make a person sick with COVID-19. Some vaccinated people do indeed have reactions to the vaccines, which are short-term. Altman (2021), using survey data, reported that 36 percent of unvaccinated adults and 41 percent of unvaccinated Black people either believe or are unsure that COVID-19 vaccinations cause COVID-19.
- Myth: Several athletes were injured by COVID-19 vaccinations. Fact: Most professional athletes in the NFL, NHL, and NBA have been vaccinated and have not reported severe side effects or died because of the vaccine (Spencer et al. 2021).
- Myth: COVID-19 vaccines will affect a person's fertility. Fact: Currently, no evidence shows that any vaccines, including COVID-19 vaccines, cause fertility problems in women.
- Myth: Being near someone who received a COVID-19 vaccine will affect menstrual cycles. Fact: Being near someone who received a COVID-19 vaccine cannot affect the menstrual cycle.

- Myth: Pregnant women should not get vaccinated because the vaccines can cause congenital disabilities or have health consequences on the unborn infant. According to Hamel, Lopes, Kirzinger, Sparks, Stokes, and Brodie (2021), about four in ten have heard that pregnant women should not get the COVID-19 vaccine and think this is true (17%) or are not sure (22%). In this vein, *Health Impact News* (2021) published a claim titled "2,809 Dead Babies in VAERS Following COVID Shots as New Documents Prove Pfizer, the FDA, and CDC Knew the Shots Were Not Safe for Pregnant Women." Fact: It is safe for the expectant mother to get vaccinated, and there are no negative consequences for the unborn infant. McDonald (2021) fact-checked many vaccine claims found on VAERS, which she likened to a "vaccine mania," and found them false and unjustified.
- Myth: Getting a COVID-19 vaccine will cause a person to test positive on a viral test. Fact: None of the authorized and recommended COVID-19 vaccines can cause a person to test positive on viral tests, which are used to identify current infections.
- Myth: COVID-19 mRNA vaccines dramatically increase heart attack risk. Fact: COVID-19 vaccines administered in the United States are not known to increase the risk of a heart attack. Social media posts are misinterpreting an abstract in an American Heart Association journal as proof that the vaccine kills. Heart inflammation has been reported in rare cases, and most people recover quickly. However, COVID-19 is known to cause heart damage in some sporadic cases.
- Myth: COVID-19 vaccines contain a live virus, so a vaccinated person can "shed" (infect others around them). Fact: The COVID-19 vaccines do not contain a live virus, so a vaccinated person has no biological path to "shed" the SARS-CoV-2 spike protein to those around them. Christopher M. Zahn, M.D., the vice president of the American College of Obstetricians and Gynecologists, sent a statement to FactCheck.org that read, "This is a conspiracy that has been created to weaken trust in a series of vaccines that have been demonstrated in clinical trials to be safe and effective and that are our single best tool for confronting a global pandemic that has taken 600,000 lives in this country alone."

GENERAL AND TREATMENT MYTHS AND FALSE RUMORS

In addition to vaccines, myths and rumors have been generated focusing on other aspects of the pandemic and COVID-19. A sample of these that have been fact-checked include:

- Myth: COVID-19 is no more serious than the common cold. Fact: COVID-19, according to the CDC, was the third leading cause of death in the United States in 2020 (Ahmad and Anderson 2021; Spencer 2021a). COVID-19 is in the same family as some cold viruses (coronaviruses) but is more likely to have severe symptoms and may result in death.
- Myth: Quercetin, essential oils, and other supplements can protect a person from infection or treat COVID-19. Fact: This is false. Quercetin, zinc, vitamin D, and other nutritional supplements cannot prevent or treat COVID-19 infections. The same applies to essential oils—they are ineffective in preventing COVID-19.
- Myth: Immigrants and tourists are bringing COVID-19 into the United States. This is why there have been surges in COVID-19 cases in the United States. Fact: While surveys have found that many Americans (55% of Republicans) believe these two groups are the source of case surges, facts do not support this conclusion. Data on infections and hospitalizations show that the surge can be attributed to the emergence of the Delta variant and not tourists or immigrants, according to FactCheck.org (Farley 2021).
- Myth: Herd immunity will end the coronavirus pandemic, so vaccinations are unnecessary (Gorski 2020b). Fact: This is false. Allowing people to get COVID-19 infections would result in many people getting severely ill, developing permanent organ damage, and even dying before herd immunity would develop. In addition, some infected individuals become reinfected with COVID-19.
- Myth: An individual can protect themselves from COVID-19 by injecting, swallowing, bathing in, or rubbing onto their body bleach, disinfectants, or rubbing alcohols. Fact: This is false.
- Myth: The COVID-19 virus was manipulated. Fact: This possibility is still being investigated. According to *Nature* magazine, "Most scientists say SARS-CoV-2 (COVID-19) probably has a natural origin and was transmitted from animals to humans" (Maxmen 2021; Maxmen and Mallapaty 2021:313). Other studies and medical researchers have confirmed that COVID-19 is likely a product of nature and not a laboratory. However, this connection has not been ruled out, and many call for deeper investigation into the hypothesis that the virus emerged from the Chinese Wuhan Institute of Virology.
- Myth: Wearing a mask activates COVID-19 in the individual's body. Fact: There is no support for this myth. Instead, there is considerable evidence that masks reduce the airborne transmission of COVID-19.

RUMORS AND BEHAVIORS REGARDING IVERMECTIN AND HYDROXYCHLOROQUINE

Two drugs that have been rumored to treat COVID-19 are hydroxychloroquine and ivermectin. A widespread myth has been that the drug hydroxychloroquine is effective against COVID-19. President Trump and other mass and social media sources have promoted this rumor. Conservative media personalities have been outspoken in supporting both drugs as COVID-19 treatments. For instance, Fox News hosts have promoted alternative treatments for COVID-19, including hydroxychloroquine and ivermectin. For example, in a show on March 8, 2021, Fox News' Laura Ingraham said: "And we know that our FDA has in many ways failed us by not allowing for the use of ivermectin and hydroxychloroquine, both of which are used around the world to reduce COVID hospitalizations and deaths." Americans opposed to vaccines quickly embraced these rumors about both drugs as effective alternative treatments. However, no credible research supports either's effectiveness as a treatment for COVID-19. To the contrary, research suggests the opposite. For example, one experimental study found no evidence of benefit, but harm was possible (see *BMJ* 2020).

Ivermectin is a medicine used as a livestock dewormer and an antimalarial drug for humans. It can also be used topically on humans to treat head lice. None of these infections have any relationship to coronaviruses and, specifically, COVID-19. Irresponsible and misleading reports were circulated on social media and elsewhere that taking the drug was a safe and proven way to prevent or cure COVID-19. As a result, prescriptions for ivermectin soared for the treatment of COVID-19.

Consequently, calls to poison control centers related to ivermectin exposure increased. However, taking ivermectin for treating COVID-19 has not been approved for good reasons. Humans should not internally take medicine for horses, cows, or other animals. The formulas for animals, such as horses, vary from those of humans and can be toxic. In addition, ivermectin can interact with other medications, such as blood thinners. which can be dangerous. Large doses of ivermectin can be harmful, causing many detrimental side effects such as seizures, and its misuse by humans can lead to hospitalization and death.

According to one study by Hamel, Lopes, Kirzinger, Sparks, Stokes, and Brodie (2021), 28 percent of adults believed or were unsure whether ivermectin was a safe and effective treatment for COVID-19. According to a survey by the Annenberg Public Policy Center (APPC) of the University of Pennsylvania (Annenberg Public Policy Center 2021c), 4 in 10 Americans and 7 in 10 heavy users of conservative media indicated they would take the drug ivermectin if they had been exposed to someone who had COVID-19. Although ivermectin is approved for treating parasitic roundworm infections in humans, the Food and Drug Administration has not approved using this anti-parasitic drug to prevent or treat COVID-19. The FDA said current data do not show that ivermectin is effective against COVID-19, and using it for that purpose in humans or animals can be highly dangerous. This was consistent with an earlier survey finding in the summer of 2020 that this group was more willing to take hydroxychloroquine, which at the time was under study, and which the Food and Drug Administration later concluded was ineffective as a treatment for hospitalized COVID-19 patients. The risks of taking this drug were greater than the benefits.

Nevertheless, some have chosen to believe conservative media rumors about the effectiveness of ivermectin and hydroxychloroquine. Surveys have found that heavy users of conservative media were more willing to take ivermectin for COVID-19. However, most Americans did not buy into the rumors. According to the Annenberg Public Policy Center (2021c) survey, just 1 in 10 Americans (10%) believed the statement "Ivermectin is an effective treatment for Covid-19" was true, compared with 27 percent who said it was false. Most Americans (63%) said they were unsure whether that statement was true.

Nevertheless, when asked how likely they would be to take ivermectin if they had been exposed to someone with COVID-19 and the drug was available, 40 percent of Americans said they were somewhat or very likely to do so. Some Americans were driven more by emotions, rumors, and misinformation than by evidence. They could also be unaware of the risks of taking unproven medications.

An Annenberg Public Policy Center (2021c:n.p.) study found that the willingness to take ivermectin was influenced by where the individual obtained their news. The findings were that of those individuals relying on:

- Ultra-conservative sources such as Newsmax, One America News (OAN), Gateway Pundit, Parler, or Telegram: 75 percent said they were likely to take ivermectin;
- Conservative media sources such as Fox News, Mark Levin, or Breitbart: 70 percent said they were likely to take ivermectin;
- Social media sources such as Facebook, Instagram, or Twitter: 46 percent said they were likely to take ivermectin; and
- Mainstream print/broadcast media sources such as ABC, NBC, CBS News, the Associated Press, and the news pages of the *New York Times* or *Wall Street Journal*: 35 percent said they were likely to take ivermectin.

WHAT OTHER SURVEYS INDICATE ABOUT COVID-19 RUMORS

A large segment of the American population appears to be susceptible to myths and rumors. For example, a 2021 Kaiser Family Foundation (KFF) survey found that 35 percent of Americans either believed or were uncertain whether the government intentionally hid deaths from the COVID-19 vaccines (Hamel et al. 2021:n.p.). In the same survey, almost 31 percent believed or were unsure if COVID-19 vaccines had been shown to cause infertility. The survey also found that 1 in 4 individuals either believed or were unsure whether vaccines could give you COVID-19 or contained a microchip, and 1 in 5 believed that the vaccine could change your DNA.

Other independent organizations have conducted public surveys on COVID-19 myths and rumors. For example, the Annenberg Public Policy Center (2021) surveyed American adults in November 2021 to measure some of their belief in facts and misinformation, such as rumors. Some of the findings included (all the changes over time noted here are statistically significant):

- Vaccine safety: Nearly 4 in 5 people (79%) said it was probably true that the vaccines approved for use in the United States were safe. Of this group, 43 percent said it was true, up from June (38%) and April (34%). Just 10 percent said it was false.
- Vaccine effectiveness: Nearly 3 in 4 people (73%) said the COVID-19 vaccines were effective in preventing COVID-19, unchanged since September. The question was asked in early November before the Omicron variant appeared.
- Fetal tissue: Most of those surveyed correctly said it is false to say that the Pfizer and Moderna vaccines contained fetal tissue (56%, up from 51% in April). A small but growing minority said it was true (15%, up from 9% in April), and 30 percent of those surveyed were unsure.
- DNA: Three-quarters of those surveyed (74%) correctly said it was false to state that COVID-19 vaccines changed people's DNA, more than in April (69%). One in ten people (10%) said this was true, and 17 percent were unsure, findings consistent with a Kaiser Family Foundation survey. The vaccines do not change human DNA, according to FactCheck.org.
- Toxins: Three-quarters (77%) said it was false that childhood vaccines contained toxins such as antifreeze. Antifreeze was not used in vaccines, and vaccines with various ingredients were tested for safety and effectiveness before they were approved (licensed).

- Infertility: Two-thirds (66%) said it was probably false to state that COVID-19 vaccines caused infertility, and a growing number of those people said it was false (41%, up from 36% in June). Just 1 in 10 (10%) said this was true, similar to the Kaiser Family Foundation survey. According to FactCheck.org, no evidence exists that the COVID-19 vaccines cause infertility (Jaramillo 2021b).
- Ivermectin: 18 percent of those surveyed say it is true that ivermectin was an effective treatment for COVID-19 (up from 10% in September), while 38 percent think that was false (up from 27% in September). Clinical trials were ongoing at the time of the survey. At that time, data did not show it to be effective against the disease (Jaramillo 2021b).

These surveys and others have reported mixed results regarding COVID-19 rumors and myths. Some Americans believe in rumors and myths regardless of what the facts indicate. Others, often the majority of Americans, dismissed these rumors and myths.

CONSPIRACY THEORIES

Conspiracy theories, such as the death of Beatle Paul McCartney; weapons of mass destruction were present in Iraq; global warming is a hoax; the moon landing was staged; the U.S. government is storing an alien body collected in Roswell, New Mexico; the 2020 election was stolen (the Big Steal or opposite the Big Lie); the Holocaust never happened; and 9/11 was a government plot, have surfaced in America. Some Americans seem to be drawn to believing in conspiracies. In America, conspiracy theories have been more in vogue than ever (see Zielonka 2021:68).

The COVID-19 pandemic has had more than its fair share of conspiracy theories. For example, in the early weeks of the pandemic, some political leaders and media commentators referred to COVID-19 as a "hoax." Many popular conservative media hosts and commentators expressed doubts about the seriousness of COVID-19 (Jamieson and Albarracin 2020). They characterized the severity of COVID-19 as being overblown by a group of elites (see chapter 5). Conspiracy theories have also focused on not trusting conventional medical treatments and suppressing effective alternative remedies.

Reviewing conspiracy theories to understand some of the collective behaviors surrounding COVID-19 is essential. This point was made by Hanafi (2020:2), who wrote, "We need to understand the conspiracy theories and fake news around COVID-19 and to seek ways of mitigating the increasing discrimination against foreigners and refugees, including rising stereotypes against Chinese, and to those being accused of spreading the virus." Belief in conspiracies can be harmful and dangerous because of the direct influence on people's behavior. In the context of the COVID-19 pandemic, these beliefs also led to adverse health effects.

Leibovitz, Shamblaw, Rumas, and Best (2021) summarized some of the basic characteristics of conspiracy beliefs (theories). They observed that conspiracy beliefs are simple explanations for ambiguous or complex problems that propose that powerful groups or individuals deceive the public. For example, the pandemic is a complex and ambiguous problem that has sparked conspiracy theories about powerful elites, the deep state, and "big pharma" (large pharmaceutical companies). Leibovitz et al. further point out that conspiracy theories may not be incorrect, are not generally evidence-based, and are resistant to contradictory evidence or facts. Conspiracy theories are grounded in beliefs, emotions, and biases rather than facts (Rieger 2022). Conspiracy theories emerge when individuals are experiencing an existential threat, in this case, the pandemic, and situations of increasing uncertainty and lack of control. In the case of the COVID-19 pandemic, individuals lost control over their lives as the virus spread, and involuntary measures were taken to limit its spread to vulnerable populations.

Conspiracy theories are alternate narratives that help some people make sense of the confusion surrounding COVID-19. Regardless of the truth, believers in a conspiracy narrative will accept it as fact and act accordingly. Believers in conspiracies tend to have a confirmation bias. Confirmation bias is the tendency to find, interpret, and recall information in a way that confirms or supports their beliefs, values, and conspiracy. Believers ignore contradictory information and interpret ambiguous information in ways to support the conspiracy. Their emotions, core values and attitudes, and hope for alternative outcomes influence their degree of commitment to the conspiracy theory. They make quick judgments and form perspectives without critical thinking (see chapter 5).

During the pandemic, conspiracy theorists have promoted unhealthy advice and misinformation regarding COVID-19. COVID-19 conspiracy beliefs have been linked to unwarranted fears of vaccinations and a reluctance to get vaccinated (Hornsey et al. 2020). For example, some Americans have not been vaccinated because they believe in the vaccine conspiracy theory that vaccines are made from fetal material or metals. In addition to the narrative of the conspiracy, COVID-19 conspiracy theorists have also discredited news organizations, medical authorities, and public health agencies. This, in effect, has fueled increased political polarization in America.

The problem with challenging conspiracies is that people who believe in them are often in echo chambers where everyone else reflects the same views, values, and beliefs in conspiracies. They are in echo chambers because believers in conspiracies share and receive reinforcing information supporting them. It is common for believers in conspiracies to rely on social media sites and biased news sources for information and news. These sources have a record of generating and supporting conspiracy theories.

Conspiracies, misinformation, and rumors flourish in these information sources for several reasons. Research has shown that some people believe in conspiracies because they need to feel special, part of an in-group, or oppose the majority opinion. Conspiracy theories reflect anxieties and fears about the kind of society where people have little power over big decisions (for a discussion, see Van Bavel, Baicker, Boggio, et al. 2021). In the case of COVID-19, Americans had little control over the big decisions regarding mask-wearing, vaccines, lockdowns, and other public health mandates and recommendations.

Belief in pandemic conspiracies is widespread. One survey of nearly 800 Canadian and American adults discovered that almost half (49.7%) of the respondents believed in at least one conspiracy theory (Leibovitz et al. 2021). The survey found that those individuals with higher anxiety levels were more likely to believe in conspiracies. Those respondents who did not know anyone at high risk of infection and had higher religiosity were more prone to believing COVID-19 conspiracies.

In a different study, Romer and Jamieson (2021) surveyed 1,050 adults in March 2020 and followed up with 840 of the same respondents in July 2020. The two surveys included questions about adopting COVID-19 preventive measures, vaccination intentions, conspiracy beliefs, perceptions of threat, beliefs about vaccine safety, political ideology, and media exposure patterns. They found that three COVID-19 conspiracy theories were stable over time and inversely related to the perceived threat of the pandemic, taking preventative measures such as mask-wearing, perceptions of vaccine safety, and intent to get vaccinated.

Belief in COVID-19 conspiracy theories predicted resistance to mask-wearing and future vaccinations. In addition, Romer and Jamieson found that younger individuals, those with lower incomes, and the less educated were more likely to hold conspiracy beliefs about the origins and seriousness of the pandemic. Non-White respondents also were more likely to believe in conspiracies. Finally, powerless individuals were more inclined to believe in conspiracy theories. Similar findings to Romer and Jamieson's conclusions have been reported in countries like the United Kingdom (Freeman et al. 2020).

WHY COVID-19 CONSPIRACY THEORIES HAVE FLOURISHED

In America, conspiracies have always been present, sometimes more prevalent than others. During crises, such as pandemics, wars, and natural disasters, government authorities often move to centralize and consolidate their power, expanding their social and political control over their populations (Delanty 2021; Turner 2021; Walby 2021). During the pandemic, groups of Americans became concerned with government expansion and intrusion. They voiced concerns that executive branch overreach and the entrenchment of more restrictive rules for behavior could become permanent after the pandemic (see Honig 2009).

The influential Italian social philosopher Giorgio Agamben has been particularly concerned about how COVID-19 has resulted in governments' overreach of authority and overreaction (see Silva and Higuera 2021). He has characterized the response to COVID-19 as disproportionate to the threat posed by the disease. To Agamben, the pandemic is socially constructed more than real and has been a move by governments to gain more control. Matthew and Huppatz (2020) reviewed some issues stemming from the governmental restriction of civil liberties, such as increased surveillance, thermal scanners, facial recognition technologies, and the increasing human rights crisis during the pandemic. These and other elevated concerns over the role of government during the pandemic are themes in many of the more popular conspiracy theories.

Van Bavel, Baicker, Boggio, et al. (2021:464) summarized the literature on why conspiracy theories have thrived during the COVID-19 pandemic:

> Research suggests that people feel the need to explain large events with proportionally large causes and are more likely to believe in conspiracy theories about events with serious consequences and in times of crisis. This is likely because people are more drawn to conspiracy theories when important psychological needs are frustrated. Thus, conspiracy theories may gain more traction as COVID-19 spreads and more people isolate themselves. However, these conspiracy theories can have harmful consequences. For example, belief in conspiracy theories has been linked to vaccine hesitancy, climate denial, extremist political views, and prejudice. COVID-19 conspiracy theories may be similarly problematic. For instance, people who believe that alternative remedies can help them fight off the virus may be less likely to follow health officials' advice and instead opt for less effective (at best) or lethal (at worst) alternatives.

They also added:

> Conspiracy beliefs may also fuel hostility toward groups responsible for the virus. Some evidence suggests that giving people factual information before exposure to conspiracy theories can reduce conspiracy theory beliefs, and this strategy might work in efforts to combat conspiracy theories relevant to the current pandemic. However, because some people consume information within like-minded "echo chambers," combating conspiracy theories remains challenging.

Crises and world-changing events, such as the COVID-19 pandemic, require exceptional explanations, which helps create a climate where conspiracy theories thrive. The following is a set of some of the most famous conspiracies advanced during the pandemic. Given the vast array of conspiracy theories during the pandemic, only a sample of some major ones is possible. The following are some of the most mentioned and representative conspiracies beginning with the "plandemic" conspiracy.

"PLANDEMIC" VIDEOS AND CONSPIRACY THEORY

COVID-19 conspiracies include the misinformation videos *Plandemic: The Hidden Agenda Behind COVID-19* (released May 4, 2020) and *Plandemic: Indoctoration* (released August 18, 2020). These videos contain several false ideas about the pandemic, including the virus being activated by handwashing and wearing masks.

According to the videos, scientists planned the COVID-19 pandemic for financial profit and to strip Americans of their liberties. Other misinformation in the videos includes the effectiveness of hydroxychloroquine as a treatment. The films make further claims, such as losing individual rights, freedom of speech, and personal autonomy. Both videos hit on mandates reducing core American values and rights. In the first video (*Plandemic*), Dr. Mikovits accuses Dr. Fauci, pharmaceutical companies, and Microsoft cofounder Bill Gates of exploiting the COVID-19 pandemic for profit. It advances the conspiracy theory that there is a plan by the world's billionaires and big pharma to control the world's vaccines while earning big profits. The COVID-19 pandemic is characterized as a highly organized operation with the goal of world control. Mikovits's claims in the video were fact-checked and found to be false (see Enserink and Cohen 2020). With over a million views of the first video, Haelle (2020:n.p.) asked the questions, "Why is this video suddenly everywhere?" and "Why are so many drawn to it?" She concluded:

> This video has been extremely successful at promoting misinformation for three reasons: First, it taps into people's uncertainty, anxiety, and need for

> answers—common reasons anyone is attracted to a conspiracy theory. Second, it is packaged professionally and uses common conventions people associate with factual documentaries. Third, it successfully exploits ancient but extremely effective methods of persuasion.

Haelle (2020:np) also wrote:

> There is more uncertainty about our world now than in decades, perhaps a century, and the stakes are higher than ever. Everyone has many unanswered questions—scientists, doctors, national leaders, and others we ordinarily look to for answers. Uncertainty is uncomfortable. People want answers. Conspiracy theories can be comforting. This video appears to provide answers that fit together, make sense, that sound credible, or at least "interesting and worth considering.

The plandemic conspiracy is a textbook example of collective behavior. Elements of social uncertainty, unrest, need for information, strain, scapegoats, and misinformation are all present in the plandemic conspiracy. A willing audience for the messages in the videos was present. Although their creators were organized and produced two well-polished conspiracy videos, the public response to both fit comfortably with concepts of rumor, misinformation, true believers, and other collective behavioral understandings. Although the videos had large audiences, most Americans did not see them or dismissed them as nonsense. However, others bought into both discredited films.

COVID-19 IS A HOAX

One conspiracy theory that may outweigh them is that the COVID-19 virus does not exist (Lynas 2020). Instead, it is a "hoax." This conspiracy theory has been promoted by the political far right. Proponents of this conspiracy theory argue that COVID-19 is no worse than a case of the flu. Similarly, the deep state manipulates the pandemic to control elected officials and election outcomes. According to Lynas, another aspect of this conspiracy is that big pharma is trying to milk money out of the general public with an exaggerated pandemic. As Lynas (2020) observed, proponents of the big pharma conspiracy are happy to discredit conventional medicine and have unproven products they are willing to sell as miracle cures (similar to snake oil remedies) to combat COVID-19.

Following the same conspiracy theme, COVID-19 pandemic deniers use the term "casedemic," referring to the theory that COVID-19 is harmless and that case counts of the virus are simply the result of testing (Gorskia 2020:n.p.). The casedemic is a term embraced by those individuals and groups opposed to vaccines and other public health pandemic efforts. They contend that COVID-19 is not as dangerous as public health and government authorities would suggest. Thus, there is no need for masks, social distancing, lockdowns, vaccinations, and other public health interventions. COVID-19 deniers believe the COVID-19 pandemic is fake and a swindle. Deniers claim there are too many COVID-19 tests. To eliminate COVID-19, a strategy would be to not test for COVID-19. Fewer tests would result in fewer COVID-19 infections and the elimination of the pandemic.

Several broadcasts and publications have emerged during the pandemic that advance conspiracy theories and question existing institutions' motives. For example, Mercola and Cummins (2021) published *The Truth About COVID-19: Exposing the Great Reset, Lockdowns, Vaccine Passports, and the New Normal*. A sample of subheadings Mercola and Cummins (2021) include are "Data Show COVID-19 Is Not a Significant Threat" (p. 52) and "Mislabeled Causes of Death" (p. 53) that reflect conspiracy thinking. In the book's foreword, Robert F. Kennedy Jr., a dedicated anti-vaccine advocate, scapegoats big pharma, public health organizations, big data, big media, and financial robber barons as conspiring to profit from the pandemic. Kennedy further argues that open dialogue about restrictions and vaccines has been suppressed at the hand of big pharma and the very wealthy at a considerable cost to American society. The concept of accusing pharmaceutical companies of profiting from vaccines is not new, and it is true that they profit and are powerful political actors in American society. The problem is that conspiracies regarding big pharma get confounded with misinformation, such as how vaccines are produced or cause unintended outcomes such as autism.

The confirmed anti-vaxxer Robert F. Kennedy Jr.'s book is probably the best example of a collection of pandemic conspiracy ideas. His book *The Real Anthony Fauci: Bill Gates, Big Pharma, and the Global War on Democracy and Public Health* (2021) encapsulates many conspiracy theories that surfaced during the pandemic. In the book, Kennedy lays out multiple allegations targeting Dr. Fauci (scapegoating), whom he characterizes as a powerful technocrat who has worked against democracy. He accuses Dr. Fauci and Bill Gates of prolonging the pandemic and promoting expensive vaccinations to benefit a big vaccination cartel. In addition, the book promotes several myths, such as the effectiveness of ivermectin, that have been scientifically proven to be false. In July 2023, Kennedy drew criticism for his latest conspiracy theory that COVID-19 "ethnically targeted" Black and White people while avoiding Asian and Ashkenazi Jewish people (Pitofsky 2023). Jewish and Asian advocacy groups immediately labeled this conspiracy theory as offensive, racist, and antisemitic.

Another book similar to Mercola and Cummins's is Marc Siegel's *COVID: The Politics of Fear and the Power of Science* (2020). Siegel's book has the central premise that society has overreacted to the COVID-19 pandemic. He attributes society's fear of COVID-19 as stemming from three sources—the government, media, and our psyche. He characterizes the pandemic as full of hype and hysteria. Frijters, Foster, and Baker's *The Great Covid Panic* (2021) reflects similar themes as in the other books. The authors build from the central proposition that fear over COVID-19 has been exaggerated. Conspiracy themes are dispersed throughout the book. For example, in their conclusion, they wrote (2021:341):

> The Great Covid Panic started with fear and a primitive call for human sacrifices in the form of nonsensical lockdowns. Over time, the Panic transformed into a big push by a new coalition of politicians and big companies towards a neo-feudal society where the vast majority has little freedom in either their personal or work lives. The development towards neo-feudalism preceded the pandemic, but many additional elements were put in place during the pandemic, such as mask surveillance, mass censorship, travel restrictions for the vast majority, and the idea that freedom is something governments can give or withhold, rather than a fundamental right.

It should be noted that concerns about medical professionals being sources of disinformation and conspiracy theories have been expressed. Having medical training does not ensure that doesn't happen, as Sage and Yang (2022) commented:

> A vocal minority and their sponsors or allies have exploited their medical credentials to the detriment of the public. They have understated known risks of severe illness, challenged the safety and effectiveness of vaccines without evidence, touted unproved and risky treatments, and amplified conspiracy theories about science and scientists.

LOSS OF FREEDOM

One conspiracy theory holds that the pandemic is a public health agency and government plot to permanently remove Americans' freedom and liberties. This conspiracy dovetailed closely with traditional distrust of the government, especially of "big government." Some authorities, such as Offe (2021:38), have observed there is a "big brother narrative" that the "state is doing too much to control the pandemic." Reflecting on this conspiracy theory, Mercola and Cummins (2021:5) expressed concern over the loss of personal liberties and wrote:

> More people are now starting to wake up to the fact that the restrictions put into place under the guise of protecting public health are anything but temporary and will likely remain permanent. Instead, they're part of a much larger long-term plan, and the end goal is to usher in a new way of life with radically reduced previous freedoms. This means that, eventually, everyone must decide which is more important: personal liberty or false security?

Later they wrote (p. 34), "It may sound appealing, until you realize that they are working efficiently to strip us of our liberties."

At some level, restrictions, and mandates require Americans to live with more healthcare rules and restrictions than before the pandemic. This is not unique to the COVID-19 pandemic, as restrictions have always been a component of public health, plagues, and pandemics. These mandates and restrictions aim to protect society, not destroy the liberties Americans enjoy. When COVID-19 numbers declined, public health and government agencies quickly removed restrictions when possible. The goal of taking away individual freedoms and liberties is not a stated objective of public health or government entities. Instead, there has been a reluctance from the pandemic's start to impose public health restrictions and mandates. This resistance has been criticized by Americans who believe the government should have reacted sooner to the pandemic threat. They point to the high number of preventable COVID-19 deaths as evidence of the government's slow response.

ORIGIN OF COVID-19

From the beginning, agencies and governments have sought to identify the origin of the coronavirus. Numerous conspiracy theories on its origin have been advanced as investigations have been underway. It did not take long for the pandemic to become influenced by nationalism and conspiracy theories in the United States and China. The first reported outbreak of COVID-19 occurred in Wuhan, China, on December 31, 2019. Two days later, Chinese foreign ministry officials generated the conspiracy theory that the United States' military had developed COVID-19 to harm Chinese people (Maxmen 2022; Molter and Webster 2020; Rieger 2022). The U.S. military had participated in military world games in 2019 near Wuhan before the COVID-19 outbreak. However, there is no evidence that the U.S. military could spread or had anything to do with COVID-19. Later, conspiracy theories escalated when former president Trump named COVID-19 the "Chinese virus." This and similar expressions chilled Chinese relations with the United States and impacted the exchange of information regarding COVID-19 (Maxmen 2022). Not wanting to be blamed for COVID-19, the Chinese ceased sharing coronavirus information with the outside world.

Other origin conspiracies have emerged that fine-tune how and why COVID-19 developed and by whom. These include COVID-19 accidentally escaping from a laboratory in China (Mercola and Cummins 2021; Lynas 2020), originating from a wet (food) market in China, being introduced by Democrats to undermine the Republican president, and so forth. Mercola and Cummins (2021) concluded that the virus originated in a Chinese laboratory in Wuhan. They proposed other ideas about the origin of COVID-19, such as the virus being part of bioweapon research. According to *Science* magazine, which fact-checked this claim, it is incorrect, as relations between the laboratory in China and the U.S. Army Medical Research Institute of Infectious Diseases had stopped well before COVID-19 surfaced.

Individuals in influential positions in the American government promoted the laboratory-origin conspiracy. For example, unsubstantiated allegations that COVID-19 was made in a Chinese laboratory and accidentally leaked were made by U.S. Secretary of State Mike Pompeo on Fox News on June 14, 2021 (Blitzer 2021). Pompeo claimed substantial evidence existed, but no evidence was provided that it escaped or was intentionally introduced to the general population. The idea that a Chinese lab worker would have intentionally introduced it to the people of Wuhan does not pass any litmus test.

In 2023, the lab leak conspiracy theory reemerged when the U.S. Department of Energy confirmed a classified report that concluded with little confidence that there was evidence COVID-19 had likely leaked from the Wuhan laboratory. The news media, such as the *Wall Street Journal* (Gordon and Strobel 2023), and conspiracy theorists jumped on the story. However, other experts concluded that most scientific evidence still supported the zoonotic (natural) source of the COVID-19 virus. A few days later, contradictory evidence was released that linked the source of COVID-19 to raccoon dogs sold at the Wuhan food market (Mallapaty 2023). However, no one knows for sure.

Nevertheless, when surveyed, some Americans believed this lab leak conspiracy theory. According to 2020 survey data from the Pew Research Center, 23 percent of those Americans surveyed thought the coronavirus was developed intentionally in a lab, and 6 percent thought it was made accidentally in a lab (Mitchell and Oliphant 2020). According to a different Pew Research Center survey of 8,914 American adults, three in ten (29%) believed COVID-19 was developed in a laboratory (Schaeffer 2020). However, most respondents believed the virus developed naturally (in nature). These perceptions differed by age, educational level, and other demographic factors. An Annenberg Public Policy Center survey of American adults found that slightly over half (53%) of Americans thought the Chinese had developed the virus as a biological weapon, and 22 percent were unsure (Annenberg Public Policy Center 2021).

In addition to the Wuhan Laboratory origin theory, there have been other conspiracy theories on the source of COVID-19. These alternatives include theft from a Canadian laboratory by Chinese scientists, COVID-19 being of Jewish or Muslim origin, COVID-19 being a tool used to facilitate the installation of the 5G mobile network, and a meteor being the source. An NBC News story reported that the Russians and Chinese created a conspiracy theory that COVID-19 was developed in Ukrainian biolabs (Collins and Collier 2022). Russian authorities used this conspiracy theory to help justify the invasion of Ukraine. The purpose of this theory was clearly to undermine support for Ukraine and demonize the Ukrainians to the Russian people. However, Ukraine does not have any biolabs capable of developing viruses. In the United States, members of the far right and far-right media embraced this conspiracy and shared it on right-wing media platforms.

In this writing, some current research points to the virus being introduced via wild animals sold at a food market in Wuhan, China. Research conducted in 2020 points to bats being the probable source (Zhou et al. 2020). Maxmen (2021) reported that it is doubtful that COVID-19 was genetically engineered, but the origin conspiracy theories continue.

ELITES ARE THE PROBLEM

In much of the conspiracy theory literature, references are made to elites, such as the CEOs of big pharma. For example, in Mercola and Cummins's 2021 book, they make several references to the elite or global elite. They proposed that fear of COVID-19 is artificial and was manipulated by a global elite to their advantage. Mercola and Cummins (2021:3) described the global elite:

> This long-anticipated pandemic, officially announced by the World Health Organization on March 11, 2020, became utilized by an international network of powerful corporations and billionaires to expand their power, wealth, and control dramatically, in what can only be described as an attempted global coup d'état.

Mercola and Cummins are just two conspiracy theorists who refer to the elites (for example, see Burrowes 2022; Frijters et al. 2021). Burrowes (2022) suggested that the world's elites have undertaken a coup to control human liberties through the pandemic. Burrowes (2022:n.p.) made a statement typical of this elite conspiracy theory when he commented:

> Using COVID-19 as "cover," the global elite is conducting a coup to take vastly greater control of our lives and neutralize our humanity. This is made very easy by the compulsion to obey that most people acquire in response to the "socialization" experience they suffered as a child.

Bill Gates is one of the most visible individuals targeted as an elite. Bill Gates allegedly plans to vaccinate the world's population for personal gain. Mercola and Cummins (2021:35) wrote of Gates, "Gates, who cofounded Microsoft in 1975, is perhaps one of the most dangerous philanthropists in modern history, having poured billions of dollars into global health initiatives that stand on shaky scientific and moral ground—including the COVID-19 pandemic." As with most conspiracy theories, there is a kernel of truth in that Gates and other philanthropists have promoted vaccinations to rid the world of severe and deadly diseases. Their efforts have saved tens of millions of lives and in no way represent a plot for world dominance. However, anti-vaxxers prefer to reframe the discussion to fit their narrative that all vaccines should be avoided because microchips are embedded in the COVID-19 vaccines to track and control people (Lynas 2020).

COVID-19 MORBIDITY RATES ARE INFLATED

Another conspiracy theory believes that COVID-19 death rates are artificially inflated. This conspiracy theory surfaces on social media and cable news platforms like Twitter. For example, President Trump in August 2020 advanced a tweet that COVID-19 deaths were systematically overcounted and only 6 percent of COVID-19 identified deaths were due to the virus (Knight and Appleby 2020). The accusation was made that medical providers and hospitals overcounted COVID-19 patients to maximize profits. Knight and Appleby (2020:n.p.) wrote, "Trump's recent assertions have fueled conspiracy theories on Facebook and elsewhere that doctors and hospitals are fudging numbers to get paid more." However, leading national medical authorities, such as the president of the American Medical Association and the CEO of the American Hospital Association, were quick to challenge the president's claims as having no basis. Lynas (2020:n.p.) described this conspiracy and how it was promoted:

> Another far-right meme is the idea that COVID death rates are being inflated and therefore there is no reason to observe lockdown regulations or other social distancing measures. Prominent in promoting this myth is Dr. Annie Bukacek, whose speech warning that COVID death certificates are being manipulated has been viewed more than a quarter of a million times on YouTube. Bukacek

> appears in a white lab coat with a stethoscope around her neck, making her look like an authoritative medical source. Dig a little deeper, however, as *Rolling Stone* magazine did, and it turns out she's actually a far-right anti-vaccination and anti-abortion activist, previously noted for bringing tiny plastic fetuses into the Montana state legislature. Her insistence that COVID death rates are inflated has, of course, no basis in fact. More likely, the current death toll is a serious under-count. To further clarify the issue, the Centers for Disease Control has published information about excess deaths associated with COVID-19.

Another example of how misinformation was used was a misleading article about COVID-19 death rates published in the student publication *Johns Hopkins News-Letter* on November 22, 2020. The author claimed there was no evidence that COVID-19 resulted in any excess deaths. This article would later be retracted but was latched on to by right-wing social media to promote conspiracy theories and myths regarding COVID-19. Experts found multiple flaws in the study design and conclusions resulting in the article being withdrawn, but the misinformation was already in the public. Although wrong, the main conclusion supported the view of conspiracy theorists who believed the pandemic had been overstated. When it was withdrawn, consistent with the view of conspiracy theorists that there are evil forces at work, the false claim was made that censorship of the truth had occurred.

In their critique of how COVID-19 has been handled, Russell and Patterson (2021) wrote:

> As a result, many Americans have an overexaggerated view of certain aspects of the pandemic. One of these may well bear on school re-openings: According to polling, Americans massively overestimate the number of children who have died from the disease. Per the CDC, in the United States, children represent less than 0.1 percent of total pandemic-related deaths. While each individual death is a tragedy, the statistics remind us of a crucial, well-established feature of this virus: It is far less risky for children, with Americans above age 65 constituting 81 percent of the share of deaths.

CDC data and other research support Russell and Patterson's (2021) point (Rothwell and Desai 2020; see chapter 1). COVID-19 was and continues to be not fully understood, so concern over children dying from COVID-19 made sense at the beginning of the pandemic. As more knowledge has been gained, there appears to be an unjustified concern over child mortality rates due to COVID-19. It remains unclear why some people are asymptomatic, and others get very sick. It is also true that death rates for older Americans are higher and likely undercounted. Conspiracy theorists often neglect this point.

WHAT DO NATIONAL SURVEYS INDICATE REGARDING INFLATED DEATH ESTIMATES?

Do Americans believe the deaths due to COVID-19 have been inflated by public health, government, and big pharma? The Pew Research Center surveyed Americans during the pandemic to learn more about how media coverage is doing (Mitchell and Oliphant 2020). Most (89%) survey respondents in 2020 replied that they were following the news about the pandemic reasonably closely, and 70 percent thought the media covered the pandemic very or somewhat well. However, most (63%) also thought the media exaggerated the risks. Only 6 percent believed the media needed to take the risks more seriously. About half (48%) said they had seen some made-up news about the pandemic.

Rothwell and Desai (2020) summarized the Franklin Templeton-Gallup Economics of Recovery Study. A sample of Americans were asked about their estimates of mortality rates from COVID-19. They found that Americans overestimated the death rates for people aged 24 and younger. Specifically, Americans thought the death rate was 8 percent when it was 0.1 percent. It is important to note that the survey was conducted before Delta and Omicron variants surfaced. Rothman and Desai pointed out that the elderly accounted for 81 percent of the deaths during the survey (August 2020). In addition, political affiliation mattered, and Democrats were off further (overestimated higher) than Republicans in their estimates of mortality rates, even when other demographic factors were considered, such as gender, race, and age. Rothwell and Desai (2020:n.p.) commented on the study:

> Meanwhile, Democrats are more likely to correctly understand that COVID can be spread by people without symptoms and more accurately assess the overall mortality risk of COVID-19 as more severe than other common causes of death, such as influenza and automobile accidents. In early September, many Republicans (41%) said that flu had caused more deaths than COVID-19 during 2020, compared to just 13% of Democrats. The President of the United States suggested as much in a tweet in October. According to CDC data, even automobile accidents were said to cause more deaths, which is also untrue. Likewise, just over one in three Republicans (37%) deny that it is true that people can spread COVID without symptoms compared to only about one in four (23%) Democrats.

Kaiser Family Foundation researchers Hamel, Lopes, Kirzinger, Sparks, Stokes, and Brodie (2021) found that six in ten adults had heard that the government was exaggerating the number of COVID-19 deaths by counting deaths due to other causes, such as preexisting conditions. Thirty-eight percent of surveyed adults believed this was true, and 22 percent were unsure if it was true or false. A different national survey of adult Americans conducted in November of 2021 found that some respondents believed the threat of COVID-19 was exaggerated (Annenberg Public Policy Center 2021a). The center found that 27 percent of respondents continued to believe that staff at the CDC exaggerated the danger posed by the pandemic to damage the Trump presidency. Fifty-eight percent said this was false, and 14 percent were unsure. Those believed this was true when COVID-19 deaths continued to mount and exceeded one million Americans in 2022.

NOTE ON DENIALISM AND THE PANDEMIC

From the beginning of the pandemic, some Americans have refused to acknowledge that COVID-19 is real and have labeled it a scam (hoax). Other Americans have questioned COVID-19 infection and mortality rates and dismissed the value of public health initiatives, such as getting vaccinated, wearing a mask, and taking other public health measures. Americans that subscribed to these and different beliefs that downplayed COVID-19 and the seriousness of the pandemic can be considered deniers. According to Paul and Haddad (2023:221), during the pandemic, there has been "a stubborn will to ignorance and blatant forms of denial."

A body of thought has focused on deniers in American society. Deniers, whether it is for racial prejudice, critical race theory, climate change is not occurring, smoking does not cause cancer, election results are fake, or the COVID-19 pandemic, rely on time-proven strategies to make their points or persuade others to take desired actions. These strategies are transferrable from one issue to another, regardless of political point of view. Deniers use strategies to discredit, undermine, discount, dismiss, or otherwise negate ideas, beliefs, and facts that do not support or conform to their views. Commentators on both sides of the pandemic have used denialist strategies.

A range of motivations drives COVID-19 and all denialists. In the business world, maximizing profit is certainly a motive. Take the tobacco industry as an example. The industry has for decades denied that smoking is bad for one's health (see Proctor and Schiebinger 2008). The vaping industry has followed suit and claimed that vaping is not harmful to youth health. In addition, political ideology or religious beliefs can cause groups of adherents to reject anything incompatible with their total views or beliefs. A case occurred in South Africa, as official denial of the AIDS problem resulted in major negative health consequences (deaths) for Black South Africans (Bateman 2007). Finally, influencers and celebrities can encourage denialist thinking for various motives.

According to Carroll (2020:n.p.), there are six basic strategies in the denialist playbook (see chapters 5 and 6 for examples):

1. Doubt the Science—This was demonstrated by the "follow the science" debate as pandemic skeptics point to scientific mistakes and missteps during the pandemic and by science in general. The point that skeptics make that thoughtful dialogue and scientific review should occur is justified. The leap of faith is that this has not happened when it has occurred. Diethelm and McKee (2009) noted that denialists employ rhetorical arguments to give the appearance of a legitimate debate where there is none. They suggested that this approach aims to reject a scientific finding or idea on which a scientific consensus exists. Unfortunately, some Americans only trust the science supporting their views and are willing to abandon all science in favor of unverified claims from a collection of political pundits, quacks, and other biased sources.
2. Question Scientists' Motives and Integrity—This was reflected in the trust in science and medicine. Conspiracy theorists and pandemic skeptics question the motives of "big pharma" scientists and the goal of making profits. The Bill Gates conspiracy theories demonstrate this strategy. Denialist references to elites also reflect this denialist strategy.
3. Magnify Disagreements among Scientists and Cite Gadflies as Authorities—The videos promoting the plandemic presented experts who contradicted scientific and factual evidence.
4. Exaggerate Potential Harm—Several anti-vaccine arguments referred to the harm of the COVID-19 vaccines, such as causing deformities, infecting the unborn, and causing COVID-19. However, on the other side, a case can be made that the risk of dying from COVID-19 has been exaggerated for most people resulting in unjustified fear and stress.
5. Appeal to Personal Freedom—This was demonstrated by the many concerns that mandates and restrictions limit Americans' freedom of choice and self-determination. In addition, add to these the concept that whatever restrictions and mandates have been imposed during the pandemic will permanently deny Americans of their rights and expand the intrusion and control of the government over its citizens.
6. Reject Whatever Would Repudiate [Deny] a Key Philosophy—This surfaced in the debate over the appropriate role of public health and the government. Does the general public good outweigh personal liberties? The claim that the pandemic is a hoax or overstated falls into the philosophical approach to the pandemic. Skeptics have argued that the pandemic is exaggerated and has impacted society negatively and unnecessarily.

Pascal Diethelm and Martin McKee (2009) made critical observations about denialism. They identified five elements that characterize the denialism process. The first is the identification of conspiracies. When the overwhelming body of scientific opinion believes something is true, it is argued that this differs from those scientists who have independently studied the evidence and reached a different conclusion. Instead, they have participated in a coordinated and secretive conspiracy to reach their biased findings. The scientific peer review process is seen as a tool by which the conspirators suppress dissent rather than as a means of weeding out scientific papers and results that do not support the conspiracy. Diethelm and McKee (2009:2) observed that when

> there is an overwhelming consensus on the evidence among scientists, some vocal commentators reject this consensus, convincing many of the public, and often the media too, that the agreement is not based on "sound science" or denying that there is a consensus by exhibiting individual dissenting voices as the ultimate authorities on the topic in question.

The second is the use of fake experts. These individuals purport to be experts in a particular area but whose views are entirely inconsistent with established knowledge. The use of fake experts is often complemented by denigration of established experts and researchers, with accusations and innuendo that seek to discredit their work and cast doubt on their motivations (Diethelm and McKee 2009:2). For example, oppositional groups and right-wing-oriented social and mass media have discredited the CDC, Dr. Fauci, and the Food and Drug Administration.

The third characteristic is selectivity, drawing on isolated papers that challenge the dominant consensus or highlighting the flaws in the weakest papers among those that support it as a means of discrediting the entire field (Diethelm and McKee 2009:3). An example of the former is the much-cited *Lancet* paper describing intestinal abnormalities in 12 children with autism, which merely suggested a possible link with immunization against measles, mumps, and rubella. Inaccurate anti-vaccine and autism propaganda play on the internet to keep such concepts alive. If MMR vaccines caused autism, although they do not, the idea lingers and is used by denialists to oppose all vaccines.

According to Diethelm and McKee (2009:3), the fourth is the creation of impossible expectations of what scientific research can provide. For example, those denying the reality of climate change point to the absence of accurate temperature measurements before the thermometer's invention; thus, trends are unknowable. For deniers, any local cold wave proves that climate change is not occurring. Diethelm and McKee (2009:3) commented, "Others use the intrinsic uncertainty of mathematical models to reject them entirely as a means of understanding a phenomenon." In the case of COVID-19, the unpredictability of the coronavirus helped, and unrealistic scientific expectations formed a good mix for this approach to be used by denialists.

"The fifth is the use of misrepresentation and logical fallacies. Logical fallacies include the use of red herrings, or deliberate attempts to change the argument and straw men, where the opposing argument is misrepresented to make it easier to refute" (Diethelm and McKee 2009:3). For example, COVID-19 vaccines did not prevent infections but minimized their impact on individuals in terms of severe cases, hospitalizations, and in rare cases, deaths. A denialist strategy was to focus anti-vaccine attention on the vaccines' lack of prevention rather than on how the vaccines reduced adverse health outcomes.

Diethelm and McKee recognized other fallacies and strategies used by denialists, such as false analogies, and underscored an additional point helpful in understanding the pandemic. They wrote, "Denialists are usually not deterred by the extreme isolation of their theories, but rather see it as the indication of their intellectual courage against the dominant orthodoxy and the accompanying political correctness, often comparing themselves to Galileo" (Diethelm and McKee 2009:3). Claims of censorship, repression, and the lack of openness represent this form of scientific martyrdom in denialists' thinking.

So, understanding denialism and its playbook can be a helpful tool in making sense of much of the pandemic rhetoric, especially if the topics are misinformation and conspiracy theories. Conspiracy theorists have capitalized on the notion of censorship to their advantage. Misinformation about COVID-19 is still being spread despite being discredited or removed from public information sources. Its removal takes on a mysterious feeling of being "taboo." Consequently, it is appealing to alt-right and conspiracy theory platforms. For example, censorship crops up early in Robert F. Kennedy Jr.'s conspiracy theory book (2021).

VACCINE CONSPIRACIES

Conspiracy rumors are not new to vaccines. Recall the 1998 scandal involving the MMR vaccine and autism (see chapter 3). There have been other rumors and myths regarding vaccines. For example, another has been that infants' immune systems cannot cope with having multiple vaccines (see chapter 8). Conspiracy theorists have developed new conspiracies regarding COVID-19 vaccines, including dangerous schemes regarding microchips, the contents of the vaccines, testing of vaccines, and the consequences of being vaccinated, among others.

THE MICROCHIP CONSPIRACY

The conspiracy theory involving microchips in vaccines was promoted during the pandemic. This conspiracy proposed that vaccines contained microchips that could be used to track and possibly control individuals. As is always the case with conspiracy theories, there is a tiny element of fact, but that fact is always manipulated into unrealistic claims. A digital device company is developing gel sensors to monitor the wearer's health and potentially help detect future disease outbreaks. A broadcast about this development made it clear that the device is not a microchip that will be used to track a person's every move but a gel that will monitor the blood for disease. There is no way the gel could track a person's location. It only reports on one item, is voluntary, and relies on an application on the user's phone.

However, conspiracy theorists latched on to the concept and generated misinformation about a government conspiracy to track everyone (Spencer, 2021b). Conspiracy theorists deceptively claimed that the sensors (gels) were COVID-19-detecting microchips that would be used to track people's movements (Spencer 2021b). Believers in this conspiracy resisted vaccines and had paranoid beliefs, similar to the idea that "big brother" was watching. A representative cautionary statement of this conspiracy is, "We are being tracked and traced every moment of the day and night, and there are plans to implant biometric readers into everyone's bodies to identify who the potential risk carriers are" (Mercola and Cummins 2021:42).

The commonsense test for this conspiracy is for people to ask whether their everyday movements to fairly mundane locations, such as a grocery store, work, school, restaurant, etc., provide the government with valuable information. Does every American citizen represent a national security risk to the point that the government needs to track everyone's movements and locations? Unfortunately, these fundamental questions seem to escape those believers who believed in this conspiracy. However, that is the point about conspiracy theories; they do not have to be based on reality but are founded on emotions and a lack of critical thinking.

Another involving Bill and Melinda Gates is similar to the microchip and elite conspiracies. At a 2015 Ted Talk, Bill Gates, one of the cofounders of Microsoft and hence one of the wealthiest and most influential men in the world, commented that if anything kills 10 million people in the world over the following decades, it would be a highly infectious virus rather than a war. Bill Gates and his then-spouse Melinda had a history of generous philanthropic work supporting public health, including vaccinating lower-income people in developing countries to prevent diseases. The Bill and Melinda Gates Foundation has contributed billions of dollars worldwide to provide public health. His comment received some coverage but resurfaced during the pandemic when some skeptics questioned his motives and even proposed he was trying to depopulate the world (Wakefield 2020).

Wakefield (2020) reported that some accused Gates of making vaccines mandatory and implanting microchips in people. Other conspiracies linked to Gates include claims that he has unethically tested vaccines on African and Indian children resulting in thousands of deaths. In addition, he is wrongly accused of introducing a tetanus vaccine in Kenya that includes abortion drugs, among others.

With the internet, many of these conspiracy theories have been disseminated and shared worldwide. What would have usually been confined as a local rumor, with the internet's reach now becomes a full-blown and widely dispersed conspiracy. Wakefield (2020) raised the question of why Bill Gates, a person who has done so much for public health. She cited experts who pointed out that he was rich and famous, similar to others targeted. So, how widespread was American belief in the Gates conspiracy? The Annenberg Policy Research Center's (2021a) national survey of 1,672 adult Americans conducted in November 2021 asked respondents if they believed the Bill Gates microchip theory. Most (79%) said it was false. However, 13 percent were unsure, and 8 percent believed it was true. The old saying "No good deed goes unpunished" applies here.

5G ROLLOUT

One conspiracy theory has tied the rollout of 5G (5th-generation high-speed communications) networks for faster communications to the COVID-19 pandemic. The hypothesis was that a link between electromagnetic radiation and the coronavirus existed (Lynas 2020). Some suggest the symptoms of COVID-19 result from 5G towers and not an actual virus. Lynas (2020) noted no evidence of this being possible, and the coronavirus was thriving in areas where 5G is unavailable. This fact did not deter conspiracy theorists from promoting this idea. One related conspiracy theory held that the purpose of social distancing was to allow for the installation of 5G wireless technology. According to one national survey, only 5 percent of those surveyed believed this to be true, 15 percent were unsure, and 80 percent said it was false (Annenberg Public Policy Center 2021a).

WHAT DO NATIONAL SURVEY DATA INDICATE?

Conspiracy theories have changed and evolved throughout the pandemic. The Annenberg Public Policy Center (2021a) conducted a follow-up survey of 1,672 Americans in November 2021 to better understand and track the evolution of COVID-19 conspiracy theories. The center found that key conspiracy theories and misbeliefs continue to fuel vaccine hesitancy despite evidence to the contrary (facts). The center also found that while most Americans did not believe in COVID-19 conspiracy theories, some continued to hold on to false beliefs and conspiracies and that misinformation had changed over time.

The Annenberg Public Policy Center's Annenberg Science Knowledge (ASK) survey found that beliefs in COVID-19 conspiracies and misinformation have significantly changed. The center provided the following as examples (Annenberg Public Policy Center 2021a:1):

- Nearly a third of those surveyed in November (31%) believed the conspiracy theory that the Chinese government created the coronavirus as a biological weapon—more than in March 2020 (23%), days before the World Health Organization declared the outbreak a pandemic.
- While a growing majority (79%, up from 71% in April 2021) rejected the conspiracy theory as false that Microsoft cofounder Bill Gates supported the development of a vaccine containing microchips that can track a vaccinated person, 1 in 5 people (21%) still think it was true or were not sure (13%).
- Over half of those surveyed (56%) correctly knew that the Moderna and the Pfizer-BioNTech vaccines do not contain fetal tissue, up from 51 percent in April 2021. However, a growing minority (15%, up from 11% in September and 9% in April) said this was true, and about a third (30%) were unsure whether it was true or false.

CONCLUDING OBSERVATIONS

A favorable social environment for rumors, misinformation, and conspiracy theories was established before the pandemic. American institutions were under fire, and a climate of unrest, uncertainty, and political polarization allowed all three to thrive. Americans wanted information about COVID-19, the pandemic, and how to respond best.

Rumors, misinformation, and conspiracy theories fed the American (and world) appetite for information. The uncertainty regarding the severity and duration of the COVID-19 pandemic, the lack of control for individuals' personal lives, and public health and government agencies imposing broad restrictions all contributed to spreading misinformation, disinformation, and conspiracy theories. Americans had factual and non-factual information on which to form their opinions and beliefs and guide their behaviors. While most people relied on facts, others consciously or unconsciously fell into falsehoods and, in some cases, either became seriously ill, needed hospitalization, infected others, or in some instances, died.

It is always challenging to discern fact from fiction. In the context of the pandemic, it took much work for some Americans to distinguish scientific evidence and facts from biased sources of information. The challenge has been tough because social media and biased news sources have become experts at sounding factual, confident, and like presenters of the truth. To borrow a concept from the past, they have become the new "opiate of the masses." Fortunately, surveys have consistently found that most Americans have been skeptical of many bizarre rumors, misinformation, and conspiracy theories.

The power of misinformation, rumors, and conspiracies has been most evident with COVID-19 vaccines. However, a blend of all three can be found in vaccine hesitancy. COVID-19-vaccine-hesitant Americans have expressed concerns about getting vaccinated because vaccine development was rushed, its side effects were not fully understood, and thus it was unsafe or contained foreign substances, such as microchips or fetal tissue. However, some of these same Americans thought it was okay and safe to take drugs unrelated to COVID-19, such as ivermectin, without expert medical approval. This is the power of rumors, misinformation, and conspiracy theories, to appeal to individuals' emotions and pre-existing beliefs over facts.

Misinformation, rumors, and conspiracy theories take a toll on those groups and individuals who believe and act as if they are valid. Besides the immediate and long-term health risks to others, there is an economic side to the pandemic that seldom gets acknowledged. The financial ramifications of being unvaccinated affect the infected individuals, families, and all Americans. For example, a case reported on a CBS national news broadcast told the story of a married couple who initially saw no value in vaccination against COVID-19. They did not believe COVID-19 was serious but had changed their minds and regretted their earlier decision. The expectant mother became infected with COVID-19 and required weeks of hospitalization in intensive care. To save her unborn baby, early surgery was performed, resulting in a premature infant. An infant that required months of intensive neonatal care. When asked, how much did care for the mother and infant cost? The answer was at least three million dollars. The parents said they now wished they had been vaccinated. In so many words, the news anchor stated, "Let this be a lesson for us all." What was missing from the story was that the parents nor any insurance they might have had would ever cover the total cost of the hospital care for the mother or the infant. The hospital will pass on all the costs to other patients who can pay or have insurance, or to a federal health care program. These are financially supported by paying patients, higher insurance premiums, or taxpayers. The bottom line is that in some way or another, all Americans will pay for the decision not to take COVID-19 seriously and be vaccinated.

Chapter 8

Controversy and COVID-19 Restrictions

"In just four months, thanks to the American people,

we have made incredible progress getting people vaccinated quickly, efficiently, and equitably.

Nearly 170 million Americans of every party, every background, every walk of life

have stepped up, rolled up their sleeves, and gotten the shot."

June 2, 2021, White House Briefing, President Joseph Biden

"The trouble with the world is not that people know too little,

it is that they know so many things that are not so."

Attributed to Mark Twain

HISTORY OF CONTROVERSY AND RESISTANCE REGARDING VACCINATIONS

Since the world first became aware of COVID-19, public health agencies and governments recommended or required mask-wearing, quarantines, vaccinations, social distancing, and lockdowns. They took other preventive measures that were difficult for everyone. All prevention efforts involved a degree of self-sacrifice and commitment. Individuals gave up personal freedoms, choices, and resources. As expected, some Americans, out of a concern for themselves and others, readily conformed to restrictions and directives and embraced these preventive measures. However, others either saw no need, ignored them, or resisted them.

One of the most contentious public health efforts involved COVID-19 vaccinations. Resistance to COVID-19 vaccinations or, for that matter, any type of vaccination is not new. Both acceptance and resistance mark the history of inoculation and vaccination (see chapter 3). Isaacs (2021) observed that there have always been doubters regardless of the medical fact that vaccines work. Likewise, there have always been groups of people and individuals who question the safety and motives behind vaccinations, and COVID-19 was no exception.

A common theme with all of the vaccine resisters is that of personal liberty. For example, in the early nineteenth century, when smallpox vaccinations were made mandatory for the military and the impoverished, vaccine resisters viewed mandatory vaccinations as an infringement on their liberty (Conis n.d.). Nevertheless, the question of liberty was only sometimes raised. For example, General George Washington mandated that all his troops be vaccinated (inoculated) for smallpox during the Revolutionary War. However, it seemed at the time that sacrificing the soldiers' personal liberties came secondary to making them available to fight for liberty.

Nevertheless, smallpox is the first example of controversy and resistance to inoculations in America. Smallpox was a devastating but preventable disease for people who were not vaccinated. As described in chapter 3, the value of smallpox vaccinations is well established, and the disease has been virtually eliminated from the world's population. However, as effective as the smallpox vaccinations have proven to be since the 1800s, in the 1950s, there were Americans opposed to smallpox vaccinations. The Anti-Vaccination Society of America was founded in 1879 as a movement against mandatory smallpox vaccinations. It was part of a more significant movement questioning the motives behind promoting the smallpox vaccine (McNamara 2021). The Anti-Vaccination Society of America challenged data released by health authorities and accused politicians, doctors, and pharmaceutical companies of being motivated more by profit than concern about patients' health (McNamara 2021). In addition, the Society formed anti-vaccine spinoff organizations and wrote to newspapers expressing its opposition. The smallpox vaccine hesitancy movement was based on a concern over the vaccine's safety and a belief that vaccination requirements violated individual liberty and personal freedoms (Domachowske and Suryadevara 2013). McNamara (2021) observed the anti-vaxxer slogan of the time, "Liberty cannot be given;

it must be taken," which sounds similar to the COVID-19 vaccine resistance witnessed today.

Almost a century later, when the first polio vaccine was introduced in 1955, it was only available to children of wealthy families due to their having better access to the healthcare system (Reich 2021). As the vaccine became more publicly available, health professionals had to put forth effort in getting people vaccinated. When polio vaccines were available, most Americans readily welcomed them, as polio was a dreaded childhood disease. Consequently, anti-vaccination efforts were not publicly prominent. Most Americans were happy to get their children and themselves vaccinated. However, over time anti-vaccination movements gained momentum. The movement questioned the government's authority in requiring parents to get their children vaccinated based on requirements as being too authoritarian. This idea combined opposition to national health insurance and concerns over socialism. This latter concern was reflected during the rollout of the Salk polio vaccine when President Eisenhower's Secretary of Health, Education, and Welfare, Oveta Culp Hobby, saw no role for the federal government in distributing the polio vaccine, as she viewed it as socialism.

Lang and Lang (1961:270–271) summarized the collective reaction to the rollout of the Salk polio vaccine in America:

> When the development of the Salk vaccine was first publicly announced, many persons opposed the desirability of mass inoculation against polio. Some scientists were skeptical; they argued that there was not yet conclusive proof of the vaccines providing lifelong immunity against all kinds of polio; that many people had already developed a lasting immunity; that there was always the risk of mishaps, of triggering an outbreak in a person already exposed. Having critically appraised the situation, they urged utmost caution. A second group of people had no firm evidence on which to base their opinion against vaccination. Still, they refused to go along because none of their friends seemed to think it worth the trouble to get a vaccination. Still other persons clambered against mass inoculations on the assumption that this was a plot—on the part of Roosevelt supporters active in the anti-polio drive or of profit-greedy laboratories or of the Russians—to push Americans into accepting a risky policy. They may further have expressed generalized distrust of authority and of medical authority in particular.

Lang and Lang's observations written over 60 years ago, in some regards, sound remarkably contemporary to the implementation of COVID-19 vaccinations.

The rollout of the polio vaccine was not flawless. Just a few weeks after a press conference announcing the success of the vaccine trials, an Idaho doctor reported a case of paralytic polio in a recently vaccinated girl. In the following few weeks, similar reports occurred. All noted that paralysis began in the vaccinated arm rather than the legs, which was more common in regular polio cases. On May 5, 1955, the U.S. Surgeon General halted the polio vaccination program to investigate vaccine safety. It soon was evident that most of the cases of paralytic polio occurred in children inoculated with a vaccine prepared by Cutter Laboratories.

Known as the Cutter Incident, it was revealed that Cutter Laboratories likely did not follow Salk's procedures correctly and failed to kill Type 1 of the polio virus. According to Isaacs (2021), 40,000 of the 200,000 children who received vaccines prepared by Cutter developed polio, 200 were paralyzed, and 10 or 11 died. By all measures, this was a major disaster. Once the problem was identified as not being the vaccine per se, production and distribution of polio vaccines restarted without incident, but some fears and misconceptions about polio vaccines continue today. Oldstone (2020:xvi) noted that common threads of fear, superstition, and irrational behavior continue. He surmised that false rumors that the polio vaccine would cause HIV infections and infertility have resulted in polio outbreaks that have reached epidemic levels. This also could be apathy, as current younger generations have no experiences or memories of the disease. Polio vaccines have slipped through the cracks in some areas.

In the 1960s, based on the social acceptance of polio vaccines, health professionals assumed that the public would welcome new vaccinations, such as the MMR vaccine for measles, mumps, and rubella, pertussis, and other childhood diseases. This would be the case for most Americans but not others. Because some families had experienced some of these childhood-associated diseases without severe consequences, they did not see a need for vaccinations. This resistance pattern led some governments and public health agencies to mandate vaccines for children attending public schools. Controversy over the measles, mumps, and rubella vaccine (MMR) stemmed from a published study in the respected British medical journal *The Lancet.* The study's author claimed that his research showed a relationship between MMR vaccines and autism which was found to be untrue (see chapter 3 for details). The study led some to avoid MMR vaccinations. However, there is no evidence that the MMR causes autism but a "great deal" of evidence that it does not. Nevertheless, anti-vaccine groups continue to ignore the evidence and oppose MMR vaccines.

Other myths fueling MMR vaccine hesitancy include that there have been no measles outbreaks. This belief is incorrect. According to the Infectious Diseases Society of America (2022), in 2019, the United States experienced the most significant number of measles cases reported since the disease was proclaimed eliminated from this country in 2000. Another myth is that the measles vaccine does not prevent severe illness or death. The number of deaths due to measles dropped long before the vaccine was introduced, and it is no longer deadly. Although rare, deaths from measles infections do kill some individuals. Even with the documented successes of the MMR vaccination program, outbreaks have occurred due to resistance to the vaccine. For example, a measles outbreak occurred in London among unvaccinated nursery school children and their siblings (Morgan et al. 2003). Some of the unvaccinated children's parents had anti-MMR vaccination views and resisted having their children vaccinated. Measles outbreaks have occurred in other locations, such as California (McNamara 2021) and New York in 2022.

Despite overwhelming supportive evidence of their safety, effectiveness, and benefits, Kavanagh and Rich (2018) linked recent skepticism about vaccine safety to the discredited and retracted MMR vaccine study. In addition, they also attributed current skepticism to celebrities who lobbied against vaccines and called more attention to the issue (Kavanagh and Rich 2018). While vaccine skeptics have always existed (see chapter 3), public opinion shifted within certain population segments. Kavanagh and Rich (2018:23) wrote:

> Now, decreasing numbers of Americans report that getting their children vaccinated is "extremely important." In a 2015 Gallup survey, 54 percent of respondents reported that it is extremely important for parents to get their children vaccinated, down from 64 percent in 2001. This might not seem like a large decrease, but the shift has been significantly greater among specific demographic groups, including younger parents.

They noted that this skepticism and hesitancy has occurred at both ends of the political spectrum. They use wealthy and liberal Southern California parents as an example of a segment resisting vaccines for their children.

Medical historian Conis (2015:n.p.) traced the "vaccination skepticism of today as being rooted in the social movements of the postwar era, which prompted a new generation of parents (and their children) to question drugs, doctors, and authority in general" (see also chapters 3 and 5). She added (2015:n.p.), "Moreover, today's vaccination skepticism is an understandable response to late-twentieth-century trends in childrearing, a steadily growing mandatory vaccination schedule, and continually expanding rationales for vaccinating against disease." Conis identified the rise of environmentalism, feminism, and the women's health movement as essential factors in how parents viewed vaccines.

In the 1970s, magazines began to raise issues about vaccines, such as their necessity, since no one contracted the diseases and they questioned whether they were still needed. Parents increasingly began to question the safety of vaccines and wanted to know more about side effects. Parents wanted to know what substances were contained in vaccines, such as heavy metals and hidden chemicals. The 1970s saw an upsurge of social movements that challenged authority and questioned traditional institutions and sources of information, such as the medical establishment. Women's rights movements fought against gender repression, for equal pay, and for civil rights. Their fight for equality spread to other social movements, such as gay rights and rights for people with disabilities. Environmental movements advanced recycling and preservation of the environment and were anti-pollution.

In 1976, a controversy surfaced over the swine flu. A group of Fort Dix, New Jersey, army recruits were seriously sick from the flu. Tests indicated that the influenza virus was similar to the 1918 virus that killed millions. The government held a massive vaccination campaign that resulted in 45 million Americans being vaccinated. A pandemic never materialized. However, approximately 450 vaccinated Americans developed the rare Guillain-Barré syndrome. Guillain-Barré syndrome is a disorder in which the body's immune system attacks the nerves. As a result, people with the syndrome experience weakness and tingling in their extremities that may eventually paralyze the whole body. Although very few people developed the syndrome, concerns about vaccinations causing the syndrome followed.

In 1982 an anti-vaccine film titled *DPT: Vaccine Roulette* aired, and three years later, the book *DPT: A Shot in the Dark* was published (Coulter and Fisher 1985). Both films questioned the safety of DPT (diphtheria-pertussis-tetanus) vaccinations. In addition, the movie blamed some of the DPT vaccines for permanent brain damage. The films generated considerable public controversy, led to congressional hearings on vaccine safety, and gave rise to anti-vaccine organizations throughout the United States. Anti-vaccination organizations formed, including the National Vaccine Information Center/Dissatisfied Parents Together, Determined Parents to Stop Hurting Our Tots, Concerned Health Professionals and Others, and Parents Concerned About the Safety of Vaccines. All of these were dedicated to unveiling the risks of vaccinations.

In 1986, Congress passed the National Childhood Vaccine Injury Act (Public Law 99–660) to address safety concerns about childhood vaccines and to mitigate the economic impact of lawsuits against drug companies that threatened the integrity of childhood immunization programs. The act permitted children to be compensated for harm caused by vaccines and protected vaccine manufacturers from legal action. Besides a compensation program, the act mandated reporting adverse events following immunizations against diphtheria, tetanus, pertussis, measles, mumps, rubella, and polio. The act also established various agencies tasked with monitoring vaccinations and programs.

COVID-19 ANTI-VAXXERS

These earlier developments set the stage for resistance and hesitancy regarding COVID-19 vaccines. Individuals who resist, are hesitant, or refuse to get vaccinated are called anti-vaxxers. Vaccine resisters have identified reasons they do not want or need to be vaccinated for COVID-19. For example, anti-vaxxers question that if vaccines are roughly 90 percent effective, why do so many vaccinated people still get COVID-19 infections? Referred to as "breakthrough" infections, vaccine-resistant groups have used these occurrences to question the effectiveness of vaccines. Initially, breakthrough infections among the vaccinated only occurred among the immunocompromised. However, as variants emerged, such as Omicron, COVID-19 was better able to circumvent vaccinations. For some, these breakthrough cases were a reason to resist vaccinations. They resisted, although data showed that unvaccinated individuals were about six times more likely to catch COVID-19 and 14 times more likely to die from it.

REASONS FOR HESITANCY/ RESISTANCE TO VACCINES

For various reasons, a collective group of people have resisted, not seen a need for, or refused COVID-19 vaccinations. As memories of diseases such as measles and polio fade, some Americans' mistrust of vaccines has grown. For instance, decades have passed between disease outbreaks that are often highly localized. Consequently, individuals who have never been confronted with the reality of polio or measles may tend to devalue the protection vaccines offer. Younger generations do not have any experience with polio or measles. They have never known anyone with these diseases or witnessed their symptoms. Thus, they do not see the value in getting vaccinated for diseases that are rare or not likely to affect their lives. Ironically, these diseases would still be very present if it were not for vaccines. This is only one of the reasons why vaccination rates never approach 100 percent.

Misinformation about vaccines contributes to resistance, hesitance, and refusal. For example, Robert F. Kennedy Jr.'s Children's Health Defense is a non-profit that is an anti-vaccination organization. It produced an hour-long video and released it on March 11, 2021, titled *Medical Racism: The New Apartheid*. The video targeted the Black community with misinformation about COVID-19 vaccines. The film presented misinformation about vaccines and highlighted historical cases of medical maltreatment of Black Americans. The film presented no evidence that COVID-19 vaccines are unsafe (Kiely et al. 2021). Given the health inequities and heavy consequences of COVID-19 on Black Americans (see chapter 2 and Joseph 2021), the film likely harmed this high-risk population more than responsibly informing them of vaccines. When fact-checked, the video was found to repeat misrepresentations of COVID-19 and other vaccines (Spencer and Fichera 2021).

There are other reasons why individuals and groups are hesitant to get vaccinated (see also chapters 3 and 5). Some of the reasons include:

- A sense of invincibility and belief that "It cannot happen to me." Some believe they are in great health and can overcome any infection. Some may think they're at low risk for negative events such as accidents, diseases, and misfortune. Examples include drivers not wearing seat belts, people driving while intoxicated, not having health insurance out of choice, taking unnecessary risks, and so forth.
- A general lack of trust in science and medicine. One of the main propositions Goldenberg (2020) makes is that it is less about misunderstanding medical science and more about the lack of trust in medicine, specifically vaccine research, that causes vaccine hesitancy. She observed that scientific and pharmaceutical institutions were occasionally fraudulent, marked by scandals, and motivated by profit. This, coupled with the spread of misinformation on social media, has fueled distrust in medical science, specifically vaccines.

Other studies have found that most Americans do not trust pharmaceutical companies (see Reh et al. 2021). For example, Singh, Eisenberg, and Sood (2023) studied a nationally representative sample of individuals at risk of cardiovascular disease to see what factors influenced their trust in pharmaceutical companies. They found that about 60 percent of respondents did not trust pharmaceutical companies. Those individuals with better health and regular sources of medical care had higher levels of trust. Individual political affiliation did not affect the level of trust. They also found that levels of trust had no significant relationship "to their gender, race and ethnicity, age, income, or educational level" (Singh et al. 2023:2).

- A concern for the safety of the vaccines and possible side effects. Some individuals indicate they will wait and see how vaccines work and whether they are safe (see Montgomery 2021; Rothwell and Desai 2020). For example, the pharmaceutical company AstraZeneca/Oxford's clinical trials had data gaps that fueled distrust in the safety of its COVID-19 vaccine (see Paul and Haddad 2023:227).
- Freedom of personal choice and control over their lives.

- Valid medical reasons, such as adverse reactions or allergies, as determined by trained physicians.
- Resistance to government involvement in their lives.
- A belief that a COVID-19 infection is similar to a common cold and, therefore, vaccinations are not needed. During the pandemic, individuals have had friends and family members who showed no signs of infection or minor symptoms that they quickly overcame. As President Trump stated following his hospitalization for COVID-19, "It's not really as bad as they say."
- Belief in misinformation about the risks of getting vaccinated. The false idea is that getting vaccinated is riskier than getting COVID-19, and the vaccines cause other health problems.
- Faith in natural remedies, such as vitamins, aspirin, and others believed to be safer and more effective than vaccines. A belief that there is no need for the vaccine in the first place, as natural diets and healthy living will prevent serious illness.
- An assumption is that natural immunity resulting from an infection protects an individual better than any vaccination. Therefore, given enough time, herd immunity will develop, and vaccines will not be needed.
- An association of the vaccine to the political motives of elected leaders and the financial motives of big pharma (Montgomery 2021).
- A concern about how fast the vaccines were developed (Montgomery 2021; Rothman and Desai 2020).
- Getting a vaccination is a low priority, and the individual will get around to it.
- Government and the power elites want to track individuals to control them through vaccines. In some social circles, it is known as the "plandemic" or a plot by billionaires to take control over the world.
- Employers will not allow paid time off for those negatively reacting to the vaccine. Reich (2021:7) noted that in a recent survey, "80 to 85 percent of Black and Hispanic respondents who indicated that they want to wait before getting a vaccine said they were worried about the vaccine side effects, including those that would require them to miss work" (85 and 66 percent, respectively).
- People have forgotten that vaccines can effectively control diseases (Gorski 2020a). These include measles, polio, smallpox, rubella, and tetanus.

WHAT NATIONAL SURVEYS INDICATE

Independent research organizations have surveyed adult Americans to determine why they are reluctant to get vaccinated. According to a 2019 multiple-wave panel survey by the Annenberg Public Policy Center (2020), most adult Americans support pro-vaccination policies. However, as many as 20 percent have negative views about vaccines. Misinformation about vaccines drove most negative views over partisan political views, education, religion, or other socio-demographic factors. Another Annenberg Public Policy Center (2021c.) survey identified the top reasons selected by the group who said they were unlikely to be vaccinated were:

- 61% – It is still too untested/I am waiting to see what happens (up significantly from 48% in April).
- 53% – I do not trust the government (up significantly from 40% in April).
- 51% – I do not trust the scientists and companies that make the vaccine (up significantly from 36% in June and 30% in April).
- 49% – I am worried about allergies and side effects (up significantly from 35% in April).
- 28% – I am just not concerned about coronavirus/COVID-19.
- 26% – I never get vaccines, generally.
- 15% – I had coronavirus/COVID-19, so I think I am immune (up significantly from 7% in June and April)

Note: The total exceeds 100 percent because respondents were allowed more than one response.

Other early pandemic surveys found that roughly 25–27 percent of Americans said they would "definitely or most likely not get it [vaccinated]" (see Reich 2021:7). Later, Reich reported this percentage rose to around 50 percent of the unvaccinated when the vaccine became politicized. She added that despite messaging, "vaccines are a community level solution, people make decisions based on personal experience, values, and goals, believing at core that they are on their own when it comes to their health." She observed, "Individual perceptions are shaped by peers and social networks, which can be seen in the ways childhood vaccine refusal clusters. For COVID–19 vaccines, it appears that knowing someone who has been vaccinated predicts wanting a vaccine" (Reich 2021:7).

A Kaiser Family Foundation public opinion survey, conducted in December 2020, found that slightly over a quarter (27%) of the American public was vaccine-hesitant, indicating they would likely not get vaccinated whether the vaccine was free or not and determined to be safe (Hamel et al. 2020).

Vaccine hesitancy was highest (42%) among Republicans responding to the survey. About 15 percent of the population indicated they would "definitely not" get the vaccine. These findings almost replicate findings from other independent research organizations. For example, the Annenberg Public Policy Center (2021c) conducted a study in May 2020 found that 18 percent of Americans said they would be "not at all likely" to get a COVID-19 vaccine if it became available.

Similar survey results from the Pew Research Center were revealed in a study by Funk and Gramlich (2021). They investigated how vaccination patterns among 10,348 adults in the United States differ by demographic, religious, regional, and political factors. The data were collected in August 2021. They found, consistent with CDC data, that most Americans at the time of the survey had received at least one dose of the vaccine. They discovered that Americans have mixed views about vaccine requirements in public settings. They also found that Democrats (86%) were "far more" likely to have been vaccinated than Republicans (roughly 6 in 10). For those surveyed, older people with higher levels of education were more likely to have been vaccinated. White and Black respondents reported the same vaccination rates, a change from earlier in the pandemic when Black Americans were more hesitant and had less access to the vaccines than White Americans. Other ethnic groups followed the same pattern of reporting higher vaccination rates.

Vaccination patterns differed among religious groups. Funk and Gramlich (2021) found that 82 percent of Catholic adults said they were at least partially vaccinated as of August. For Protestants, 73 percent of White non-evangelicals and 70 percent of those who are Black said they had received at least one dose. However, White evangelical Protestants' percentage was considerably lower (57%). For those unaffiliated, roughly three-quarters said they were at least partially vaccinated. The important role the Black church has played in Black Americans getting vaccinated has been documented (Kramer 2021).

The majority of adults they surveyed favored requiring adults to show proof of COVID-19 vaccination when traveling by airplane (61%), attending public colleges or universities in person (57%), or attending a sporting or entertainment event (56%). However, fewer supported showing proof of vaccination when dining at an indoor restaurant, 50 percent were for it, and 50 percent were opposed. A slightly higher percentage (54%) opposed showing proof of vaccination to shop or conduct business indoors. Respondents were divided on how businesses should approach vaccinations. A minority (39%) thought businesses should require all employees to be vaccinated, 35 percent indicated businesses should encourage vaccinations, and 25 percent said businesses should do nothing. The respondents' views were tied to political party affiliation. Most Democrats were in favor of requiring proof of vaccination status in five public settings, while the majority of Republicans were opposed to requirements in all locations. In addition, vaccinated adults tended to favor requiring proof of vaccination status, and of course, unvaccinated adults were overwhelmingly opposed.

Vaccination status was linked to confidence in vaccine research and development. Ninety-one percent of those vaccinated had a great deal or a fair amount of confidence in the vaccine research and development process. This compared with 21 percent of unvaccinated adults who lacked confidence. Those not vaccinated expressed a range of concerns about the vaccines. Among the concerns expressed were having too much pressure on them to get vaccinated (88%), concern over health risks (81%), lack of trust in public health officials (80%), and confusion over all of the information regarding vaccines (78%).

Two years into the pandemic, Parker, Horowitz, and Minkin (2022) surveyed 5,889 American adults working part- or full-time who had only one job or a job they consider their primary job. Parker et al. (2022) found that most workers (69%) said their employer should not mandate vaccines for adults not working from home. Roughly a third said vaccines should be required of all workers. Of those in favor of no mandates, 39% said their employer should encourage vaccinations, and 30% said they should neither mandate nor encourage vaccinations. Black workers were more likely (55%) to say their employer should encourage vaccinations than Hispanic (43%) and White (37%) workers. Democratic and Democratic-leaning workers (47%) think employers should require vaccines, compared to 10 percent of Republican or Republican-leaning workers.

The United States is not unique in vaccine hesitancy. Researchers in other countries, such as Australia, have identified similar reasons why people resist or avoid getting vaccinated (Attwell et al. 2017). In addition, anti-vaccine protests have occurred in various countries, including in Europe. For example, far-right anti-vaccine protests and pro-vaccination counterprotests have been observed in Berlin (Griesher 2022).

PRO-VACCINATION/VACCINE ACCEPTANCE

Most Americans have been vaccinated for COVID-19. To those in favor of vaccinations, the idea that someone would resist getting vaccinated can be perplexing (Reich 2021), especially when clinical studies report that the vaccines were very effective (ranging from 65 to 95%) in preventing severe illness or death. Some view vaccinations as a "magic bullet" to solve the pandemic (see Paul and Haddad 2023:227). In response to hesitancy, non-governmental organizations have undertaken projects to promote public health measures, such as vaccinations. For example, the Ad Council initiated a campaign in the United States promoting COVID-19 vaccinations. While the campaign tried to reach everyone, it focused on people of color disproportionately impacted by COVID-19 (see chapter 2). Research has found that communities of color were especially hesitant to get vaccinated due to health inequities and negative experiences with health care (Montgomery 2021). For example, the Tuskegee syphilis research conducted on Black men without their consent in the 1930s and the years following continues to influence some Black Americans' trust in medicine and the government.

GOVERNMENT PANDEMIC EFFORTS

Although COVID-19 vaccine benefits are well understood, vaccination rates, even in higher-income countries, such as the United States, only range between 70 and 75 percent. Government agencies became convinced that the fear of catching COVID-19 and possibly getting severely ill or disabled, dying, or infecting others, including family members, was insufficient to compel some individuals to get vaccinated. Consequently, the U.S. and local governments implemented various strategies to persuade Americans to get vaccinated, such as running promotional campaigns, outreach events, and celebrity testimonials. Public health and government agencies offered incentives, such as cash, tickets to sporting events, gift cards, movie tickets, and lottery tickets, if people would get vaccinated. In addition, government agencies, such as the Food and Drug Administration, Centers for Disease Control and Prevention, Department of Health and Human Services, and Government Accountability Office, public health agencies, and elected officials, have researched COVID-19. Government agencies collected much-needed data on the pandemic. Government agencies have played essential roles in COVID-19 mitigation, prevention, education, and the development of vaccines and treatments. Governments also actively distributed ventilators, medical supplies, and vaccines nationwide and to other countries.

How effective were these incentives? Campos-Mercade, Meler, Schneider, Meier, Pope, and Wengström (2021) conducted a study of 8,286 Swedish adults to determine the effectiveness of monetary incentives on vaccination rates. They also investigated behavioral nudges, such as reminders to get vaccinations. They found that, as would be expected, monetary incentives increased vaccination rates. However, gains in vaccination rates were small, around 4 percent, and encouraging nudges even smaller. Overall, non-monetary nudges had little impact on motivating people to get vaccinated. Gains may be so small that they do not outweigh the costs of administering incentive programs. Campos-Mercade et al. (2021) concluded that monetary incentives were effective but had limited value. The interesting question is why the potentially catastrophic consequences of COVID-19 did not motivate some individuals to get vaccinated but small incentives were sufficient.

VACCINE MANDATES, LAWS, AND CASES

Governments and private employers used another approach to increase vaccination rates by mandating vaccinations. The history of vaccine mandates and court cases is lengthy. The state of Massachusetts was the first to impose compulsory smallpox vaccinations in 1809. Washington, DC, and eight other states soon required infant vaccinations. The states have different rules for various vaccines in different contexts, with some making exemptions on religious, medical, or philosophical grounds (Reich 2021). The result is variations in rules among the states. Most states (35) have allowed local authorities to regulate vaccine requirements (mandates). For example, California passed a law eliminating personal and religious exemptions to mandated vaccines based on measles and pertussis (whooping cough) outbreaks and other vaccine-preventable infections. Different states have opposed vaccination mandates, and in 1930, Arizona, Utah, North Dakota, and Minnesota passed laws against their residents' vaccination requirements.

Many of these vaccine mandates have been challenged in the courts. In the 1905 case of *Jacobson v. Massachusetts*, 197 U.S. 11 (1905), the U.S. Supreme Court set a legal precedent by finding that individual liberty does not supersede actions required for the public good. The court ruled:

> The liberty secured by the Constitution of the United States does not import an absolute right in each person to be at all times, and in all circumstances, wholly freed from restraint, nor is it an element in such liberty that one person, or a minority of persons residing in any community and enjoying the benefits of its local government, should have the power to dominate the majority when supported in their action by the authority of the State. (Justia 2022:n.p.)

With this decision, the Court upheld the authority of states to enforce compulsory vaccination laws. The Court's decision expressed the view that individual liberty is not absolute and is subject to the police power (authority) of the state. This case also has served as the foundation for COVID-19 face-mask and stay-at-home orders.

President Biden's administration mandated that large employers require vaccinations for all employees. On November 5, 2021, the Occupational Safety and Health Administration (OSHA) published an emergency temporary standard for all employers with 100 or more employees. The standard required covered employers to "develop, implement, and enforce a mandatory COVID-19 vaccination policy." If they preferred, employers could allow employees to avoid being vaccinated if they wore face masks and were tested weekly.

Section 264 of the Public Health Services Act of 1944 defined the CDC's statutory authority. It gives the agency the right to promulgate regulations aimed at "identifying, isolating, and destroying" diseases. Section 264 (a) has two sentences that provide the agency the power to issue regulations necessary "to prevent the spread of communicable diseases." The second sentence illustrates the kinds of policies that would or could be necessary. They include "inspection, fumigation, disinfection, sanitation, pest extermination and destruction of contaminated animals and articles."

This large-employer mandate was soon challenged in the courts because the federal government overstepped its authority. The U.S. Supreme Court would hear and issue a decision on January 13, 2022, on the *National Federation of Independent Business v. OSHA* case. The U.S. Supreme Court ruling of 595 US ____ (2022) prevented the administration (OSHA) from enforcing a rule that would require businesses employing 100 or more workers to insist (require) that their employees who work in settings conducive to the spread of COVID-19 either be vaccinated or wear masks and undergo regular coronavirus testing. The U.S. Supreme Court agreed and ruled that the administration had overstepped its authority.

In a related case, *Biden v. Missouri*, the Supreme Court allowed a different rule to proceed. The government mandated COVID-19 vaccination, absent a medical or religious exemption, for all healthcare workers in institutions receiving federal funding for Medicare or Medicaid patients. The court ruled that the administration had the authority to impose a vaccination requirement for all employers receiving federal Medicaid or Medicare funds. Mandates for healthcare workers were legal, but mandates for ordinary employees of large businesses were not.

Controversy immediately surfaced, with some applauding the decisions and others bemoaning them. Opponents thought the January 13, 2022, Supreme Court decision defied common sense, as deadly and highly infectious diseases may not be controlled unless mandates are in place (Kamarck 2022). It is essential to acknowledge that with epidemics and pandemics, social perceptions matter, and the unethical infringements on civil liberties and stigmatization of the infected and those who care for them occur. Some Americans have argued that any mandate restricting their freedom, such as choosing to be unvaccinated or being unmasked, infringes on their rights.

The large-employer mandate was not the only challenge to government mandates. In January 2022, thousands of protestors gathered on the National

Mall in Washington, DC, to protest COVID-19 vaccine mandates. They protested under the general banner of personal freedoms. Protestors chanted "No more mandates" and carried "Don't Tread on Me" flags. The event was sponsored by the Children's Health Defense Fund, the political wing of Robert F. Kennedy Jr.'s anti-vaccine organization. In a speech at the protest, Kennedy referred to the mandates as "a *coup d'état* to democracy" and compared vaccine passports to "slavery" (cited by Voght 2022).

The United States is not alone in resistance to mandates, as other countries have experienced similar protests. For example, on May 10, 2020, groups of protestors gathered in Melbourne and Sydney, Australia, to protest lockdowns, exposure tracking, vaccines, and the public health philanthropy of Bill Gates (Attwell 2020). In several French cities and Berlin, Germany, protests against lockdowns surfaced (Zielonka 2021). It was reported that China experienced protests against restrictive policies and lockdowns in 2022 (Kang and Wu 2022).

SURVEYS OF COMMUNITY PERCEPTIONS OF VACCINATIONS

Parker, Horowitz, and Minkin (2021) surveyed 9,676 American adults in October 2021 to better understand American views on the impact of COVID-19 prevention efforts on local communities. The Pew Research Center survey focused on mask-wearing, vaccines, and restrictions on public activities. Roughly half of the adults surveyed indicated they lived in communities where people had mixed views on these prevention measures. For example, regarding the importance of getting vaccinated, 12 percent indicated it was not important, and 5 percent were unsure. Concerning mask-wearing in public, 23 percent thought it was important, and 22 percent said it was not and should not be done. Finally, regarding public restrictions, 26 percent thought tight restrictions were unimportant and should not be imposed, and 13 percent thought they were important.

Parker et al. (2021) also found that perceptions of these public health COVID-19 prevention measures differed by community type, a few demographic variables, and political party identification (see chapter 6). Rural residents were less likely than urban or suburban residents to say that most community members think any mitigation steps to limit COVID-19 are important and should be taken. Case in point, only 3 percent of rural residents, compared to 23 percent of suburban and 34 percent of urban residents, believed wearing masks in public was important. Thirty-two percent of rural residents said most people in the community believe mask-wearing is unimportant and should not be done. This percentage compares to 21 percent of suburban and 15 percent of urban residents.

Race and ethnicity were also associated with community views on prevention efforts (Parker et al. 2021). For mask-wearing, Asian (49%), Black (29%), and Hispanic (32%) adults were more likely than White adults (18%) to say most people in their community think wearing a mask was important. White adults were more likely than other groups to say that most people where they live believe it is not essential to wear a mask or that masks should not be worn. However, 54 percent of White, 47 percent of Black, and 44 percent of Hispanic adults said their community has differing views. These patterns were similar for vaccines and restrictions on public activities.

Other patterns were found for political identification, income level, and level of education. College graduates and upper-income adults were much more likely than those with less education or income to have said most people in their community think getting a COVID-19 vaccine was important. In addition, political identification was found to be critical. Thirty-one percent of Democrats, compared to 14 percent of Republicans, said most people in their area think wearing masks is essential. This compares to 28 percent of Republicans and 18 percent of Democrats saying most in their community think this was unimportant or should not be done. Finally, regarding vaccines, a higher percentage of Republicans than Democrats indicated a mix of views in their community (Parker et al. 2021). Parker et al.'s (2021) research has been echoed in other national surveys, such as those conducted by the Kaiser Family Foundation, which found important and increasingly strong relationships between political partisanship and vaccine status (Kirzinger et al. 2021).

Finally, communities struck by recent COVID-19 deaths had different perceptions of the importance of preventative measures (Parker et al. 2021). Adults living in communities hard-hit by COVID-19 deaths reported less support among their fellow community members for vaccines, mask-wearing, and tight restrictions on public activities. This suggests that communities with lower opinions of the value of COVID-19 preventative measures tended to have higher death rates than those with more positive community perceptions of such actions.

The theme of mixed views on COVID-19 prevention measures surfaces in other studies. A Pew Research Center study of American adults by Tyson and Funk (2022) found diverse support for pandemic control measures. The majority (58%) of Americans surveyed favored requiring proof of vaccination for air travel, but approval for attending sporting events and concerts decreased to 53 percent and 46 percent, respectively. Americans expressed less support for proof of vaccination for more routine activities, such as going to a restaurant (53%), and most (59%) opposed proof of vaccination when shopping. Political party membership and vaccination status influenced opinions on whether proof of vaccination should be required. Republicans tended to be less supportive, and Democrats more supportive of proof of vaccination. As expected, vaccinated adults tended to approve of requirements, and unvaccinated adults tended to disapprove.

FACE MASK WEARING

One of the most controversial mandates during the COVID-19 pandemic has been using face masks. Face mask wearing, specifically face mask mandates, pros and cons, have been the grounds for collective behavior. Spontaneous groups have formed on both sides, particularly regarding public schools and transportation. One topic of controversy has been requiring schoolchildren to wear face masks at school. Parents have advocated and protested for the end of school mask mandates. Sides have been divided between parents that demand that face mask mandates be eliminated and parents who want to continue face mask requirements. Opponents of face mask wearing contend that mask-wearing harms students educationally, socially, and psychologically. In addition, they argue that vulnerable children can wear face masks regardless of their medical condition. Pro-mask-wearing parents argue that medically vulnerable students are at high risk of becoming very ill from COVID-19. One media account described a school board meeting in Minnesota where a fight broke out regarding mask mandates in schools due to the risk of COVID-19 cases (WCCO-TV 2021). The story noted that school districts have been forced to change due to recent spikes in COVID-19 cases. Each school district handles COVID-19 differently, and bullying occurs on both sides.

Since COVID-19 became a public health crisis in 2020, different cities and states have responded with preventative measures, many of them including a recommendation or a requirement to wear a face mask when in proximity to other people. These mandates have drawn protests from opponents, many of whom feel that face masks are unnecessary, ineffective, or violate individual rights. However, not wearing face masks can have health consequences. It should be recalled that during the 1918 influenza pandemic, when San Francisco authorities relaxed mask requirements and lockdowns, a resurgence of influenza occurred soon after. A similar pattern was observed in Saint Louis (see chapter 3).

Deadly diseases, like COVID-19 and other SARS viruses, are spread through the air. For example, measles lives in an infected person's nose and throat mucus and can easily be spread through coughing or sneezing. Influenza viruses are also spread through respiratory droplets, thus are passed through the air. Given prior experiences with coronaviruses, health officials relied on face masks to limit the spread of COVID-19. Face masks have been an important strategy for controlling the expansion of COVID-19 from the beginning of the pandemic (see chapter 1).

The wearing of face masks is an ancient tradition in medicine, even if it was not fully understood. Strasser and Schlich (2020:19) summarized how face masks were used in early modern Europe, such as when the black plague hit much of the continent:

> Covering the nose and mouth had been part of traditional sanitary practices against contagious diseases in early modern Europe. This protection was primarily about neutralizing so-called miasma in the air through perfumes and spices held under a mask, such as the plague doctors' bird-like masks. Such practices, however, had become marginal by the 18th century. Instead, face masks, as they are used today in health care and the community, can be traced back to a more recent period when a new understanding of contagion based on germ theory was applied to surgery.

The COVID-19 pandemic is not the first American public-mandated use of face masks to prevent the spread of infections. For example, during the 1918 influenza pandemic, cloth masks were worn by many Americans in and outside of the health care system. During the 1918 influenza pandemic, face mask wearing became mandatory for certain occupations, such as police and medical workers, and in some cities, for citizens in general, but it was often controversial (Strasser and Schlich 2020). San Francisco provides a case example of collective resistance to face mask requirements. The city had tried other efforts to curb the spread of the disease, such as curfews, banning gatherings, and closing schools. Instead, the city required people who had direct contact with the public, such as medical personnel, barbers, bank tellers, and others, to wear face masks. Violators of the mandate could be fined, warned, and possibly jailed. The ordinance would last a month and be repealed due to political pressure and a decline in cases.

Later, with an upsurge in influenza cases, city officials passed a new mask-wearing ordinance on October 25, 1919. The city ordinance required everyone in San Francisco to wear a face mask in public or in a group of two or more people, except at mealtime. Most residents initially complied with the requirement and wore masks without resistance. However, groups of citizens complained about the new requirement, and thus, resistance and opposition to the ordinance quickly surfaced. In the city, the Anti-Mask League of San Francisco formed to protest the face mask requirement (see chapter 3).

The league was comprised of physicians and civil libertarians, among others. The league questioned the requirement on scientific grounds and its impingement on civil liberties. According to a newspaper report, an estimated

4,000 to 5,000 people attended a meeting to protest the ordinance in January 1919 (Logansport et al. 1919:8). In 1918, a study of the effectiveness of face masks was conducted. The study concluded that mandatory mask mandates did not make any difference while observing that a likely reason for their ineffectiveness was that masks were worn outdoors and not inside gatherings where the risk for transmission would be greatest. It also noted that most masks needed to be correctly constructed of adequate materials, otherwise rendering them ineffective. However, according to later medical historians, the decline in deaths from influenza in San Francisco can be partly attributed to its mandatory mask-wearing policies (Strasser and Schlich 2020).

Researchers have studied the factors influencing whether individuals are likely or unlikely to wear face masks during the COVID-19 pandemic. For example, Stosic, Helwig, and Ruben (2021) studied if and how an individual's belief in science directly impacted reported face mask wearing behavior. Their survey of 1,050 adults included questions on face mask wearing behavior, general beliefs in science, and belief in face masks' effectiveness in reducing the spread of COVID-19. Their findings indicated there was evidence that greater belief in science predicted greater belief in the efficacy of face masks in reducing the spread of COVID-19. This transferred into actual public face mask wearing behavior. The study showed that people with greater faith in science and the scientific process are likelier to comply with health mandates, wear face masks, and get vaccinated. In addition, Stosic et al. (2021) found that gender, age, race, ethnicity, region, and political ideology were significant predictors of face mask wearing.

A different study by Rothwell and Desai (2020) concluded that those people who denied the asymptomatic spread of COVID-19 or believed the flu was more deadly than the coronavirus were less likely to wear face masks and isolate. Specifically, even when individual characteristics, such as age, race, education, and individuals denying were factored in, individuals denying the asymptomatic spread of COVID-19 were 27 percent less likely to wear a face mask indoors and out in public. The same pattern (13%) held for those believing the flu was more serious than COVID-19.

During the COVID-19 pandemic, false claims about face masks have been commonplace and fueled resistance to wearing them. For example, Kiely (2021) identified a conservative website referencing a Stanford study claiming that face masks were unsafe and ineffective against COVID-19. According to Kiely, in April of 2021, the conservative website *The Gateway Pundit* carried the headline "Stanford Study Results: Facemasks are Ineffective to Block Transmission of COVID-19 and Actually Can Cause Health Deterioration and Premature Death." However, the paper's author had no affiliation with Stanford University and it was later withdrawn from the *Medical Hypotheses* journal. The content of the article was also found to be inaccurate.

It is important to recognize the role culture plays in face mask wearing. In some cultures, face mask wearing is more common and accepted, whether amid pandemics or not. The cultural connection to mask-wearing is important. The sociologist Jens Zinn (2021:605) observed the following about culture and face mask wearing:

> The socio-cultural patterns were well established before the COVID-19 pandemic. For example, public mask wearing in Japan and other east Asian countries is accepted and widespread, thus when citizens were asked to wear masks in public, there was no resistance. Such was different in European and North American countries. Mask wearing, for some, became an issue of personal liberty versus the health of the larger community (society). While there is little evidence that a facemask can protect an individual over time, wearing them does reduce the transmission of COVID-19 to the community.

Socio-cultural patterns surface when scientific experts debate and provide evidence to inform political decision-making. A compelling example was the debate about recommending wearing face masks in public, which can be interpreted as a negotiation of culturally mediated practices and values. However, wearing face masks is a common and widely accepted means of response to infectious diseases in many Asian countries. However, it is sometimes seen as a cultural oddity in the global North and lacks scientific evidence for efficacy (Fleming 2020). Therefore, the World Health Organization (WHO) did not recommend it by the end of March 2020 (Howard 2020). However, the recommendations soon shifted. For example, the U.S. Centers for Disease Control and Prevention (CDC) recommended wearing "cloth face coverings" in public on April 3, 2020 (Jingnan 2020). Zinn (2021:612) wrote:

> After face-mask wearing has been proven to be an efficient means to slow the spread of the virus, it would be desirable to integrate face-mask wearing into the general behavioral repertoire in the global West, where prejudice and doubts have been strongest about their effectiveness. At the same time, people still felt uncomfortable wearing them.

Controversy about the value of face masks continued to thrive in 2023, sparked by a reputable Cochrane Library investigation of studies on the effectiveness of handwashing and face mask wearing in limiting the spread of respiratory viruses. The Cochrane Library, a respected British research organization, conducted an extensive study of face mask mandates and concluded that face mask mandates had little value in controlling COVID-19. The study (meta-analysis) identified COVID-19 studies that concluded face masks had minimal value in preventing the spread of influenza and COVID-19 (Jefferson et al. 2023).

Conservative columnists and news outlets, and anti-maskers, quickly embraced the study results. For example, *New York Times* columnist Bret Stephens (2023), using the study's findings, wrote, "Mask mandates were a bust" and a "Fool's errand from the start." Stephens also raised the issues of following science, incompetent government, and the tendency to do something (whether it makes sense or not).

His opinion was soon rebutted by other columnists, government officials, and scientists. *Los Angeles Times* columnist Michael Hiltzik, in a column titled "COVID Deniers Think a New Study Says Mask Mandates Do Not Work. They Should Try Reading It," accused Stephens of not reading the study (Hiltzik 2023). Hiltzik counter-argued that the survey reached tentative conclusions based on limited studies and was misinterpreted. Hiltzik noted that the study's lead author had little involvement with the study, and Stephens's comments contradicted the actual findings. Hiltzik stated that only six of the studies reviewed dealt with COVID-19, and of those, only two with mask-wearing. The two studies of COVID-19 face mask wearing reported benefits. In addition, the reviewed studies did not consider individual compliance with mask-wearing, and one study concluded it had limited value based on a tiny sample. Hiltzik identified other studies, such as one conducted on the USS *Theodore Roosevelt*, that demonstrated a 70% reduction in the risk of infection. His point is that commentators should be careful in drawing conclusions that are not well-supported and may contradict political ideologies.

The Annenberg Public Policy Center (McDonald 2023) fact-checked the study and concluded that study was uncertain whether masks helped slow the spread of COVID-19. According to McDonald, the study was misinterpreted, and even the Cochrane Review agreed it was. This case and corresponding controversy is another example of how anti-masking, political biases, denialism, and misinterpreting information continue about face masks.

SOCIAL DISTANCING

Early in the pandemic public health officials recommended social distancing be implemented to control the spread of COVID-19. In some locations, public health officials limited the size of social gatherings (number of people allowed) in indoor settings and recommended spatial distances be maintained between people in public spaces. In addition, quarantine timeframes were also implemented. In some locations, officials mandated and enforced these restrictions. Furthermore, some businesses implemented their social distancing restrictions.

If properly implemented, social distancing can effectively prevent the spread of COVID-19. Nevertheless, some people view the practice as detrimental to healthy social relationships, work, and sectors of the economy, such as entertainment, travel, and businesses requiring face-to-face interaction (Ferreira et al. 2020).

Like other COVID-19 prevention measures, protests against social distancing public health orders surfaced in Michigan, Colorado, Maryland, Minnesota, North Carolina, Virginia, Pennsylvania, Maine, and Kentucky. Similar to other protests, the restrictions and human rights themes surfaced at these gatherings. Interwoven in the protests were political messages, including pro–gun rights, from right-wing groups, and for reelecting Donald Trump. In the United States, COVID-19 protests became "entwined" with other political and social issues, with both extremes of the political continuum represented at protests, including the far left (Delanty 2021b:1). Some of the far-right protesters carried automatic rifles as symbols of power and intimidation.

Social protests occurred in different countries throughout the world. The spread or repetition of similar campaigns, events, and gatherings occurred across other geopolitical states, communities, or locations within weeks or months. Collective behaviorists refer to this social pattern as a "wave" (Miller 2014:55). Waves are precisely what occurred with protests regarding mandates, masks, vaccines, and other COVID-19 requirements.

LOCKDOWNS

Public health and elected officials have relied on lockdowns of public spaces, such as businesses and public buildings, to control the spread of COVID-19. However, academic research has sent mixed messages regarding the value of lockdowns. Take the case of research on the effectiveness of lockdowns in reducing COVID-19 mortality rates. Herby, Jonung, and Hanke (2022) conducted a systematic review (meta-analysis) of research studies on COVID-19 lockdowns to determine if there was valid evidence that lockdowns reduced COVID-19 mortality rates. They (Herby et al. 2022:2) defined lockdown as "an imposition of at least one compulsory, non-pharmaceutical intervention (NPI)." NPIs are government mandates restricting people's actions, such as closing schools or businesses or limiting internal movement. They screened over 18,000 studies and narrowed them down to 34 that met their standards for analysis. For three types of lockdowns, they concluded that "lockdowns have little to no effect on COVID-19 mortality" (Herby et al. 2022:2). Lockdowns in Europe and the United States only reduced mortality on average by 0.2 percent. This was less than a one percent reduction in mortality rates, and they concluded (Herby et al. 2022:2):

> While this meta-analysis concludes that lockdowns have had little to no public health effects, they have imposed enormous economic and social costs where they have been adopted. Consequently, lockdown policies could be better founded and rejected as a pandemic policy instrument.

They also noted, "Overall, our meta-analysis fails to confirm that lockdowns have had a large, significant effect on mortality rates" (Herby et al. 2022:40). However, they did acknowledge that "closing non-essential businesses seems to have had some effect (reducing COVID-19 mortality by 10.6%), which is likely to be related to the closure of bars." Herby et al. (2022:43) concluded:

> The use of lockdowns is a unique feature of the COVID-19 pandemic. Lockdowns have not been used to such a large extent during pandemics of the past century. However, lockdowns during the initial phase of the COVID-19 pandemic have had devastating effects. They have contributed to reducing economic activity, raising unemployment, reducing schooling, causing political unrest, contributing to domestic violence, and undermining liberal democracy. These costs to society must be compared to the benefits of lockdowns, which our meta-analysis has shown are marginal at best. Such a standard benefit-cost calculation leads to a strong conclusion: lockdowns should be rejected out of hand as a pandemic policy instrument.

Latching on to this study's conclusions, at least one opinion columnist (Kafer 2022) wrote an opinion, titled "Lockdowns—Tremendous Cost, Few Lives Saved." Kafer's opinion questioned the value of lockdowns in light of the costs to society. However, not everyone agrees with the Herby, Jonung, and Hanke (2022) study's conclusions and contend that it was flawed (see Joszt 2022).

Other researchers have provided evidence that lockdowns have had negative consequences. Studies have examined the adverse psychological effects of state-imposed lockdowns. (see Solomou and Constantinidou 2020). Bagus, Peña-Ramos, and Sánchez-Bayón (2021:4), citing previous research, covered the issue of lockdowns and concluded that lockdowns were a source of unnecessary psychological strain. They wrote:

> If, and to what extent, the world has been suffering from mass hysteria or mass psychogenic illness during the COVID-19 crisis is open to future research, even though some observers have made that claim. It is clear, in any case, that the population has been under tremendous psychological strain during the COVID-19 crisis. Lockdowns have especially contributed to a surge in anxiety and stress, which are important ingredients for the development of mass hysteria.

Zielonka (2021) concluded that politicians on both sides of restrictions and lockdown policies presented statistics in favor of their position. Politicians favoring these measures pointed to how many lives were saved by "prudent measures." Politicians in favor of lifting restrictions and lockdowns relied on statistics showing how many jobs had been saved and the economic benefits of more "sensible" approaches to COVID-19 (Zielonka 2021:62). In the end, the public is faced with conflicting claims and resulting confusion on what are the best ways to address COVID-19.

VACCINE PROTESTS

In 2021, the *Los Angeles Times* ran a news story regarding anti-mandate protests. In the report, Solis and Branson-Potts (2021) described how thousands of protestors gathered in front of Los Angeles City Hall to protest implementing COVID-19 vaccine verification rules for businesses. The city had started requiring individuals to provide proof of COVID-19 vaccinations before entering indoor restaurants, museums, movie theaters, and other public spaces. Similar requirements have been implemented in foreign countries, such as France.

Other mandates have required vaccinations for schoolchildren and government workers. These requirements were controversial from the beginning. Protestors carried signs with messages such as "Job Mandate—Vaccinations without exemptions are a violation of our 14th constitutional amendment!" "Vaccines Kill," "Freedom not Force!" and "Vaccines are Toxic." Some protestors wore hats supporting the Proud Boys and other alt-right groups. Some protestors interviewed indicated they would rather quit their jobs than get vaccinated. Others promoted using ivermectin and hydroxychloroquine (both proven ineffective) as alternatives to vaccinations. Some protestors claimed that getting vaccinated would strip away their freedom. Similar protests occurred in New York, Salt Lake City, Minneapolis, Salem (Oregon), and countries including New Zealand, England, and Australia.

A journalistic account of a 2022 protest in a San Francisco suburb represents another example of an anti-mandate protest (Frenkel 2022). Protestors carried signs reading, "Defeat the Mandates," "No Vaccines," "Protect Our Kids," and "Our Kids, Our Choice." According to the report, parents opposed masks, school closures, and vaccines. The protestors used social media platforms like Facebook to organize what might evolve into a beginning social movement. The report noted several anti-vaccine and anti-mandate Facebook groups have materialized in some states, including New York, New Jersey, and Connecticut. A central concern of the protest groups was school closures, which they viewed as traumatic for children. In addition, some interviewed indicated that pandemic issues had moved to the front of their political thinking and would drive their voting patterns.

One of the most publicized protests occurred on the U.S.-Canadian border. The "Freedom Convoy" protests surfaced in Canadian border towns, including Toronto and Ottawa, in February 2022. Protesters blocked traffic at the Ambassador Bridge that connects Windsor, Ontario, to Detroit, shutting down one of the busiest international border crossings. The protestors parked trucks on major bridges to block traffic. The protests focused on proof of vaccination mandates required to cross the Canadian and U.S. border. The protests rapidly expanded beyond vaccination mandates to include other public health measures. One protestor reflected the group's thoughts, "We just want to go back to normal without having to take into our veins the poison which they call vaccines" (Paperny and Gable 2022:n.p.). The leadership of the protestors threatened to overthrow the current government unless restrictions were lifted. Some protestors waved Confederate or Nazi flags, and some said they wanted to dissolve Canada's government. These blockades and protests successfully halted trade between the two countries at the border crossings.

In contrast, other Canadians were frustrated with the protests and tired of the incessant honking, property damage, and being harassed for wearing masks. They criticized the police for not doing more to stop the blockade. Eventually, law enforcement was able to break up the protests. Ironically, the Canadian and U.S. governments were already moving toward reducing mandates independent of the demonstrations.

A similar type of protest occurred in the United States. A U.S. Department of Homeland Security document, marked for official use only, noted that as of its release on February 8, 2022, a U.S. trucker convoy "appears to be purely aspirational because the event is only being discussed online," although it warned that "this could change quickly." It did change quickly. A loosely planned protest by a group of far-right-wing truckers drove across the country to protest COVID-19 mandates. A trucker convoy drove around Washington, DC, for a few days. "Make America Great Again" banners and signs marked some trucks. Some of the supporters and participants of the protest were involved in the January 6, 2021, assault on the U.S. Capitol Building. The threat was to shut down the national capital, but that never materialized.

Right-wing groups supported the U.S. trucker convoy. This alliance should not come as a surprise, as true believers can shift from one cause to another with little difficulty. There is merit in Hoffer's (Hoffer 1951:17) propositions that "since all mass movements draw their adherents from the same types of humanity and appeal to the same types of mind, it follows: (a) all mass movements are competitive, and the gain of one in adherents is the loss of all the others; (b) all mass movements are interchangeable. One mass movement rally transforms into another."

Another COVID-19 protest was described in a *Time* magazine report that interviewed vaccine mandate protestors at a "Defeat the Mandates" rally in North Carolina (Bergengruen 2022). According to those at the rally, the government had overreached its authority by mandating vaccines. Bergengruen (2022:n.p.) described the thoughts and feelings of the protesters:

> The spectacle was part Trump rally, part conspiracy convention, part protest. Groups of teachers and nurses mingled with firefighters and church groups. The yellow Gadsden flags adopted by the Tea Party a decade ago mixed with Trump 2020 placards, "Stop the Steal" signs, and "F—Joe Biden" flags. A group of men wearing the insignia of the far-right Proud Boys lingered on the crowd's edges, near a group of women wearing flower crowns and flashing peace signs as they took selfies with a "Mama Bears Against Mandates" board.

At the protest, comparisons between the U.S. vaccination policies and Nazi Germany and the Soviet Union (no longer a country) were made. Signs declaring "Best practices in health care = Natural Immunity" and "Doctors against mandates" were present. Social media podcasts and right-wing political groups promoted the event.

Finally, public celebrities, such as tennis star Novak Djokovic and football quarterback Aaron Rodgers, have resisted mandates and drawn attention to the anti-vaccination movement. In the case of Djokovic, his stance was tested in the Australian civil courts. Firmly committed to his opposition, he voluntarily withdrew or was prohibited from playing in some tennis tournaments, such as the 2022 US Open. Other celebrities have spoken out against COVID-19 vaccinations, including Jenny McCarthy, Jim Carrey, Bill Maher, and Eric Clapton.

COVID-19 SOCIAL MOVEMENTS

Social unrest, insecurity, frustration, the sudden changes that COVID-19 introduced to the world, and other factors made conditions ripe for pre-existing and new social movements to gain traction. The pre-existing anti-vaccination movement was re-energized with the pandemic and became more active nationally. In addition, some public health resistance organizations re-energized and formed new alliances. Gorski (2020b) observed that anti-vaxxers, anti-maskers, COVID-19 pandemic minimizers, deniers, and others opposed to public health mandates joined together to resist any public health requirements. Other social movements and organizations jumped on the pandemic bandwagon furthering their causes, such as QAnon conspiracy theorists, eliminationists, and other anti-government groups. Consequently, as previously described, a mix of groups with differing agendas was often present at mandate protests.

All active mass movements, such as the anti-vaxxers, claim that the ultimate and absolute truth is already embodied in their doctrine, and there is no truth outside it. Eric Hoffer's concept of the true believer has value in making sense of what is occurring with these protests for some, but not all, participants. According to Hoffer, the facts on which true believers base their conclusions must not be derived from experience or observation but from doctrine (Hoffer 1951:79). Absurd ideas, trivial nonsense, and sublime truths are equally potent and readying people for self-sacrifice if accepted as the truth (Hoffer 1951:80). To be effective, a doctrine must not be understood but only has to be believed in. True believers can be sure only about things they do not understand. The true believer can deny and not be open to facts. Hoffer (1951:80) wrote, "He [or she] cannot be frightened by danger or disheartened by obstacles nor baffled by contradictions because he denies their existence." Hoffer continued, "Its truth, applicability, and complexity should not judge the effectiveness of a doctrine but how thoroughly it insulates the individual from his [or her] self in the world as it is." These observations seem remarkably appropriate for some protestors who have resisted what medical research has found or what is best for public health. It should be noted that there are true believers on the other side of these issues who also mindlessly adhere to their COVID-19 doctrines.

Of particular interest is what some scholars have labeled the eliminationist movement. Eliminationist rhetoric and views are typical in some Americans' thoughts. According to Miller (2014:103), "Eliminationist rhetoric is hate rhetoric, and some rumors are stated through the use of eliminationist rhetoric." Miller further wrote, "Hateful rants and rumors about liberals, gays, Muslims, Teabaggers, Occupy Wall Street, Democrats and Republicans alike, the government, unions, and illegal immigrants abound." He added, "Eliminationist rhetoric portrays groups as evil and dangerous and implicitly or explicitly advocates the elimination of these groups by violent or civil means."

With COVID-19, eliminationist rhetoric targeted people of Asian ancestry, whether they were Americans or not. The former president's comments about "Kung Flu" and accusing China of being the source of the pandemic moved some predisposed individuals to attack Americans of Asian ancestry. These Americans became scapegoats, a typical pattern for understanding and responding to mass contagions. The eliminationist movement also targeted public health officials and the government in general. Hence, it is not surprising that some COVID-19 protestors called for the overthrow of the government.

Similar eliminationist patterns have surfaced in other countries. For example, in Germany, the Querdenker movement has protested COVID-19 restrictions (Denny 2022). In German, Querdenker means someone who thinks outside of the box. Initially, the movement was formed to oppose pandemic mandates, but it has evolved into a radicalized movement that seeks to demonize German media and government. It began as small local protests, which eventually were taken over by right-wing extremists with broader political objectives. The movement shares with American conspiracy theorists ideas, such as the coronavirus is relatively harmless—no worse than the common flu. It characterizes German efforts to control COVID-19 as a hygiene dictatorship. The groups have become increasingly violent over the past two years towards COVID-19 restrictions. Even as those restrictions have been reduced, it has moved toward a far-right agenda. In doing so, some have seen it as threatening German democracy.

Social movements are embodied in ideologies that offer simplified perspectives in which people can make sense of complex events, such as the COVID-19 pandemic. Social movements find certainty and structure in otherwise ambiguous situations. Ideologies often drive social movements. Ideologies are normative worldviews that provide a simplified frame of reference for understanding events and people. Ideologies differ from scientific theories in that they are based on unfounded assumptions and use paranoid rather than scientific logic. Participants in social movements believe what they are doing is best for society. Ideologies may conspire against the general good for their interest. For example, some militant groups adhere to the ideology that the existing government is the villain. Some militant groups view their purpose as to restore, protect, modify, or create norms in the name of generalized beliefs. These generalized beliefs blame specific groups and their policies for unacceptable social conditions that need change. Social conditions, such as COVID-19 mandates and restrictions, are viewed as unacceptable. Specifically, militant (patriot) groups blame the Bureau of Alcohol, Tobacco, Firearms and Explosives (ATF), Central Intelligence Agency (CIA), or Federal Bureau of Investigation (FBI) for their loss of liberty. In the case of COVID-19, they blame the federal government, CDC, Food and Drug Administration (FDA), and public health departments for taking away their freedom.

COVID-19 FATIGUE AND APATHY

Initially, COVID-19 restrictions were adhered to, and Americans had a sense of unity. However, as Vandenberghe and Verán (2021:181) observed, a few weeks into lockdowns and restrictions, this unity began to "fracture." Some people started to question the value of these restrictions and requirements that were seen as unnecessary. Others became tired of lockdowns, face masks, and restrictions. COVID-19 fatigue and apathy are real, as people have grown weary of mandates such as wearing masks and lockdowns (Sheikh and Seo 2022). Evidence of COVID-19 fatigue and apathy can be found in a March 2022 Associated Press poll that found 44 percent of survey respondents said they often or always wear a face mask around people outside of their homes, a decrease from 65 percent who said they did in January (Bynum and Swanson 2022). Forty percent said they avoided nonessential travel, compared with 60 percent in January 2022. Forty-seven percent said they regularly stayed away from large groups, down from 65 percent in January. The waning of COVID-19 infections is also a reason for less concern and compliance with mandates, restrictions, and recommendations.

Public opinion regarding COVID-19 mandates has shifted throughout the pandemic from acceptance and compliance for some measures to less tolerance. A Monmouth University survey of 809 adults taken in March of 2022 indicated a shift in support for some COVID-19 preventative measures (Monmouth University 2022). Public support for face mask wearing and social distancing dropped from about half to one-third of the respondents. COVID-19 fatigue developed as some people have become tired of living restricted lives. The survey found that 77 percent of Americans favored relaxing face mask and social distancing recommendations in areas with low COVID-19 infection rates. However, support for showing vaccination cards had remained steady (about 43–44%). Some respondents (50%) indicated they preferred flexible guidelines depending on changes in COVID-19, others wanted stable protocols (14%), and some wanted to do away with all COVID-19 regulations (34%). Most respondents (73%) believed that COVID-19 was here to stay (endemic). Support for booster vaccines declined as more respondents were less likely to get a booster shot (33%). These attitudes toward newly required mask-wearing, social distancing, lockdowns, and vaccines will pose formidable challenges to public health and government agencies if a new and dangerous version of COVID-19 arises.

Another dimension of COVID-19 fatigue is the decline of data collection efforts and information sources of public health agencies, governments, and research organizations. The increased reliance on home (self-administered) tests, which do not require public health reporting, has decreased the number of cases known to authorities. Data collection on COVID-19 cases, tests, and deaths has diminished in the United States and other countries. For example, Johns Hopkins University, a reliable source of COVID-19 data, shut down COVID-19 data collection efforts, although an estimated 900 to 1,000 people worldwide die from the virus daily. There has been a numbing to the daily death toll attributed to COVID-19. In addition, local and national news outlets have not continued reporting on the coronavirus, as was once the case.

CONCLUDING OBSERVATIONS

Resistance to government and public health authority is not new to American society. Negative responses to pandemic requirements and mandates should come as no surprise. Much controversy and resistance have focused on vaccinations, face masks, social distancing, and lockdowns. Most Americans have been vaccinated, but some have been hesitant or refused. Major reasons for resistance include vaccine safety, medical pre-conditions, belief in myths and conspiracies, and political partisanship. To address these concerns, concerted efforts have been made to promote vaccinations. Pro-vaccine groups, public health agencies, and the government have implemented marketing and public health initiatives to encourage vaccinations. The government has been able to mandate some COVID-19 vaccine requirements but has faced resistance and legal challenges when it has overstepped its authority. National surveys have found general support for and compliance with COVID-19 vaccinations. However, a group of Americans remains highly resistant to vaccinations.

While science guides what the public should do to respond to COVID-19 and the pandemic, there is a human side to medical interventions that can be overlooked. Human beliefs, values, culture, and behaviors must also be considered. Science may offer a straightforward course of action that may only sometimes be taken because human factors have yet to be considered (for discussion, see Larson 2020; Ofri 2021). For example, international public health workers have been killed for vaccinating impoverished children against polio based on repressive religious beliefs despite the proven effectiveness of polio vaccines. Ultimately, the human dimension needs to be considered in addition to what science indicates.

Inconsistent implementation of mandates, lockdowns, vaccinations, social distancing, and mask-wearing practices have led to the spread of COVID-19 (Siegel 2020:168). In addition, the government's timing of these preventative measures was too late, as COVID-19 was already the "cat out of the bag." These public health initiatives have proven inconvenient, involved individual sacrifice, have affected social relationships, and have not been easy to live with. Mask-wearing has affected social relationships and communications in meaningful and lasting ways.

COVID-19 policies have had positive consequences in controlling the spread of the virus but also negative economic, religious, social, business, family, financial, and employment consequences (see chapter 2 and Offe 2021). Lockdowns have had a powerful impact on schools, businesses, work, and families. Likewise, without such public health interventions, COVID-19 would have taken more lives and made many more people seriously ill at a significant cost. Researchers are only now discovering what the long-term consequences are of COVID-19 infections. At this juncture, it is evident that long COVID will have major lasting impacts on some Americans and the healthcare system.

Americans have taken sides, pros and cons, on implementing these public health measures. Protests for and against these and other COVID-19 public health requirements have surfaced nationwide. Some of these led to social movements and the melding of political and COVID-19 protest movements. However, regardless of the positions taken, all would agree that American society has forever changed. It is also apparent that COVID-19 is now endemic and likely to be present from this point forward. With COVID-19 fatigue widespread, the challenges of having Americans comply with new mandates, restrictions, and recommendations will be immense when the following pandemic surfaces. In addition, the risks of the next pandemic being highly politicized are great. If it is politicized, the harm to American society in terms of loss of life could be enormous.

Finally, as was the case with COVID-19, responses to pandemics must be approached globally and avoid nationalistic and isolationist political impulses. The world is so interconnected that epidemics and outbreaks of new diseases will put everyone at risk, regardless of where they live. The belief that nations can isolate themselves from external pandemics is not realistic. If history provides any lessons, these diseases will most likely first occur in regions that are least capable of responding. However, medical and scientific responses to new diseases will likely emerge from more developed countries. As world citizens, people must begin to view diseases as a human rather than a national or political problem. Information, policies, data, and responses must be shared across borders to address effectively what some predict will be an increase in new human diseases.

References

Aassve, A., Cavalli, N., Mencarini, L., Plach, S., and M. Livi Bacci. 2020. The COVID-19 pandemic and human fertility. *Science* 369 (6502):370–371. https://www.science.org/doi/10.1126/science.abc9520?url_ver=Z39.88-2003&rfr_id=ori:rid:crossref.org&rfr_dat=cr_pub%20%200pubmed.

Ahmad, F. and R. Anderson. 2021. The leading causes of death in the US for 2020. *JAMA* 325 (18):1829–1830. https://jamanetwork.com/journals/jama/fullarticle/2778234.

Ahmad, F.B., Cisewski, J.A., Xu, J., and R.N. Anderson. 2023. Provisional mortality data—United States, 2022. *Morbidity and Mortality Weekly Report* 72 (18):488–492. https://www.cdc.gov/mmwr/volumes/72/wr/mm7218a3.htm#:~:text=During%202022%2C%20the%20three%20leading,218%2C064)%20(Figure%202).

Allport, G. and L. Postman. 1947/1965. *The psychology of rumor*. New York: Henry Holt.

Altman, D. 2021. Persistent vaccine myths. Kaiser Family Foundation. https://www.kff.org/coronavirus-covid-19/perspective/persistent-vaccine-myths/.

Anderson, M., Faverio, M., and C. McClain. 2022. How teens navigate school during COVID-19. Pew Research Center. https://www.pewresearch.org/internet/2022/06/02/how-teens-navigate-school-during-covid-19/?utm_source=Pew+Research+Center&utm_campaign=ad2458f7fe-EMAIL_CAMPAIGN_2022_06_03_02_53&utm_medium=email&utm_term=0_3e953b9b70-ad2458f7fe-400075373.

Angeny, G. L. n.d. *Precautions against influenza*. United States Navy.

Annenberg Public Policy Center. 2020. How misinformed vaccine beliefs affect policy views. https://www.annenbergpublicpolicycenter.org/how-misinformed-vaccine-beliefs-affect-policy-views/.

Annenberg Public Policy Center. 2021a. Millions embrace Covid-19 misinformation, which is linked to hesitancy on vaccination and boosters. https://www.annenbergpublicpolicycenter.org/millions-embrace-covid-19-misinformation-which-is-linked-to-hesitancy-on-vaccination-and-boosters/.

Annenberg Public Policy Center. 2021b. Misplaced trust: When trust in science fosters pseudoscience. https://www.annenbergpublicpolicycenter.org/misplaced-trust-when-trust-in-science-fosters-pseudoscience/.

Annenberg Public Policy Center. 2021c. Heavy users of conservative media more willing to take Ivermectin for Covid-19. https://www.annenbergpublicpolicycenter.org/heavy-users-of-conservative-media-more-willing-to-take-ivermectin-for-covid-19/.

Annenberg Public Policy Center. 2022. Confidence declines in CDC and Dr. Anthony Fauci. https://www.annenbergpublicpolicycenter.org/confidence-declines-in-cdc-and-dr-anthony-fauci/.

Arias, E., Tejada-Vera, B., Ahmad, F., and K.D. Kochanek. 2021. Provisional life expectancy estimates for 2020. Report No. 015, U.S. Department of Health and Human Services Centers for Disease Control and Prevention, National Center for Health Statistics. National Vital Statistics System. https://www.cdc.gov/nchs/data/vsrr/vsrr015-508.pdf.

Arnold-Foster, A. 2021. Vaccine rollout: History shows us that it's always a bit shambolic. https://theconversation.com/vaccine-rollout-history-shows-us-that-its-always-a-bit-shambolic-153120.

Arora, T., Grey, I., Östlundh, L., Lam, K.B.H., Omar, O.M., and D. Arone. 2020. The prevalence of psychological consequences of COVID-19: A systematic review and meta-analysis of observational studies. *Journal of Health Psychology* 27 (4):805–824. https://journals.sagepub.com/doi/pdf/10.1177/1359105320966639.

Ash, E., Galletta, S., Hangartner, D., Margalit, Y., and M. Pinna. 2020. The effect of Fox News on health behavior during COVID-19. *SSRN*. https://papers.ssrn.com/sol3/papers.cfm?abstract_id=3636762.

Attwell, K. 2020. Coronavirus anti-vaxxers aren't a huge threat yet: How do we keep it that way? https://theconversation.com/coronavirus-anti-vaxxers-arent-a-huge-threat-yet-how-do-we-keep-it-that-way-138531.

Attwell, K., Leask, J., Meyer, S.B., Rokkas, P., and P. Ward. 2017. Vaccine rejecting parents' engagement with expert systems that inform vaccination programs. *Journal of Bioethical Inquiry* 14:65–76.

Bach, K. 2022a. Is "long Covid" worsening the labor shortage? Brookings Institution. https://www.brookings.edu/research/is-long-covid-worsening-the-labor-shortage/.

Bach, K. 2022b. New data shows long Covid is keeping as many as 4 million people out of work. Brookings Institution. https://www.brookings.edu/research/new-data-shows-long-covid-is-keeping-as-many-as-4-million-people-out-of-work/?utm_campaign=brookings-comm&utm_medium=email&utm_content=224094088&utm_source=hs_email.

Baddeley, M. 2020. Hoarding in the age of COVID-19. *Journal of Behavioral Economics for Policy* 4:69–75. https://opus.lib.uts.edu.au/bitstream/10453/147087/2/JBEP-4-S-9.pdf.

Bagus, P., Peña-Ramos, J.A., and A. Sánchez-Bayón. 2021. COVID-19 and the political economy of mass hysteria. *International Journal of Environmental Research and Public Health* 18 (4):1376. https://www.ncbi.nlm.nih.gov/pmc/articles/PMC7913136/.

Barbosa, C., Dowd, W., Barnosky, A., and K. Karriker-Jaffe. 2021. *Assessing pandemic-driven changes in alcohol consumption.* Bethesda, MD: National Institute on Alcohol Abuse and Alcoholism.

Barr, A. and A.G. Shiro. 2022. The pandemic showed why social and structural determinants of health matter: Now it's time for policymakers to act. Brookings Institution. https://www.brookings.edu/blog/how-we-rise/2022/02/18/the-pandemic-showed-why-social-and-structural-determinants-of-health-matter-now-its-time-for-policymakers-to-act/.

Bateman, C. 2007. Paying the price for AIDS denialism. *South American Medical Journal* 97 (10):913–914. http://www.samj.org.za/index.php/samj/article/viewFile/606/131.

Bauer, L., Edelberg, W., Estep, S., and B. Hershbein. 2023. Who's missing from the post-pandemic labor force? Brookings Institution. https://www.brookings.edu/2023/04/04/whos-missing-from-the-post-pandemic-labor-force/?utm_campaign=Economic%20Studies&utm_medium=email&utm_content=253842535&utm_source=hs_email.

Benjamin, J.C., Ali, S.T., Ng, T.W.Y., Tsang, T.K., Li, J.C.M., Fong, M.W., Liao, Q., Kwan, M.Y., Lee, S.L., Chiu, S.S., Wu, J.T., Wu, P., and G.M. Leung. 2020. Impact assessment of non-pharmaceutical interventions against coronavirus disease 2019 and influenza in Hong Kong: An observational study. *The Lancet Public Health*. https://doi.org/10.1016/S2468-2667(20)30090-6.

Bergengruen, V. 2022. How the anti-vax movement is taking over the right. *Time*. January 26, 2022. https://time.com/6141699/anti-vaccine-mandate-movement-rally/.

Best, L.E. 2021. Understanding the pandemic's impact on Black Americans' health from a life course perspective. *Footnotes* 49 (2):10–11. https://www.asanet.org/sites/default/files/attach/footnotes/footnotes_spring-2021.pdf.

Biden, J. 2021. Remarks by President Biden on the COVID-19 response and vaccination program. https://www.whitehouse.gov/briefing-room/speeches-remarks/2021/06/02/remarks-by-president-biden-on-the-covid-19-response-and-vaccination-program/.

Blitzer, R. 2021. Pompeo: COVID-19 leaked from Wuhan lab. Fox News. June 14, 2021. https://www.foxnews.com/politics/pompeo-covid-leaked-wuhan-lab.

Blumer, H. 1975. Outline of collective behavior. In *Readings in collective behavior*, 2nd edition, ed. R.R. Evans, 22–45. Chicago: Rand McNally.

Blundell, R., Dias, M.C., Joyce, R., and X. Xu. 2020. Covid-19 and inequalities. *Fiscal Studies: The Journal of Applied Public Economics* 41 (2):291–319. https://onlinelibrary.wiley.com/doi/full/10.1111/1475-5890.12232.

BMJ. 2020. Further evidence does not support Hydroxychloroquine for patients with covid-19: Adverse events were more common in those receiving the drug. *BMJ*. https://www.bmj.com/company/newsroom/further-evidence-does-not-support-hydroxychloroquine-for-patients-with-covid-19/.

Borenstein, S. and H. Fingerhut. 2022. Poll: Americans' trust in science now deeply polarized. *The Associated Press*. January 27, 2022.

Boss, L. 1997. Epidemic hysteria: A review of the published literature. *Epidemiologic Reviews* 19 (2):233–243.

Brafman, O., and R. Brafman. 2008. *Sway: The irresistible pull of irrational behavior*. New York: Broadway Books.

Brennen, J.S., Simon, F., Howard, P.N., and R.K. Nielsen. 2020. Types, sources, and claims of COVID-19 misinformation. The Reuters Institute for the Study of Journalism. https://reutersinstitute.politics.ox.ac.uk/types-sources-and-claims-covid-19-misinformation.

Brink, S. 2021. Can't help falling in love with a vaccine: How polio campaign beat vaccine hesitancy. National Public Radio (NPR). May 3, 2021. https://www.npr.org/sections/health-shots/2021/05/03/988756973/cant-help-falling-in-love-with-a-vaccine-how-polio-campaign-beat-vaccine-hesitant.

Brooks, D. 2020. The first invasion of America: And the cultural earthquake it's unleashing. *The New York Times.* May 21, 2020. https://www.nytimes.com/2020/05/21/opinion/us-coronavirus-history.html.

Buckner, H.T. 1975. A theory of rumor transmission. In *Readings in collective behavior,* 2nd edition, ed. R.R. Evans, 86–102. Chicago, IL: Rand McNally.

Bullock, J. and A. Korinek. 2022. @elonmusk and @twitter: The problem with social media is misaligned recommendation systems, not free speech. Brookings Institution. https://www.brookings.edu/research/elonmusk-and-twitter-the-problem-with-social-media-is-misaligned-recommendation-systems-not-free-speech/?utm_campaign=Brookings%20Brief&utm_medium=email&utm_content=213598880&utm_source=hs_email.

Burrowes, R.J. 2022. The elite's COVID-19 coup: Fighting for our humanity, our liberty and our future. *Nation of Change.* https://www.nationofchange.org/2020/05/29/the-elites-covid-19-coup-fighting-for-our-humanity-our-liberty-and-our-future/.

Busette, C. 2022. Covid-19 takes its toll on American life. Brookings Institution. https://www.brookings.edu/blog/how-we-rise/2022/03/30/covid-19-takes-its-toll-on-american-life/?utm_campaign=brookings-comm&utm_medium=email&utm_content=208755605&utm_source=hs_email.

Butler, K. 2022. Hunting the plague. *American Experience*. https://www.pbs.org/wgbh/americanexperience/features/plague-golden-gate-hunting-plague/.

Bynum, R. and E. Swanson. 2022. Americans ease up on masks, virus safeguards: AP-NORC poll. Associated Press. March 29, 2022. https://abcnews.go.com/Health/wireStory/americans-ease-masks-virus-safeguards-ap-norc-poll-83743697.

Calvillo, D.P., Ross, B.J., Garcia, R.J.B., Smelter, T.J., and A.M. Rutchick. 2020. Political ideology predicts perceptions of the threat of COVID-19 (and susceptibility to fake news about it). *Social Psychological and Personality Science* 11 (8):1119–1128. https://journals.sagepub.com/doi/pdf/10.1177/1948550620940539.

Campos-Mercade, P., Meler, A.N., Schneider, F.H., Meier, S., Pope, D., and E. Wengström. 2021. Monetary incentives increase COVID-19 vaccinations. *Science* 374 (6569): 879–882.

Camus, A. 1991. *The plague,* trans. S. Gilbert. New York: Vintage Books.

Cantril, H. 1940. *The invasion from mars: A study in the psychology of panic.* Princeton, NJ: Princeton University Press.

Carroll, S.B. 2020. The denialist playbook: On vaccines, evolution, and more, rejection of science has followed a familiar pattern. *Scientific American.* https://www.scientificamerican.com/article/the-denialist-playbook/.

Cartwright, M. 2020. Black death. *World history encyclopedia.* https://www.worldhistory.org/Black_Death/.

Cave, D. 2022. Why Australia's death rate is one-tenth of the U.S. level. *The New York Times.* May 15, 2022. https://www.nytimes.com/2022/05/15/world/australia/covid-deaths.html.

Centers for Disease Control and Prevention. 2018a. 1918 pandemic influenza historic timeline. https://www.cdc.gov/flu/pandemic-resources/1918-commemoration/pandemic-timeline-1918.htm.

Centers for Disease Control and Prevention. 2018b. The 1918 Flu Pandemic: Why It Matters 100 Years Later. *Public Health Matters Blog.* https://blogs.cdc.gov/publichealthmatters/2018/05/1918-flu/.

Centers for Disease Control and Prevention. 2021a. COVID-19 pandemic planning scenarios. https://www.cdc.gov/coronavirus/2019-ncov/hcp/planning-scenarios.html.

Centers for Disease Control and Prevention. 2021b. Myths and facts about COVID-19 vaccines. https://www.cdc.gov/coronavirus/2019-ncov/vaccines/facts.html?s_cid=10495:covid%20vaccine%20facts:sem.ga:p:RG:GM:gen:PTN:FY21.

Centers for Disease Control and Prevention. 2021c. History of smallpox. https://www.cdc.gov/smallpox/history/history.html.

Centers for Disease Control and Prevention. 2022a. CDC Museum COVID-19 timeline. https://www.cdc.gov/museum/timeline/covid19.html.

Centers for Disease Control and Prevention. 2022b. New CDC data illuminate youth mental health threats during the COVID-19 pandemic. https://www.cdc.gov/media/releases/2022/p0331-youth-mental-health-covid-19.html.

Centers for Disease Control and Prevention. 2022c. Disease burden of flu. https://www.cdc.gov/flu/about/burden/index.html.

Centers for Disease Control and Prevention. 2022d. Daily updates of totals by week and state: Provisional death counts for coronavirus disease 2019 (COVID-19). https://www.cdc.gov/nchs/nvss/vsrr/covid19/index.htm.

Centers for Disease Control and Prevention. 2023a. End of the federal COVID-19 public health emergency (PHE) declaration. https://www.cdc.gov/coronavirus/2019-ncov/your-health/end-of-phe.html#:~:text=The%20federal%20COVID%2D19%20PHE,share%20certain%20data%20will%20change.

Centers for Disease Control and Prevention. 2023b. Living with long COVID can be hard, especially when there are no immediate answers of solutions. Long COVID or Post-COVID Conditions. Washington, DC: Centers for Disease Control and Prevention. https://www.cdc.gov/coronavirus/2019-ncov/long-term-effects/index.html.

Cheng, M. 2022. Polio in US, UK and Israel reveals rare risk of oral vaccine. *The Washington Post.* August 21, 2022. https://www.ny1.com/nyc/all-boroughs/news/2022/08/21/polio-in-us--uk-and-israel-reveals-rare-risk-of-oral-vaccine.

Cherlin, A.J. 2021. The family and COVID-19: What can we say so far? *Sociology in the News.* September 2020. https://www.mheducation.com/highered/ideas/sociology-in-the-news/the-family-and-covid-19-what-can-we-say-so-far.

Chomsky, N. and M. Waterstone. 2021. *Consequences of capitalism: Manufacturing discontent and resistance.* Chicago, IL: Haymarket Books.

Cohn, S.K. 2012. Pandemics: Waves of disease, waves of hate from the plague of Athens to A.I.D.S. *History Journal* 85 (230):535–555. https://www.ncbi.nlm.nih.gov/pmc/articles/PMC4422154/.

Collins, B. and K. Collier. 2022. Russian propaganda on Ukraine's non-existent "bio-labs" boosted by U.S. far right. NBC News. March 14, 2022. https://www.nbcnews.com/tech/internet/qanon-ukraine-biolabs-russian-propaganda-efforts-boosted-us-far-right-rcna19392.

Colloca, L. 2017. Nocebo effects can make you feel pain. *Science* 358 (6359):44. https://www.ncbi.nlm.nih.gov/pmc/articles/PMC5754642/pdf/nihms924496.pdf.

Conis, E. 2015. Vaccination resistance in historical perspective. *The American Historian.* https://www.oah.org/tah/issues/2015/august/vaccination-resistance/.

Connell, R. 2020. COVID-19/sociology. *Journal of Sociology* 56 (14):675–683. https://journals.sagepub.com/doi/full/10.1177/1440783320943262.

Coulter, H.L. and B.L. Fisher. 1985. *DPT: A shot in the dark.* New York: Warner Books.

Covey, H.C. 2007. *African American slave medicine: Herbal and non-herbal treatments.* Lanham, MA: Lexington Books.

Cutler, D.M. and L.H. Summers. 2020. The COVID-19 pandemic and the $16 trillion virus. *JAMA Network* 324 (15):1495–1496. https://jamanetwork.com/journals/jama/fullarticle/2771764.

Czeisler, M.E., Lane, R.I., Petrosky, E., Wiley, J.F., Christensen, A., Njai, R., Weaver, M.D., Robbins, R., Facer-Childs, E.R., Barger, L.K., Czeisier, C.A., Howard, M.E., and S.M.W. Rajaratnam. 2020. Mental health, substance use, and suicidal ideation during the COVID-19 pandemic—United States, June 24–30, 2020. *MMWR Morbidity and Mortality Weekly Report* 69:1049–1057. https://www.ncbi.nlm.nih.gov/pmc/articles/PMC7440121/.

Deane, C., Parker, K., and J. Gramlich. 2021. A year of U.S. public opinion on the coronavirus pandemic. Pew Research Center. https://www.pewresearch.org/2021/03/05/a-year-of-u-s-public-opinion-on-the-coronavirus-pandemic/.

Defoe, D. 1722/1978. *A journal of the plague year.* Norwalk, CT: Easton Press.

Delanty, G. (Ed.) 2021a. *Pandemics, politics, and society: Critical perspectives on the Covid-19 crisis.* Berlin, Germany: De Gruyter.

Delanty, G. 2021b. Introduction: The pandemic in historical and global context. In *Pandemics, politics, and society: Critical perspectives on the Covid-19 crisis,* ed. G. Delanty, 1–21, Berlin, Germany: De Gruyter.

Denny, S. 2022. Trouble is brewing in Germany. *Lawfare.* https://www.lawfareblog.com/trouble-brewing-germany?utm_campaign=Brookings%20Brief&utm_medium=email&utm_content=209847252&utm_source=hs_email.

Diamond, J. 2005. *Collapse: How societies choose or fail to survive.* New York: Penguin.

Diethelm, P. and M. McKee. 2009. Denialism: What is it and how should scientists respond? *European Journal of Public Health* 19 (1):2–4. https://academic.oup.com/eurpub/article/19/1/2/463780.

Dingwall, R., Hoffman, L.M., and K. Staniland. 2013. Introduction: Why a *sociology* of pandemics? *Sociology of Health & Illness* 35 (2):167–173.

Dobson, E., Graham, C., Hua, T., and S. Pinto. 2022. Despair and resilience in the US: Did the COVID pandemic worsen mental health outcomes? Brookings Global Working Paper #171. https://www.brookings.edu/wp-content/uploads/2022/03/Despair-and-Resilience.pdf.

Doggett, L. 2022. Timeline of Trump's coronavirus responses. https://doggett.house.gov/media/blog-post/timeline-trumps-coronavirus-responses.

Dolan, B. 2020. Unmasking history: Who was behind the anti-mask league protests during the 1918 influenza epidemic in San Francisco? *Perspectives in Medical Humanities.* May 19, 2020. https://escholarship.org/uc/item/5q91q53r.

Domachowske, J.B. and M. Suryadevara. 2013. Practical approaches to vaccine hesitancy issues in the United States: 2013. *Human Vaccines and Immunotherapeutics* 9 (12):2654–2657.

Enserink, M. and J. Cohen. 2020. Fact-checking Judy Mikovits, the controversial virologist attacking Anthony Fauci in a viral conspiracy video. *Science*. May 12, 2020. https://www.science.org/content/article/fact-checking-judy-mikovits-controversial-virologist-attacking-anthony-fauci-viral.

Evans, R.R. 1975. *Readings in collective behavior*, 2nd ed. Chicago, IL: Rand McNally.

Farley, R. 2021. Migrants not responsible for latest COVID-19 surge. FactCheck.org. October 8, 2021. https://www.factcheck.org/2021/10/scicheck-migrants-not-responsible-for-latest-covid-19-surge/.

Federal Communications Commission. 2021. COVID-19 text scams. https://www.fcc.gov/covid-19-text-scams.

Ferreira, C.M., José Sá, M., Martins, J.G., and S. Serpa. 2020. The COVID-19 contagion-pandemic dyad: A view from social sciences. *Societies*. 10 (4):77. https://www.mdpi.com/2075-4698/10/4/77.

Finkel, E.J., Ball, C.A., Cikara, M., Ditto, P.H., Iyengar, S., Klar, S., Mason, L., McGrath, M.C., Nyhan, B., Rand, D.G., Skitka, L.J., Tucker, J.A., Van Bavel, J.J., Wang, C.S., and J.N. Druckman. 2020. Political sectarianism in America: A poisonous cocktail of othering, aversion, and moralization poses a threat to democracy. *Science* 370 (6516):533–536.

Fischer, M. and E. Bubola. 2020. As coronavirus deepens inequality, inequality worsens its spread. *New York Times.* March 15, 2020. https://www.nytimes.com/2020/03/15/world/europe/coronavirus-inequality.html.

Fleming, A. 2020. Our face mask future: Do they really help beat flu, coronavirus and pollution? *The Guardian.* January 31, 2020. https://www.theguardian.com/world/2020/jan/31/our-face-mask-future-do-they-really-help-beat-flu-coronavirus-and-pollution.

Flores, A., Cole, J.C., Dickert, S., Eom, K., Jiga-Boy, G.M., Kogut, T., Loria, R., Mayorga, M., Pedersen, E.J., Pereira, B., Rubaltelli, E., Sherman, D.K., Slovic, P., Västfjäll, D., and L. Van Boven. 2022. Politicians polarize and experts depolarize public support for COVID-19 management policies across countries. *Proceedings of the National Academy of Sciences of the United States of America* 119 (3). January 18, 2022. https://doi.org/10.1073/pnas.2117543119.

Freeman, D., Waite, F., Rosebrock, L., Petit, A., Causier, C., East, A., Jenner, L., Teale, A.L., Carr, L., Mulhall, S., Bold, E., and S. Lambe. 2020. Coronavirus conspiracy beliefs, mistrust, and compliance with government guidelines in England. *Psychological Medicine* 52:251–263.

Frenkel, S. 2022. How some parents altered their politics in the pandemic. *The New York Times*. August 1, 2022. https://www.nytimes.com/2022/08/01/technology/anti-vax-parents-political-party.html.

Frey, W.H. 2022a. New census data shows a huge spike in movement out of big metro areas during the pandemic. Brookings Institution. https://www.brookings.edu/blog/the-avenue/2022/04/14/new-census-data-shows-a-huge-spike-in-movement-out-of-big-metro-areas-during-the-pandemic/?utm_campaign=brookings-comm&utm_medium=email&utm_content=210153679&utm_source=hs_email.

Frey, W.H. 2022b. Big cities saw historic population losses while suburban growth declined during the pandemic. Brookings Institution. https://www.brookings.edu/research/big-cities-saw-historic-population-losses-while-suburban-growth-declined-during-the-pandemic/?utm_campaign=brookings-comm&utm_medium=email&utm_content=220518669&utm_source=hs_email.

Frijters, P., Foster, G., and M. Baker. 2021. *The great Covid panic: What happened, why, and what to do next*. Austin, TX: Brownstone Institute.

Funk, C. and J. Gramlich. 2021. 10 facts about Americans and coronavirus vaccines. Pew Research Center. https://www.pewresearch.org/fact-tank/2021/09/20/10-facts-about-americans-and-coronavirus-vaccines/.

Funk, C., Tyson, A., Pasquini, G., and A. Spencer. 2022. Americans reflect on nation's COVID-19 response. Pew Research Center. https://www.pewresearch.org/science/2022/07/07/americans-reflect-on-nations-covid-19-response/?utm_source=Pew+Research+Center&utm_campaign=41cecefa0e-Weekly_2022_07_09&utm_medium=email&utm_term=0_3e953b9b70-41cecefa0e-400075373.

Goldenberg, M.J. 2021. *Vaccine hesitancy: Public trust, expertise, and the war on science*. Pittsburgh, PA: University of Pittsburgh Press.

Goldin, C. 2022. Understanding the economic impact of COVID-19 on women. The Brookings Institution. https://www.brookings.edu/bpea-articles/understanding-the-economic-impact-of-covid-19-on-women/?utm_campaign=Brookings%20Brief&utm_medium=email&utm_content=207798069&utm_source=hs_email.

Goode, E. and N. Ben-Yehuda. 2009. *Moral panics: The social construction of deviance,* 2nd ed. Chichester, UK: Wiley Blackwell. https://onlinelibrary.wiley.com/doi/book/10.1002/9781444307924.

Gordon, M.R. and W. P. Strobel. 2023. Lab leak most likely origin of Covid-19 pandemic, Energy Department now says. *The Wall Street Journal.* February 26, 2023. https://www.wsj.com/articles/covid-origin-china-lab-leak-807b7b0a.

Gorski, D. 2020a. There is no COVID-19 "casedemic": The pandemic is real and deadly. *Science-Based Medicine*. https://sciencebasedmedicine.org/no-covid-19-casedemic/.

Gorski, D. 2020b. Antivaccine leader Del Bigtree on COVID-19: "Let's catch this cold!" Why antivaxxers and coronavirus conspiracy theorists are often one in the same. *Science-Based Medicine*. https://sciencebasedmedicine.org/antivaccine-leader-del-bigtree-on-covid-19-lets-catch-this-cold-why-antivaxxers-and-coronavirus-conspiracy-theorists-are-often-one-in-the-same/.

Gramlich, J. and C. Funk. 2020. Black Americans face higher COVID-19 risks, are more hesitant to trust medical scientists, get vaccinated. Pew Research Center. https://www.pewresearch.org/fact-tank/2020/06/04/black-americans-face-higher-covid-19-risks-are-more-hesitant-to-trust-medical-scientists-get-vaccinated/.

Granovetter, M. 1978. Threshold models of collective behavior. *American Journal of Sociology* 83 (6):1420–1443.

Graso, M., Henwood, A., Aquino, K., Dolan, P., and F.X. Chen. 2022. The dark side of belief in Covid-19 scientists and scientific evidence. *Personality and Individual Differences* 193: 111594.

Griesher, K. 2022. Activists rise up to counter vaccine skeptics. *The Associated Press*. January 30, 2022.

Haelle, T. 2020. Why it's important to push back on "Plandemic"—And how to do it. *Forbes*. May 8, 2020. https://www.forbes.com/sites/tarahaelle/2020/05/08/why-its-important-to-push-back-on-plandemic-and-how-to-do-it/?sh=581736435fa3.

Hamel, L., Kirzinger, A., Muñana, C., and M. Brodie. 2020. KFF COVID-19 vaccine monitor: December 2020. Kaiser Family Foundation. https://www.kff.org/coronavirus-covid-19/report/kff-covid-19-vaccine-monitor-december-2020/.

Hamel, L., Lopes, L., Kirzinger, A., Sparks, G., Stokes, M., and M. Brodie. 2021. KFF COVID-19 vaccine monitor: Media and misinformation. Kaiser Family Foundation. https://www.kff.org/coronavirus-covid-19/poll-finding/kff-covid-19-vaccine-monitor-media-and-misinformation/.

Hammond, R.A. and M. Kasman. 2022. How the Omicron response can prepare us for the next wave. Brookings Institution. https://www.brookings.edu/blog/up-front/2022/05/25/how-the-omicron-response-can-prepare-us-for-the-next-wave/?utm_campaign=brookings-comm&utm_medium=email&utm_content=215333931&utm_source=hs_email.

Hanafi, S. 2020. Post-COVID-19 sociology. ISA Digital Platform. April 2020. https://www.isa-sociology.org/frontend/web/uploads/files/Post-COVID-19%20Sociology.pdf.

Hardy, A. 2021. Average costs for a COVID-19 hospital stay top $400,000 in some states: Study. *Money*. October 25, 2021. https://money.com/covid-19-hospital-cost-by-state/.

Harris, D.N. and F. Chen. 2022. How has the pandemic affected high school graduation and college entry? Brookings Institution. https://www.brookings.edu/blog/brown-center-chalkboard/2022/05/10/how-has-the-pandemic-affected-high-school-graduation-and-college-entry/?utm_campaign=brookings-comm&utm_medium=email&utm_content=213060894&utm_source=hs_email.

Hastie, C.E., Lowe, D.J., McAuley, A., Winter, A.J., Mills, N.L., Black, C., Scott, J.T., O'Donnell, C.A., Blane, D.N., Browne, S., Ibbotson, T.R., and J.P. Pell. 2022. Outcomes among confirmed cases and a matched comparison group in the long-COVID in Scotland study. *Nature Communications* 13:5663. https://www.nature.com/articles/s41467-022-33415-5.

Health Impact News. 2021. 2,809 dead babies in VAERS following COVID shots as new documents prove Pfizer, the FDA, and the CDC knew the shots were not safe for pregnant women. *Health Impact News.* December 4, 2021. https://archive.ph/E4o36#selection-795.0-795.148.

Herby, J., Jonung, L., and S.H. Hanke. 2022. A literature review and meta-analysis of the effects of lockdowns on COVID-19 mortality. *Studies in Applied Economics* 200:1–61. https://sites.krieger.jhu.edu/iae/files/2022/01/A-Literature-Review-and-Meta-Analysis-of-the-Effects-of-Lockdowns-on-COVID-19-Mortality.pdf.

Hillis, S.D., Blenkinsop, A., Villaveces, A., Annor, F.B., Liburd, L., et al. 2021. COVID-19-associated orphanhood and caregiver death in the United States. *Pediatrics*. October 7, 2021. https://pubmed.ncbi.nlm.nih.gov/34620728/.

Hiltzik, M. 2023. COVID deniers think a new study says mask mandates don't work. They should try reading it. *Los Angeles Times*. February 24, 2023. https://www.latimes.com/business/story/2023-02-24/covid-deniers-celebrate-a-study-that-claims-mask-mandates-dont-work-but-the-study-says-the-opposite.

Hochman, D. 2023. Three years in, how the pandemic has changed our lives (and how it hasn't). *AARP Bulletin* March: 8–10, 12.

Hoffer, E. 1951. *The true believer: Thoughts on the nature of mass movements*. New York: Harper Collins.

Homola, S. 1963. Chiropractors and poliomyelitis. Chirobase. https://quackwatch.org/chiropractic/rb/bcc/9-2/.

Honig, B. 2009. *Emergency politics: Paradox, law, democracy.* Princeton, NJ: Princeton University Press.

Hopkins, D.R. 2002. *The greatest killer: Smallpox in history.* Chicago: University of Chicago Press.

Hornsey, M., Finlayson, M., Chatwood, G., and C.T. Begeny. 2020. Donald Trump and vaccination: The effect of political identity, conspiracist ideation and presidential tweets on vaccine hesitancy. *Journal of Experimental Social Psychology* 88, May 2020. https://www.researchgate.net/publication/341080858_Donald_Trump_and_vaccination_The_effect_of_political_identity_conspiracist_ideation_and_presidential_tweets_on_vaccine_hesitancy.

Horowitz, J.M. 2020. Views on why Black Americans face higher COVID-19 hospitalization rates vary by party, race and ethnicity. Pew Research Center. https://www.pewresearch.org/fact-tank/2020/06/04/black-americans-face-higher-covid-19-risks-are-more-hesitant-to-trust-medical-scientists-get-vaccinated/.

Horowitz, J.M., Brown, A., and R. Minkin. 2021. A year into the pandemic, long-term financial impact weighs heavily on many Americans. Pew Research Center. https://www.pewresearch.org/social-trends/2021/03/05/a-year-into-the-pandemic-long-term-financial-impact-weighs-heavily-on-many-americans/.

Howard Community College. 2016. *Sociology: Understanding and changing the social worlds*. Minneapolis, MN: Pressbooks. https://pressbooks.howardcc.edu/soci101/chapter/21-1-types-of-collective-behavior/.

Howard, J. 2020. To help stop coronavirus, everyone should be wearing face masks. The science is clear. *The Guardian.* April 4, 2020. www.theguardian.com/commentisfree/2020/apr/04/why-wear-a-mask-may-be-our-best-weapon-to-stop-coronavirus.

Howick, J. and G. Ongaro. 2020. Coronavirus: Could reading about the pandemic cause harm? *The Conversation.* April 20, 2020. https://theconversation.com/coronavirus-could-reading-about-the-pandemic-cause-harm-135585.

Hurt, M. C. 2022. Distrust of public health's response to the COVID-19 pandemic. *American Journal of Nursing* 122 (6):53–56.

Infectious Diseases Society of America. 2022. Measles vaccination: Myths and facts. March 24, 2022. https://www.idsociety.org/public-health/measles/myths-and-facts/.

Innerarity, D. 2021. Political decision-making in a pandemic. In *Pandemics, politics, and society: Critical perspectives on the Covid-19 crisis,* ed. G. Delanty, 93–104. Berlin, Germany: De Gruyter.

International Labour Organization. 2020. Youth & COVID-19: Impacts on jobs, education, rights and mental well-being. https://www.ilo.org/global/topics/youth-employment/publications/WCMS_753026/lang--en/index.htm.

Isaacs, D. 2021. From smallpox to polio, vaccine rollouts have always had doubters. But they work in the end. https://theconversation.com/from-smallpox-to-polio-vaccine-rollouts-have-always-had-doubters-but-they-work-in-the-end-161803.

Jamieson, K.H. and D. Albarracin. 2020. The relation between media consumption and misinformation at the outset of the SARS-CoV-2 pandemic in the US. *The Harvard Kennedy School Misinformation Review*, Volume 1: Special Issue on COVID-19 and Misinformation. https://www.researchgate.net/publication/340720014_The_Relation_between_Media_Consumption_and_Misinformation_at_the_Outset_of_the_SARS-CoV-2_Pandemic_in_the_US.

Jaramillo, C. 2021a. No credible evidence COVID-19 mRNA vaccines "dramatically increase" heart attack risk, contrary to flawed abstract. FactCheck.org. December 16, 2021. https://www.factcheck.org/2021/12/no-credible-evidence-covid-19-mrna-vaccines-dramatically-increase-heart-attack-risk-contrary-to-flawed-abstract/.

Jaramillo, C. 2021b. No evidence vaccines impact fertility. FactCheck.org. August 16, 2021. https://www.factcheck.org/2021/02/scicheck-no-evidence-vaccines-impact-fertility/.

Jefferson, T. 1785. Letter to Peter Carr. August 19, 1785. https://tjrs.monticello.org/letter/2249.

Jefferson, T., Dooley, L., Ferroni, E., et al. 2023. Physical interventions to interrupt or reduce the spread of respiratory viruses. Cochrane Library. https://www.cochranelibrary.com/cdsr/doi/10.1002/14651858.CD006207.pub6/full.

Jingnan, H. 2020. Why there are so many different guidelines for face masks for the public. National Public Radio (NPR). April, 10, 2020. www.npr.org/sections/goatsandsoda/2020/04/10/829890635/whythere-so-many-different-guidelines-for-face-masks-for-the-public.

John, H. 2020. A world without vaccines: A history of smallpox. *BioLogos.* July 29, 2020. https://biologos.org/articles/a-world-without-vaccines-a-history-of-smallpox

?gclid=Cj0KCQiAosmPBhCPARIsAHOen-NSezDbYMGoFma9iJzaHX-SqVDvTo0GNau5HskgK7cnW6Ol9foGf68aAtEpEALw_wcB.

Jones, A. and R. Allen. 1794. *A narrative of the proceedings of the black people, during the late awful calamity in Philadelphia, in the year 1793.* Philadelphia, PA: William W. Woodward. https://www.loc.gov/resource/rbc0001.2019hazard13737/?sp=5&r=0.156%2C0.813%2C0.504%2C0.282%2C0&st=pdf&pdfPage=3.

Jones, B. 2022. The changing political geography of COVID-19 over the last two years. Pew Research Center. https://www.pewresearch.org/politics/2022/03/03/the-changing-political-geography-of-covid-19-over-the-last-two-years/?utm_source=Pew+Research+Center&utm_campaign=14487cd394-Weekly_2022_03_05&utm_medium=email&utm_term=0_3e953b9b70-14487cd394-400075373.

Joseph, T.D. 2021. How vaccine rollout reveals another failure of U.S. public health infrastructure and implications for marginalized populations. *Footnotes* 49 (2):8. https://www.asanet.org/sites/default/files/attach/footnotes/footnotes_spring-2021.pdf.

Joszt, L. 2022. Working paper finds COVID-19 lockdowns had little public health effect and draws criticism of being flawed. *Managed Care Executive*. https://www.managedhealthcareexecutive.com/view/working-paper-finds-covid-19-lockdowns-had-little-public-health-effect-and-draws-criticism-of-being-flawed.

Jurkowitz, M. and A. Mitchell. 2021. Americans who relied most on Trump for COVID-19 news among least likely to be vaccinated. Pew Research Center. https://www.pewresearch.org/fact-tank/2021/09/23/americans-who-relied-most-on-trump-for-covid-19-news-among-least-likely-to-be-vaccinated/.

Justia. 2022. Jacobson v. Massachusetts, 197 U.S. 11 (1905). *Justia: US Supreme Court*. https://supreme.justia.com/cases/federal/us/197/11/.

Kafer, K.L. 2022. Lockdowns—tremendous cost, few lives saved. *The Denver Post.* March 13, 2022: 20.

Kamarck, E. 2022. The mask mandate decision defies common sense. Brookings Institution. https://www.brookings.edu/blog/fixgov/2022/04/27/the-mask-mandate-decision-defies-common-sense/?utm_campaign=Governance%20Studies&utm_medium=email&utm_content=212043846&utm_source=hs_email.

Kang, D. and H. Wu. 2022. Crowd, angered by lockdowns, calls for leader Xi to step down. The Associated Press. November 27, 2022. https://apnews.com/article/taiwan-health-fires-social-media-50d7515e5fae00f5054062209e9306cc.

Kavanagh, J. and M.D. Rich. 2018. Truth decay: An initial exploration of the diminishing role of facts and analysis in American public life. Rand Corporation. https://www.rand.org/pubs/research_reports/RR2314.html.

Kennedy, B., Tyson, A. and C. Funk. 2022. Americans' trust in scientists, other groups declines: Republicans' confidence in medical scientists down sharply since early in the coronavirus outbreak. Pew Research Center. https://www.pewresearch.org/science/2022/02/15/americans-trust-in-scientists-other-groups-declines/.

Kennedy, R.F., Jr. 2021. *The real Anthony Fauci: Bill Gates, big pharma, and the global war on democracy and public health.* New York: Skyhorse Publishing.

Kiely, E., Robertson, L., Rieder, R., and D. Gore. 2020. Timeline of Trump's COVID-19 comments. The Annenberg Public Policy Center. https://www.factcheck.org/2020/10/timelines-of-trumps-covid-19-comments/.

Kiely, E. 2021. Misinformation about face masks. The Annenberg Public Policy Center. https://www.factcheck.org/2021/08/scicheck-misinformation-about-face-masks/.

Kiely, E., Farley, R., and D. Gore. 2021. The whoppers of 2021. The Annenberg Public Policy Center. https://www.factcheck.org/2021/12/the-whoppers-of-2021/.

Kirzinger, A., Kearney, A., Hamel, L., and M. Brodie. 2021. KFF COVID-19 vaccine monitor: The increasing importance of partisanship in predicting COVID-19 vaccination status. Kaiser Family Foundation. https://www.kff.org/coronavirus-covid-19/poll-finding/importance-of-partisanship-predicting-vaccination-status/.

Klapp, O. 1972. *Currents of unrest: An introduction to collective behavior*. New York: Holt, Rinehart and Winston.

Knight, V. and J. Appleby. 2020. How COVID death counts become the stuff of conspiracy theories. *Kaiser Health News*. https://khn.org/news/how-covid-death-counts-become-the-stuff-of-conspiracy-theories/.

Kochhar, R. and S. Sechopoulos. 2022. COVID-19 pandemic pinches finances of America's lower- and middle-income families. Pew Research Center. https://www.pewresearch.org/social-trends/2022/04/20/covid-19-pandemic-pinches-finances-of-americas-lower--and-middle-income-families/?utm_source=Pew+Research+Center&utm_campaign=917f4ab92f-SDT_2022_04_21&utm_medium=email&utm_term=0_3e953b9b70-917f4ab92f-400075373.

Kolbert, E. 2020. Pandemics and the shape of human history. *The New Yorker*. March 30, 2020. https://www.newyorker.com/magazine/2020/04/06/pandemics-and-the-shape-of-human-history.

Kramer, S. 2021. In historically Black Protestant churches, regular attenders more likely to have received COVID-19 shot. Pew Research Center. https://www.pewresearch.org/fact-tank/2021/10/15/in-historically-black-protestant-churches-regular-attenders-more-likely-to-have-received-covid-19-shot/.

Kuhfeld, M., Soland, J., Lewis, K., and E. Morton. 2022. The pandemic has had devastating impacts on learning. What will it take to help students catch up? Brookings Institution. https://www.brookings.edu/blog/brown-center-chalkboard/2022/03/03/the-pandemic-has-had-devastating-impacts-on-learning-what-will-it-take-to-help-students-catch-up/?utm_campaign=Brookings%20Brief&utm_medium=email&utm_content=205750379&utm_source=hs_email.

Kuhfeld, M., Soland, J., and K. Lewis. 2022. Test score patterns across three COVID-19- impacted school years. The Annenberg Public Policy Center. https://edworkingpapers.com/sites/default/files/ai22-521.pdf.

Lang, K. and G.E. Lang. 1961. *Collective dynamics*. New York: Thomas Y. Crowell.

Larson, H.J. 2020. *Stuck: How vaccine rumors start and why they don't go away*. New York: Oxford University Press.

Lazarsfeld, P.F. and R.K. Merton. 1954. Friendship as a social process: A substantive and methodological analysis. In *Freedom and control in modern society*, eds. M. Berger, T. Abel, and C.H. Page, 18–66. New York: D. Van Nostrand.

Leibovitz, T., Shamblaw, A.L., Rumas, R., and M.W. Best. 2021. COVID-19 conspiracy beliefs: Relations with anxiety, quality of life, and schemas. *Personality and Individual Differences* 175:110704. https://www.sciencedirect.com/science/article/pii/S0191886921000799.

Lempert, R. 2022. The vaccine mandate cases, polarization, and jurisprudential norms. Brookings Institution. https://www.brookings.edu/blog/fixgov/2022/01/15/the-vaccine-mandate-cases-polarization-and-jurisprudential-norms/.

Lewis, D. 2022. Why the WHO took two years to say COVID is airborne. *Nature.* April 6, 2022. https://www.nature.com/articles/d41586-022-00925-7.

Lewis, T. 2021. How the U.S. pandemic response went wrong—and what went right—during a year of COVID. *Scientific American.* March 11, 2021. https://www.scientificamerican.com/article/how-the-u-s-pandemic-response-went-wrong-and-what-went-right-during-a-year-of-covid/.

Lindberg, L.D., VandeVusse, A., Mueller, J., and M. Kirstein. 2020. Early impacts of the COVID-19 pandemic: Findings from the 2020 Guttmacher survey of reproductive health experiences. Guttmacher Institute. https://www.guttmacher.org/report/early-impacts-covid-19-pandemic-findings-2020-guttmacher-survey-reproductive-health.

Logansport Daily Tribune. 1919. Big mass meeting condemns masks. *Logansport Daily Tribune.* February 14, 1919, 8.

Loomis, J.S. 2018. *Epidemics: The impact of germs and their power over humanity.* Nashville, TN: Turner Publishing.

Lynas, M. 2020. COVID: Top 10 current conspiracy theories. Alliance for Science. April 20, 2020. https://allianceforscience.cornell.edu/blog/2020/04/covid-top-10-current-conspiracy-theories/.

Maestripieri, L. 2021. The Covid-19 pandemics: Why intersectionality matters. *Frontiers in Sociology* 6. https://doi.org/10.3389/fsoc.2021.642662.

Mallapaty, S. 2023. Covid-origins study links raccoon dogs to Wuhan market: What scientists think. *Nature.* https://www.nature.com/articles/d41586-023-00827-2.

Maragakis, L. and G. Kelen. 2021. Covid-19—myth versus fact. Johns Hopkins Medicine. https://www.hopkinsmedicine.org/health/conditions-and-diseases/coronavirus/2019-novel-coronavirus-myth-versus-fact.

Mark, J.J. 2020a. Medieval cures for the black death. *World history encyclopedia.* https://www.worldhistory.org/article/1540/medieval-cures-for-the-black-death/.

Mark, J.J. 2020b. Plague in the ancient & medieval world. *World history encyclopedia.* https://www.worldhistory.org/article/1528/plague-in-the-ancient--medieval-world/.

Mark, J.J. 2020c. Religious responses to the black death. *World history encyclopedia.* https://www.worldhistory.org/article/1541/religious-responses-to-the-black-death/.

Marx, G.T. and D. McAdam. 1994. *Collective behavior and social movements.* Upper Saddle River, NJ: Prentice Hall.

Masroor, S. 2020. Collateral damage of COVID-19 pandemic: Delayed medical care. *Journal of Cardiac Surgery* 35 (6):1345–1347. https://www.ncbi.nlm.nih.gov/pmc/articles/PMC7276840/.

Masters, R.K., Aron, L.Y., and S.H. Woolf. 2022. Changes in life expectancy between 2019 and 2021: United States and 19 peer countries. *MedRxiv*. https://www.medrxiv.org/content/10.1101/2022.04.05.22273393v2.full.pdf.

Matthewman, S. and K. Huppatz. 2020. A sociology of Covid-19. *Journal of Sociology* 56 (4):675–683.

Maxmen, A. 2021. US COVID origins report: Researchers pleased with scientific approach. *Nature* 597 (September 9):159–160. https://www.nature.com/articles/d41586-021-02366-0.

Maxmen, A. 2022. Scientists struggle to probe COVID's origins amid sparse data from China. *Nature* 603:773–775. https://www.nature.com/articles/d41586-022-00732-0.

Maxmen, A. and S. Mallapaty. 2021. The COVID lab-leak hypothesis: What scientists do and don't know. *Nature* 594:313–315. https://www.nature.com/articles/d41586-021-01529-3.

Mayo Clinic. 2023. Myocarditis—Symptoms and causes. https://www.mayoclinic.org/diseases-conditions/myocarditis/symptoms-causes/syc-20352539#:~:text=Myocarditis%20is%20inflammation%20of%20the%20heart%20muscle%20(myocardium).,is%20one%20cause%20of%20myocarditis.

McDonald, J. 2021. Increase in COVID-19 VAERS reports due to reporting requirements, intense scrutiny of widely given vaccines. Annenberg Public Policy Center. https://www.factcheck.org/2021/12/scicheck-increase-in-covid-19-vaers-reports-due-to-reporting-requirements-intense-scrutiny-of-widely-given-vaccines/.

McDonald, J. 2023. What the Cochrane Review says about masks for COVID-19—and what it doesn't. Annenberg Public Policy Center. https://www.factcheck.org/2023/03/scicheck-what-the-cochrane-review-says-about-masks-for-covid-19-and-what-it-doesnt/.

McLuhan, M. and Q. Fiore. 1967. *The medium is the massage: An inventory of effects.* New York: Random House.

McNamara, D. 2021. History does repeat: Pandemic vaccine uproar is nothing new. WebMD. https://www.webmd.com/vaccines/covid-19-vaccine/news/20211014/vaccine-opposition-not-new.

McNeill, W.H. 1976. *Plagues and peoples.* New York: Quality Paperback Book Club.

McPhail, C. and R.T. Wohlstein. 1983. Individual and collective behaviors within gatherings, demonstrations, and riots. *Annual Review of Sociology* 9:579–600. https://www.academia.edu/31111351/_1983_Individual_and_Collective_Behaviors_within_Gatherings_Demonstrations_and_Riots_.

McPherson, M., Smith-Lovin, L., and J.M. Cook. 2001. Birds of a feather: Homophily in social networks. *Annual Review of Sociology* 27:415–444.

Mercola, J. and R. Cummins. 2021. *The truth about COVID-19: Exposing the great reset, lockdowns, vaccine passports, and the new normal.* White River Junction, VT: Chelsea Green.

Mervosh, S. 2022. Test results take a large hit: Pandemic erases two decades of progress in math and reading. *The New York Times*. September 1, 2022. https://www.nytimes.com/2022/09/01/us/national-test-scores-math-reading-pandemic.html.

Miller, D.L. 2014. *Introduction to collective behavior and collective action.* Long Grove, IL: Waveland Press.

Mitchell, A. and J. Liedke. 2021. About four-in-ten Americans say social media is an important way of following COVID-19 vaccine news. Pew Research Center. https://www.pewresearch.org/fact-tank/2021/08/24/about-four-in-ten-americans-say-social-media-is-an-important-way-of-following-covid-19-vaccine-news/.

Mitchell, A. and B. Oliphant. 2020. Americans immersed in COVID-19 news; Most think the media are doing fairly well covering it. Pew Research Center. https://www.pewresearch.org/journalism/2020/03/18/americans-immersed-in-covid-19-news-most-think-media-are-doing-fairly-well-covering-it/#knowledge-misperceptions-and-made-up-news.

Molter, V. and G. Webster. 2020. Virality project (China): Coronavirus conspiracy claims. Stanford Internet Observatory. https://fsi.stanford.edu/news/china-covid19-origin-narrative.

Monmouth University. 2022. Shifting support for some, but not all, Covid mandates. Monmouth University Polling Institute. https://www.monmouth.edu/polling-institute/reports/monmouthpoll_us_032822/.

Montgomery, D. 2021. How to sell the coronavirus vaccines to a divided, uneasy America. *The Washington Post Magazine*. April 26, 2021. https://www.washingtonpost.com/magazine/2021/04/26/coronavirus-vaccines-ad-council/.

Morgan, O.W., Meltzer, M., Muir, D., Hogan, H., Seng, C., Hill, J., and J. Beckford. 2003. Specialist vaccination advice and pockets of resistance to MMR vaccination: Lessons from an outbreak of measles. *Communicable Disease and Public Health* 6 (4):330–333.

Moyer, M.W. 2022. Long COVID sufferers are struggling with exercise. *The New York Times.* March 25, 2022. https://www.nytimes.com/2022/02/12/well/move/long-covid-exercise.html.

Mueller, B. and S. Nolen. 2022. WHO: Deaths far exceed what countries reported. *The New York Times*. May 5, 2022. https://www.nytimes.com/2022/05/05/health/covid-global-deaths.html.

Munro, A. 2023. Populism: Political program or movement. *Encyclopedia Britannica.* https://www.britannica.com/topic/populism.

Nature. 2020. A four-year timeline of Trump's impact on science. *Nature.* https://www.nature.com/articles/d41586-020-02814-3.

Nayak, S. and M.E. Reynolds. 2022. How has Congress responded to issues surrounding vaccinations? Brookings Institution. https://www.brookings.edu/blog/fixgov/2022/05/13/how-has-congress-responded-to-issues-surrounding-vaccinations/?utm_campaign=Brookings%20Brief&utm_medium=email&utm_content=213077505&utm_source=hs_email.

Neal, K. 2020. The collateral damage of COVID-19. *Journal of Public Health* 42 (4):659. https://www.ncbi.nlm.nih.gov/pmc/articles/PMC7717275/.

Needham, J. 2000. *Science and civilization in China: Volume 6, biology and biological technology, Part 6, Medicine*. Cambridge, UK: Cambridge University Press.

Neiwert, D. 2009. *The Eliminationists: How hate talk radicalized the American right.* Sausalito, CA: Poli Point Press.

Ng, R. and N. Indran. 2021. Reframing aging during COVID-19: Familial role-based framing of older adults linked to decreased ageism. *Journal of the American Geriatric Society* 70 (1):60–66. https://agsjournals.onlinelibrary.wiley.com/doi/pdfdirect/10.1111/jgs.17532.

Niederhuber, M. 2014. The fight over inoculation during the 1721 Boston smallpox epidemic. Harvard University: The Graduate School of Arts and Sciences. https://sitn.hms.harvard.edu/flash/special-edition-on-infectious-disease/2014/the-fight-over-inoculation-during-the-1721-boston-smallpox-epidemic/.

O'Brien, T.C., Palmer, R., and D. Albarracin. 2021. Misplaced trust: When trust in science fosters belief in pseudoscience and the benefits of critical evaluation. *Journal of Experimental Social Psychology* 96:104184. https://www.asc.upenn.edu/sites/default/files/2021-08/misplaced%20trust.pdf.

Offe, C. 2021. Corona pandemic policy: Exploratory notes on its "epistemic regime." In *Pandemics, politics, and society: Critical perspectives on the Covid-19 crisis,* ed. G. Delanty, 25–41. Berlin, Germany: De Gruyter.

Ofri, D. 2021. Heidi Larson, vaccine anthropologist. *The New Yorker.* June 12, 2021. https://www.newyorker.com/science/annals-of-medicine/heidi-larson-vaccine-anthropologist.

Oldstone, M.B.A. 2020. *Viruses, plagues, and history,* 2nd edition. New York: Oxford University Press.

Organization for Economic Co-operation and Development (OECD). 2020. Transparency, communication and trust: The role of public communication in responding to the wave of disinformation about the new coronavirus. https://www.oecd.org/coronavirus/policy-responses/transparency-communication-and-trust-the-role-of-public-communication-in-responding-to-the-wave-of-disinformation-about-the-new-coronavirus-bef7ad6e/.

Oshinsky, D.M. 2006. *Polio: An American story.* New York: Oxford University Press.

Paperny, A.M. and B. Gable. 2022. Canadian cities see anti vaccine mandate protests spread. *Reuters.* February 5, 2022. https://nationalpost.com/pmn/health-pmn/canadian-cities-see-anti-vaccine-mandate-protests-spread.

Parker, K., Horowitz, J.M., and A. Brown. 2020. About half of lower-income Americans report household job or wage loss due to COVID-19. Pew Research Center. https://www.pewresearch.org/social-trends/2020/04/21/about-half-of-lower-income-americans-report-household-job-or-wage-loss-due-to-covid-19/.

Parker, K., Horowitz, J.M., and R. Minkin. 2021. Americans are less likely than before COVID-19 to want to live in cities, more likely to prefer suburbs. Pew Research Center. https://www.pewresearch.org/social-trends/2021/12/16/americans-are-less-likely-than-before-covid-19-to-want-to-live-in-cities-more-likely-to-prefer-suburbs/.

Parker, K., Horowitz, J.M., and R. Minkin. 2022. Covid-19 pandemic continues to reshape work in America. Pew Research Center. https://www.pewresearch.org/social-trends/2022/02/16/covid-19-pandemic-continues-to-reshape-work-in-america/.

Paul, K.T. and C. Haddad. 2023. The pandemic as we know it: A policy studies perspective on ignorance and nonknowledge in COVID-19 governance. In *Routledge international handbook of ignorance studies*, 2nd edition, eds. M. Gross and L. McGoey, 221–233. London: Routledge.

Paz, C. All the president's lies about the coronavirus: An unfinished compendium of Trump's overwhelming dishonesty during a national emergency. *The Atlantic*. https://www.theatlantic.com/politics/archive/2020/11/trumps-lies-about-coronavirus/608647/.

Pei, S., Kandula, S., and J. Shaman. 2020. Differential effects of intervention timing on COVID-19 spread in the United States. *Science Advances* 6 (49). https://www.science.org/doi/10.1126/sciadv.abd6370.

Perlstadt, H. 2016. The plague of Athens and the cult of Asclepius: A case study of collective behavior and a social movement. *Sociology and Anthropology* 4 (12):1048–1053.

Pescosolido, B.A. and B. Lee. 2021. COVID-19 and sociology's mental health moment. *Footnotes* 49 (2):1–13. https://www.asanet.org/news-events/footnotes/apr-may-jun-2021/features/covid-19-and-sociologys-mental-health-moment.

Petri, A.E. 2022. Medical experts urge Spotify to crack down. *The New York Times*. January 14, 2022. https://www.nytimes.com/2022/01/27/business/media/medical-professionals-urge-spotify-to-crack-down-on-covid-misinformation.html.

Pew Research Center. 2021. Public trust in government: 1958-2021. https://www.pewresearch.org/politics/2021/05/17/public-trust-in-government-1958-2021/.

Pickersgill, M. 2020. Pandemic sociology. *Engaging Science, Technology, and Society* 6:347–350.

Pitofsky, M. 2023. "Abhorrent": Groups call Robert F. Kennedy Jr.'s COVID theory antisemitic and racist. *USA Today*, July 16, 2023. https://www.usatoday.com/story/news/politics/2023/07/16/robert-kennedy-ashkenazi-jewish-chinese-covid/70418041007/.

Pleyers, G. 2020. A plea for global sociology in times of the coronavirus. ISA Digital Platform. https://www.isa-sociology.org/frontend/web/uploads/files/Global%20Sociology%20in%20Times%20of%20the%20Coronavirus.pdf.

Pollard, M.S. and L.M. Davis. 2021. Decline in trust in the Centers for Disease Control and Prevention during the COVID-19 pandemic. Rand Corporation. https://www.rand.org/pubs/research_reports/RRA308-12.html.

Pollard, M.S., Tucker, J.S., and H.D. Green. 2020. Changes in adult alcohol use and consequences during the COVID-19 pandemic in the US. *JAMA Network Open*. https://www.ncbi.nlm.nih.gov/pmc/articles/PMC7525354/.

Prasad, V. and J.S. Flier. 2020. Scientists who express different views on Covid-19 should be heard, not demonized. *STAT*. https://www.statnews.com/2020/04/27/hear-scientists-different-views-covid-19-dont-attack-them/.

Priniski, J.H. and K.J. Holyoak. 2022. A darkening spring: How preexisting distrust shaped COVID-19 skepticism. *PLOS One*. https://journals.plos.org/plosone/article?id=10.1371/journal.pone.0263191.

Proal, A.D. and M.B. VanElzakker. 2021. Long COVID or post-acute sequelae of COVID-19 (PASC): An overview of biological factors that may contribute to persistent symptoms. *Frontiers of Microbiology*. https://doi.org/10.3389/fmicb.2021.698169.

Proctor, R.N. and L. Schiebinger. (Eds.). 2008. *Agnotology: The making & unmaking of ignorance*. Stanford, CA: Stanford University Press.

Rabin, R.C. and T. Arango. 2022. Gun deaths surged in pandemic's first year. *The New York Times*. May 10, 2010. https://www.nytimes.com/2022/05/10/health/cdc-gun-violence-pandemic.html.

Randall, D.K. 2019. *Black death at the golden gate*. New York: Norton.

Reh, G., Ronte, H., Gupta, L., and H. Varia. 2021. Overcoming biopharma's trust deficit: Why people mistrust the biopharma industry—and what to do about it. *Deloitte Insights.* https://www2.deloitte.com/us/en/insights/industry/life-sciences/trust-in-biopharmaceutical-companies-covid.html.

Reich, J.A. 2021. All in this together?: Inequalities and hesitancy surrounding the COVID-19 vaccine. *Footnotes* 49 (2): 6–7. https://www.asanet.org/sites/default/files/attach/footnotes/footnotes_spring-2021.pdf.

Richmond, T. 2022. GOP targets race as a factor in treatment. *The Associated Press.* January 24, 2022. https://www.pressreader.com/usa/the-denver-post/20220124/281676848291800.

Rieger, M.O. 2022. Uncritical patriotism and belief in COVID-19 conspiracies. *Frontiers in Sociology.* 7: April 27, 2022. https://www.frontiersin.org/articles/10.3389/fsoc.2022.777650/full.

Robertson, L., McDonald, J., and E. Kiely. 2021. Aaron Rodgers' inaccurate COVID-19 claims. FactCheck.org. https://www.factcheck.org/2021/11/scicheck-aaron-rodgers-inaccurate-covid-19-claims/.

Robinson, K.R. 2021. Comparing the Spanish flu and COVID-19 pandemics: Lessons to carry forward. *Nursing Forum* 56:350–357. https://onlinelibrary.wiley.com/doi/epdf/10.1111/nuf.12534.

Romer, D. and K.H. Jamison. 2020. Conspiracy theories as barriers to controlling the spread of COVID-19 in the U.S. *Social Science & Medicine* 263:113356. https://doi.org/10.1016/j.socscimed.2020.113356.

Roosevelt, T. 1903. *Letter to his son Kermit,* January 17, 1903.

Rothwell, J. and S. Desai. 2020. How misinformation is distorting COVID policies and behaviors. Brookings Institution. https://www.brookings.edu/research/how-misinformation-is-distorting-covid-policies-and-behaviors/.

Ruiz, N.G., Horowitz, J.M., and C. Tamir. 2020. Many Black and Asian Americans say they have experienced discrimination amid the COVID-19 outbreak. Pew Research Center: https://www.pewresearch.org/social-trends/2020/07/01/many-black-and-asian-americans-say-they-have-experienced-discrimination-amid-the-covid-19-outbreak/.

Russell, J.H. and D. Patterson. 2021. America's smug elite is harming our kids: The push to decouple skepticism from science turns children into victims. *Tablet.* https://www.tabletmag.com/sections/science/articles/americas-ham-fisted-elite-harming-kids-wrecking-scientific-debate-dennis-patterson-jacob-hale-russell.

Sabin, N. 2022. The new war on science: 4 reasons people reject good data. *WebMD Health News*. https://www.webmd.com/a-to-z-guides/news/20220805/war-on-science-why-people-reject-good-data.

Sage, W.M., and Y.T. Yang. 2022. Reducing "COVID-19 misinformation" while preserving free speech. *Journal of the American Medical Association* 327 (15):1443–1444. https://jamanetwork.com/journals/jama/fullarticle/2790859.

Sanchez, G.R., Gilbert, K.L., and C. Busette. 2022. Living with COVID-19 will not be easy for many Americans suffering from long COVID-19, particularly those from diverse communities. Brookings Institution. https://www.brookings.edu/blog/how-we-rise/2022/06/21/living-with-covid-19-will-not-be-easy-for-many-americans-suffering-from-long-covid-19-particularly-those-from-diverse-communities/?utm_campaign=Brookings%20Brief&utm_medium=email&utm_content=217394132&utm_source=hs_email.

Schaeffer, K. 2020. Nearly three-in-ten Americans believe COVID-19 was made in a lab. Pew Research Center. https://www.pewresearch.org/fact-tank/2020/04/08/nearly-three-in-ten-americans-believe-covid-19-was-made-in-a-lab/.

Shear, M.D., Stolberg, S.G., LaFraniere, S., and N. Weiland. 2022. Issues persist in battle vs. virus. *The New York Times*. January 24, 2022. https://www.pressreader.com/usa/the-denver-post/20220124/281483574763480.

Sheikh, K. and H. Seo. 2022. How to live with Covid-19 when you are tired of living with Covid-19. *The New York Times*. August 2, 2022. https://www.nytimes.com/2022/07/25/well/live/covid-ba5-precautions.html.

Siegel, M. 2020. *COVID: The politics of fear and the power of science.* Nashville, TN: Turner Publishing.

Silva, G.A.D. and C.D. Higuera. 2021. Political theology and COVID-19: Agamben's critique of science as a new "pandemic religion." *Open Theology* 7 (1):501–513. https://www.degruyter.com/document/doi/10.1515/opth-2020-0177/html?=en.

Silver, L. and A. Connaughton. 2022. Partisanship colors views of COVID-19 handling across advanced economies. Pew Research Center. https://www.pewresearch.org/global/2022/08/11/partisanship-colors-views-of-covid-19-handling-across-advanced-langeconomies/?utm_source=Pew+Research+Center&utm_campaign=6c5978a866-Weekly_2022_08_13&utm_medium=email&utm_term=0_3e953b9b70-6c5978a866-400075373.

Singh, Y., Eisenberg, M.D., and N. Sood. 2023. Factors associated with public trust in pharmaceutical manufacturers. *JAMA Network Open*. https://jamanetwork.com/journals/jamanetworkopen/fullarticle/2802393.

Solis, N. and H. Branson-Potts. 2021. Thousands protest COVID-19 vaccination mandates as L.A.'s verification rules kick in. *Los Angeles Times.* November 8, 2021. https://www.latimes.com/california/story/2021-11-08/thousands-protest-covid-19-vaccine-mandates-in-l-a.

Solomou, I. and F. Constantinidou. 2020. Prevalence and predictors of anxiety and depression symptoms during the COVID-19 pandemic and compliance with precautionary measures: Age and sex matter. *International Journal of Environmental Research and Public Health* 17 (14):4924. https://www.ncbi.nlm.nih.gov/pmc/articles/PMC7400373/.

Soper, G.A. 1919. The lessons of the pandemic. *Science* 49:501–506.

Spencer, A. and C. Funk. 2022. When Americans think about science, what do they have in mind? Pew Research Center. https://www.pewresearch.org/fact-tank/2022/03/25/when-americans-think-about-science-what-do-they-have-in-mind/?utm_source=Pew+Research+Center&utm_campaign=607fe7c2a2-Weekly_2022_03_26&utm_medium=email&utm_term=0_3e953b9b70-607fe7c2a2-400075373.

Spencer, S.H. 2021a. COVID-19 far more lethal than a cold, contrary to suggestion in viral video. SciCheck Digest. https://www.factcheck.org/2021/12/scicheck-covid-19-far-more-lethal-than-a-cold-contrary-to-suggestion-in-viral-video/.

Spencer, S.H. 2021b. Health sensors misconstrued as government tracking "microchips." https://www.factcheck.org/2021/08/scicheck-health-sensors-misconstrued-as-government-tracking-microchips/.

Spencer, S.H. and A. Fichera. 2021. RFK Jr. video pushes known vaccine misrepresentations. FactCheck. https://www.factcheck.org/2021/03/scicheck-rfk-jr-video-pushes-known-vaccine-misrepresentations/.

Spencer, S.H., Jones, B., Hancock, T., and E. Kiely. 2021. Article makes unfounded claims linking athletes' injuries, deaths to vaccines. SciCheck Digest. https://www.factcheck.org/2021/12/scicheck-article-makes-unfounded-claims-linking-athletes-injuries-deaths-to-vaccines/.

Stahl, S.M. and M. Lebedun. 1974. Mystery gas: An analysis of mass hysteria. *Journal of Health and Social Behavior* 15 (1):44–50.

Stephens, B. 2023. The mask mandates did nothing—will any lessons be learned? *The New York Times*. February 21, 2023. https://www.nytimes.com/2023/02/21/opinion/do-mask-mandates-work.html.

Stosic, M.D., Helwig, S., and M.A. Ruben. 2021. Greater belief in science predicts mask-wearing behavior during COVID-19. *Personality and Individual Differences* 176:110769. https://pubmed.ncbi.nlm.nih.gov/33612904/.

Strasser, B.J. and T. Schlich. 2020. A history of the medical mask and the rise of throwaway culture. *The Lancet* 396 (10243):19–20. https://www.ncbi.nlm.nih.gov/pmc/articles/PMC7255306/.

Strong, P M. 1990. Epidemic psychology: A model. *Sociology of Health and Illness* 12 (3):249–259.

Tang, L. and H. Liu. 2010. Toward predicting collective behavior via social dimension extraction. *Social Learning* July/August:19–25.

Taquet, M., Dercon, Q., Luciano, S., Geddes, J.R., Husain, M., and P.J. Harrison. 2021. Incidence, co-occurrence, and evolution of long-COVID features: A 6-month retrospective cohort study of 273,618 survivors of COVID-19. *PLOS Medicine*. https://journals.plos.org/plosmedicine/article?id=10.1371/journal.pmed.1003773.

Tarafder, B.K., Khan, M.A.I., Islam, M.T., Mahmud, S.A.A., Sarker, M.H.K., Faruq, I., Miah, M.T., and S.M.Y. Arafat. 2016. Mass psychogenic illness: Demography and symptom profile of an episode. *Psychiatry Journal* 2016:1–5. https://www.ncbi.nlm.nih.gov/pmc/articles/PMC4884863/.

Tollerson, J. 2020. How Trump damaged science—and why it could take decades to recover. *Nature* 586:190–194. https://www.nature.com/articles/d41586-020-02800-9.

Tressler, C. Ignore bogus COVID vaccine survey. Federal Trade Commission. https://consumer.ftc.gov/consumer-alerts/2021/03/ignore-bogus-covid-vaccine-survey.

Trotochaud, M., Smith, E., Hosangadi, D., and T.K. Sell. 2023. Analyzing social media messaging on masks and vaccines: A case study on misinformation during the COVID-19 pandemic. *Disaster Medicine and Public Health Preparation* (January 10):1–9.

Trump, D. 2021. Donald Trump Cullman, Alabama rally transcript. Transcript Library. https://www.rev.com/blog/transcripts/donald-trump-cullman-alabama-rally-speech-transcript.

Tsai, J.Y., Phua, J., Pan, S., and C.C. Yang. 2020. Intergroup contact, COVID-19 news consumption, and the moderating role of digital media trust on prejudice toward Asians in the United States: Cross-sectional study. *Journal of Medical Internet Research* 22 (9):e22767. https://pubmed.ncbi.nlm.nih.gov/32924948/.

Tsampasian, V., Elghazaly, H., Chattopadhyay, R., et al. 2023. Post-COVID-19 condition: A systematic review and meta-analysis. *JAMA Internal Medicine*. https://jamanetwork.com/journals/jamainternalmedicine/fullarticle/2802877?resultClick=1.

Turner, B.S. 2021. The political theology of Covid-19: A comparative history of human responses to catastrophes. In *Pandemics, politics, and society: Critical perspectives on the Covid-19 crisis,* ed. G. Delanty, 139–156, Berlin, Germany: De Gruyter.

Turner, R.H. and L.M. Killian. 1957. *Collective behavior.* Englewood Cliffs, NJ: Prentice-Hall.

Tyson, A. and C. Funk. 2022. Increasing public criticism, confusion over COVID-19 response in U.S. Pew Research Center. https://www.pewresearch.org/science/2022/02/09/increasing-public-criticism-confusion-over-covid-19-response-in-u-s/.

Unwin, H.J.T., Hillis, S., Cluver, L., Flaxman, S., Goldman, P.S., Butchart, A., Bachman, G., Rawlings, L., Donnelly, C.A., Ratzman, O., Green, P., Nelson, C.A., Blenkinsop, A., Bhatt, S., Desmond, C., Villavecest, A., and L. Sherr. 2022. Global, regional, and national minimum estimates of children affected by COVID-19-associated orphanhood and caregiver death, by age and family circumstance up to Oct 31, 2021: An updated modeling study. *The Lancet* 6 (4):249–259. https://www.thelancet.com/journals/lanchi/article/PIIS2352-4642(22)00005-0/fulltext.

U.S. Bureau of Labor Statistics. 2022. Supplemental data measuring the effects of the coronavirus (COVID-19) pandemic on the labor market. Washington, DC: United States Bureau of Labor Statistics. https://www.bls.gov/cps/effects-of-the-coronavirus-covid-19-pandemic.htm#MayJune.

Valverde, M. 2021. Fact check: Yes, an average COVID-19 hospital stay costs about $17,000. *Detroit Free Press.* September 4, 2021. https://www.freep.com/story/news/local/michigan/2021/09/04/covid-hospital-cost-pramila-jayapal/5715191001/.

Van Bavel, J.J., Baicker, K., Boggio, P.S., et al. 2021. Using social and behavioural science to support COVID-19 pandemic response. *Nature Human Behaviour* 4 (May):460–471. https://www.nature.com/articles/s41562-020-0884-z.pdf.

Vandenberghe, F. and J-F Verán. 2021. The pandemic as a total social fact. In *Pandemics, politics, and society: Critical perspectives on the Covid-19 crisis,* ed. G. Delanty, 171–187. Berlin, Germany: De Gruyter.

Villasenor, J. 2022. The vital role of Twitter in responding to Covid. Brookings Institution. https://www.brookings.edu/blog/techtank/2022/01/04/the-vital-role-of-twitter-in-responding-to-covid/.

Voght, K. 2022. "I'm a full anti-vaxxer now": How the conspiracists are winning over fresh converts. *Rolling Stone*. https://www.rollingstone.com/culture/culture-news/anti-vaccine-rfk-jr-rally-washington-dc-1289458/.

Wachter, R.M. 2022. Nailing the nuance on COVID-19. *Science* 377 (6603):243.

Wakefield, J. 2020. How Bill Gates became the voodoo doll of Covid conspiracies. BBC. June 6, 2020. https://www.bbc.com/news/technology-52833706.

Walby, S. 2021. The COVID pandemic and social theory: Social democracy and public health in the crisis. *European Journal of Social Theory* 24 (1):22–43.

Walby, S. 2022. Crisis and society: Developing the theory of crisis in the context of COVID-19. *Global Discourse* 12 (3-4):498–516.

Walker, M. 2022. Nearly a quarter of Americans get news from podcasts. Pew Research Center. https://www.pewresearch.org/fact-tank/2022/02/15/nearly-a-quarter-of-americans-get-news-from-podcasts/.

Washington, G. 1796. *Letter to John Jay*. July 6, 1796. http://www.notable-quotes.com/w/washington_george_viii.html#:~:text=Serious%20misfortunes%2C%20originating%20in%20misrepresentation,can%20be%20dissipated%20by%20truth.&text=I%20was%20no%20party%20man,did%20exist%2C%20to%20reconcile%20them.

WCCO-TV Staff. 2021. Fight breaks out at eastern Carver County school board meeting. https://minnesota.cbslocal.com/2021/09/28/school-board-meeting-fight-chaska/.

Weiland, N. 2021. Like a hand grasping: Trump appointees describe the crushing of the CDC. *New York Times* January 15, 2021. https://www.nytimes.com/2020/12/16/us/politics/cdc-trump.html.

Wilson, C. 2022. Report: Vaccinations could have prevented quarter-million COVID deaths in U.S. https://www.aol.com/news/report-vaccinations-could-prevented-quarter-162852395.html.

Wood, D. and G. Brumfiel. 2021. Pro-Trump counties now have far higher COVID death rates. Misinformation is to blame. National Public Radio. December 5, 2021. https://www.npr.org/sections/health-shots/2021/12/05/1059828993/data-vaccine-misinformation-trump-counties-covid-death-rate.

World Health Organization Writing Group. 2006. Nonpharmaceutical interventions for pandemic influenza, national and community measures. *Emerging Infectious Diseases* 12 (1):88–94. https://doi.org/10.3201/eid1201.051371.

World Health Organization. 2023. Statement on the fifteenth meeting of the IHR (2005) Emergency Committee on the COVID-19 pandemic. World Health

Organization. May 5, 2023. https://www.who.int/news/item/05-05-2023-statement-on-the-fifteenth-meeting-of-the-international-health-regulations-(2005)-emergency-committee-regarding-the-coronavirus-disease-(covid-19)-pandemic?adgroupsurvey=%7Badgroupsurvey%7D&gclid=CjwKCAjwvdajBhBEEiwAeMh1U4UNynblqk1l6kueBu3Y_F6AKaLYmcxmbusf5xgzPTUiOzhugfUG2hoCCSEQAvD_BwE.

Zatz, M. 1987. Chicano youth gangs and crime: The creation of a moral panic. *Contemporary Crises* 11 (2):129–158.

Zhao, E., Wu, Q., Crimmins, E.M., and J.A. Ailshire. 2020. Media trust and infection mitigating behaviours during the COVID-19 pandemic in the USA. *BMJ Global Health* 5 (10):003323. https://www.ncbi.nlm.nih.gov/pmc/articles/PMC7545496/.

Zhou, P., Yang, X.L., Wang, X.G., et al. 2020. A pneumonia outbreak associated with a new coronavirus of probable bat origin. *Nature* 579:270–273. https://www.nature.com/articles/s41586-020-2012-7#citeas.

Zielonka, J. 2021. Who should be in charge of pandemics? Scientists or politicians. In *Pandemics, politics, and society: Critical perspectives on the Covid-19 crisis,* ed. G. Delanty, 59–73. Berlin, Germany: De Gruyter.

Zinn, J. O. 2021. Conclusions: Towards a sociology of pandemics and beyond. *Current Sociology Monograph* 69 (4):603–617.

Index

About the Author

Herbert C. Covey, Ph.D., worked over forty years as an administrator in human services, public policy, and juvenile justice. He also taught part-time at the University of Colorado. His scholarly works include over 22 books on African American history, methamphetamine, street gangs, and child welfare. His most recent books are *African-American Slave Medicine* (2007), *The Methamphetamine Crisis* (2007), *What the Slaves Ate* (2009), *How the Slaves Saw the Civil War* (2014), *Crips and Bloods* (2015), *Youth Gangs* (2016), *The Smallest Victims* (2018), *Street Gangs Throughout the World* (2021), *Daily Life of African Americans in Primary Documents* (2021), and *Adolescent Exposure to Violence and Adult Outcomes* (2021). He has also authored and co-authored multiple articles on social gerontology, gangs, child welfare, criminology, and criminal justice.

www.ingramcontent.com/pod-product-compliance
Lightning Source LLC
LaVergne TN
LVHW091527200926
848483LV00002B/328
* 9 7 8 1 6 6 6 9 5 4 2 9 6 *